Occupational Therapy Practice in Mental Health: Models, Conditions, Interventions, and Recovery

Edited By

Tawanda Machingura
Head of Discipline Occupational Therapy Program
University of Notre Dame Australia
Sydney, Australia

Occupational Therapy Practice in Mental Health: Models, Conditions, Interventions, and Recovery

Editor: Tawanda Machingura

ISBN (Online): 978-981-5313-71-0

ISBN (Print): 978-981-5313-72-7

ISBN (Paperback): 978-981-5313-73-4

need for a court order if at any point you breach any terms of this License Agreement. In no event will any delay or failure by Bentham Science Publishers in enforcing your compliance with this License Agreement constitute a waiver of any of its rights.

3. You acknowledge that you have read this License Agreement, and agree to be bound by its terms and conditions. To the extent that any other terms and conditions presented on any website of Bentham Science Publishers conflict with, or are inconsistent with, the terms and conditions set out in this License Agreement, you acknowledge that the terms and conditions set out in this License Agreement shall prevail.

Bentham Science Publishers Pte. Ltd.
No. 9 Raffles Place
Office No. 26-01
Singapore 048619
Singapore
Email: subscriptions@benthamscience.net

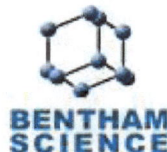

CONTENTS

FOREWORD

The Foreword is by World Federation of OT President Elect. Tecla Mlambo. PhD, MSc OT, MSc Clin Epidemiology, BSc HOT.

The purpose of this book is to enhance the understanding of occupational therapy practice in mental health for all people around the globe, including consumers, families, students, occupational therapists, and other health professionals. This book presents a diverse range of views from authors around the world and is informed by all forms of knowledge, not just Western ways of knowing. Many of the authors of the chapters of this book are themselves from ethnic minority groups. Some of them are consumers of occupational therapy and mental health services. The authors reside in different parts of the world, including Africa, Oceania, and Europe. This was a deliberate effort to ensure that those diverse voices are heard, and that a diverse range of worldviews is included.

This book intentionally uses simple English, pictures, tables, and illustrations to aid the reader, student, or occupational therapy practitioner to clearly understand the concepts. The case examples used are from different contexts around the world to give relevance to the reader. This is the goal of this book, to increase understanding of occupational and practice in mental health practice for everyone not just native English speakers or those from the dominant western cultures.

Chapters are organised in sections, with each section having been carefully crafted and coordinated by one author. Coordinating authors and specific chapter authors are identified. While the text is substantially the work of the contributing authors, a small number of additional authors were invited to contribute to specific areas. Each chapter starts with a brief synopsis of key theoretical and empirical issues to guide the reader who wishes to investigate the broader literature. Most chapters include resources, tools, and instruments that support effective practice. To ensure continuity of style and a coherent, integrated body of material, the coordinating author for each section will assume editorial responsibility for the chapters that constituted that section, and the editor reviewed the entire text for continuity and styling for the book.

Section one summarises theoretical models commonly used by mental health occupational therapists so that the reader is able to choose an appropriate model to use for their clients in their contexts. Section two builds on the theoretical models and provides practitioners with an understanding of the person's components through an introductory understanding of common mental health conditions encountered in practice. Section three delves into interdisciplinary team interventions with a focus on occupational therapy-specific interventions such as psychoeducation, cognitive behavioural therapy, dialectical behavioural therapy, solution-focused therapy, and many others. Lastly, section four discusses and critiques the concept of recovery.

Despite the sequential nature of the organisation of the book, each chapter is a standalone chapter that can be read and understood on its own. Readers can assume a smorgasbord approach and read what they need when they need it and are not bound by the order of the sections or chapters.

This is one of the most comprehensive and transformative books on mental health and occupational therapy, written by academics, clinicians and consumers of occupational therapy and mental health services from various parts of the world. The book is the beginning of an important journey of indigenisation and true globalisation of occupational therapy curricula and knowledge. An excellent resource that has been long overdue on the market, and a critical tool in the hands of an educator, student and consumer of occupational therapy and mental health services.

Tecla Mlambo
World Federation of Occupational Therapy President Elect &
Head of Occupational Therapy Program
University of Zimbabwe
Harare, Zimbabwe

PREFACE

Growing up, I have always wanted to write a book. In my mind, writing a book was the epitome of academic excellence. That was before the advent of the internet. Now, with the internet being accessible to most of the world's population, anyone can write a book and publish it themselves, so why write a book? There are many reasons **why not** to write a book, including 'it is time-consuming for very little benefit'. A colleague of mine advised me to just write an article and publish it! "It takes way less time, and you get better metrics from journal articles," they said. By the way, these so-called metrics are tied to one's promotion and career advancement opportunities. I had to write this book in my own time and in secret, without sharing what I was doing with my colleagues for fear of ridicule. So why did I write this book?

First, there were some encouraging people along the way. Notably, a colleague at Waikato Hospital in New Zealand, Dr Basil Bunting, a psychiatrist from South Africa and author of Psychiatry in Easy Steps, wrote a message in a copy of his book that he gave to me in 2002, which was as follows: *"Hi Tawanda, It is very nice working with you. It's a pleasure to have a colleague from Africa. Hope this book inspires you to write your book. Basil"*. Twenty-two years later, I have now written my book in response to this call to action.

Secondly, I am an occupational therapist working and living in Australia. The first thing you should know about me is that I identify as and am biologically male. At the time of writing this preface, there were only 9% registered male occupational therapists in Australia. Now, that is a familiar story worldwide, but the point is that I belong to the minority in this profession. The second thing you should know about me is that I am a black African of African origin born and bred in Zimbabwe. Now, without doing the maths, you get the picture that I truly belong to the minority (probably less than 1%) in this wonderful profession of occupational therapy.

'My people', meaning the group of people I am similar to or belong to, are, however, not the minority as the current population of Africa is close to 1.5 billion people or 18.2% of the world's population. Culturally, I also belong to the non-western or collectivist cultures, which constitute about 85% of the world's population. It is baffling to note that occupational therapy practice is meant to serve the world, and yet people who make up 85% of occupational therapy clients are probably less than 10% of the world's occupational therapists. This figure is far less when one looks at people who then go on to produce the knowledge that informs what occupational therapists know and do. So, the reason for writing this book is to contribute towards making the occupational therapy profession a truly global profession that is applicable to all people and representative of the views of all people, not just those who are 'privileged'. Okay, this needs a bit of explanation- I have been an occupational therapist for almost 3 decades, have a growing publication record, and my highest qualification is a PhD, but at the time of writing this book, I had never been invited to write a book chapter! My story is not dissimilar to many other people of a similar background to mine in the profession of occupational therapy. I think you would have quickly discerned that I wrote this book out of frustration and also purpose. The frustration was that I realised that I did not belong to the group of usual book contributors who often get invited to write popular occupational therapy texts. The purpose was that I felt we were being fed information from one worldview and, more specifically, from the views of academics only, most of whom had not seen or treated a single patient in two decades. By the way, this is not a criticism of academics; I am one of them. They know stuff, and they do important research. Rather, this is a call to action for academics to also value the contributions from clinicians and other minority groups, which include not only culturally and linguistically diverse people but also people with a lived experience.

Decolonising OT: Historically, occupational therapy has been referred to as 'a white middle-class female profession'. This is still the case today. Many authors of a similar background to mine are calling for the 'decolonisation' of occupational therapy. This call emanates from the 2015 'Rhodes Must Fall' campaign at UCT, which quickly spread to other universities in South Africa and sparked a worldwide debate on decolonising curricula. Some argue that this is a sensationalist or cheap way of gaining political mileage, and others argue it is a much-needed transformation in academia and, indeed, in occupational therapy. It must be noted that the concept of decolonising a curriculum was first discussed in Ngũgĩ wa Thiong'o's book, Decolonising the Mind, which argued that the annihilating 'cultural' and 'psychological' consequences of colonialism had to be taken as seriously as, though not separately from, its economic, political and military ones.

As I understand it, 'decolonisation', as used in occupational therapy literature, describes a process of critically examining the current curricula, which is Western culture dominated with the intention of removing the cultural and psychological impacts of colonialism on the axiology, ontology, and epistemology of occupational therapy. It is argued by many in the profession of occupational therapy that occupational therapy is based on Western culture because of the existing structures, processes, and systems in the profession that continue to perpetuate the status quo. There are no deliberate efforts by occupational therapy professional bodies to seriously change the status quo, and in fact, some are becoming an occupational therapy out of reach for most minorities by constantly raising the bar and increasing the level of qualification and years of training needed to become an occupational therapist. Such practices are precipitants for some to call for 'decolonisation' of the profession.

Let me be very clear here, I totally agree with the intent of 'decolonisation'. Whilst I agree with the intent of 'decolonisation', I tend to disagree with the use of the term 'decolonisation' to describe this noble intent. Let me explain a bit more about myself, *i.e.*, my positionality. I was born in Zimbabwe, then Southern Rhodesia, a British colony at the time. I grew up during the time of the liberation struggle in Zimbabwe. I experienced colonisation as a brutal matter of life and death, and I am living with the after-effects of the war and the colonisation practices of the time today. Colonisation should never be minimised, and using the term 'decolonisation' when referring to curricula is minimising the real evil nature of colonisation. For lack of better words, 'globalisation' and 'indigenisation' to me seem more appropriate terms to spark the transformation that is needed in the profession. To me, these words are more in line with the principles of 'allyship', and that is what we need rather than the revolutionary message that is latent in 'decolonisation'.

Occupational therapy is a relatively new profession, new to the world and new to non-Western cultures, so yes, there is a lack of non-white voices, and we certainly need to be heard. To me, this is about inclusivity and making the profession more applicable and relevant to all people. I think, as people, we should refrain from divisive and sensationalism and instead focus on progressive and inclusive talk whilst acknowledging our history. As occupational therapists, we want our beloved profession to be more relevant to all people, more encompassing of diverse views of people around the world, and to be informed by all forms of knowledge, not just Western ways of knowing. Here is a fun fact: not all black people or people from minority groups think the same; it is racist to assume they do. So, my views are my views, and I am not representing any other person or group's views here.

Many of the authors of the chapters of this book are themselves from ethnic minority groups. Most authors of this book are practising clinicians, and some of them are consumers of occupational therapy and mental health services. The authors reside in different parts of the world, including Africa, Australia, India, North America, and Europe. This was a deliberate effort to ensure that those diverse voices are heard, and their diverse worldviews included.

Occupational therapy theory and practice is complex. For many people from around the world, the concepts do not have meaning in their own cultures and contexts. This book deliberately uses simple English, pictures, tables, and illustrations to aid the student or occupational therapy practitioner to clearly understand the concepts. The case examples used are from different contexts around the world to give relevance to the reader. This is the goal of this book, to increase understanding of occupational theory and practice in mental health practice for everyone not just native English speakers or those from the dominant western cultures. Although this book can be read sequentially, this is not a necessity. In fact, I anticipate that this book will be read like a smorgasbord where each person will pick what they wish to devour first according to their taste.

To conclude, I hope that every reader will reflect on their values, their way of thinking, knowing, and practice and, to some extent, motivate them to question, adapt, change, confirm, or re-affirm it and consequently move them towards a new understanding. To me, through critical thinking and reflection, being truly person-centred and value-driven and deliberately being inclusive in our ways of knowing and doing, we can actively eliminate the remnants of colonialism and globalise occupational therapy.

Yes, to responsible transformation as we march together in this journey towards doing, being, and/ or becoming evidence-based, value-driven global occupational therapists. Let this book be a vehicle for transformation and the first to many more editions to come.

BIBLIOGRAPHY

Bunting, B. (2002). *Psychiatry in easy steps.*. Hamilton, New Zealand: Bunting Books.

Gopal, P. (2021). On Decolonisation and the University. *Textual Pract., 35*(6), 873-899. [http://dx.doi.org/10.1080/0950236X.2021.1929561]

Ngũgĩ wa Thiong'o, (1981).. *Decolonising the Mind: The Politics of Language in African Literature.*, London: James Currey.4.

Rhodes Must Fall in Oxford Founding Statement', (2018). In Rhodes Must Fall Oxford (eds.), *Rhodes Must Fall: the Struggle to Decolonise the Racist Heart of Empire.*, London: Zed Books.4.

Tawanda Machingura
Head of Discipline Occupational Therapy Program
University of Notre Dame Australia
Sydney, Australia

DEDICATION

This book is dedicated to all my clients, whose insights and experiences have profoundly shaped my understanding of mental health practice. Without their trust and collaboration, I would not have been able to share the knowledge that informs my teaching and writing today.

I also dedicate this work to future occupational therapy clients and therapists across the globe, as it is for them that this journey of exploration and learning is truly intended.

To all therapists and clients, may we always remember that our greatest strength lies in collaboration, where collective efforts illuminate the path to healing and growth.

ACKNOWLEDGEMENTS

Firstly, I would like to acknowledge the encouragement from my mentor and PhD supervisor, who encouraged me to get into research many years ago. I would also like to acknowledge the belief in me by Jenni Tregoweth (Manager in Mental Health Rehab at Waitemata District Health in New Zealand), who, as my master's lecturer at Auckland University of Technology, predicted that I was going to write a book and gave me the belief and encouragement to do so. I have now done so. I would also like to acknowledge my fellow section editor, Professor Pamela Meredith (University of Sunshine Coast, Australia), who reviewed most of my own work and was my sounding board through and through. I would also like to acknowledge all the authors who contributed to this book and those who will contribute to future editions of this book. Thank you so much. I would like to specifically acknowledge those with a lived experience who shared their expertise and stories and co-authored chapters in this book, as without their input, the whole ethos of this book would have been lost. Thank you. Lastly, I would like to thank my wife, children, and the entire extended family for their unwavering and ongoing support.

List of Contributors

Ben Milbourn	Faculty of Health Sciences, Curtin School of Allied Health, Curtin University, Perth, Australia
Bex Symons	Department of Occupational Therapy, Coventry University, Coventry, England, United Kingdom
Clement Nhunzvi	Occupational Therapy Program, Bond University, Gold Coast, Australia
Catherine Hurley	Discipline of Occupational Therapy, University of Notre Dame Australia, Sydney, Australia
Charleen Machingura	Department of Mental Health Services, Gold Coast Hospital and Health Service, Gold Coast, Queensland, Australia
Edwin Mavindidze	Department of Occupational Therapy, University of Zimbabwe, Harare, Zimbabwe
Jessica Levick	School of Health Sciences, University of Southern Queensland, Occupational Therapy Program Ipswich, Queensland, Australia
Last Machingura	Occupational Therapist, Unworthy Therapeutic Services, Cape Town, South Africa
Michelle Fair	Department of Occupational Therapy, University of Tasmania, Tasmania, Australia
Moffat Makomo	Occupational Therapist, Manchester University NHS Foundation Trust, Manchester, England, United Kingdom
Maya Hayden-Evans	Faculty of Health Sciences, Curtin School of Allied Health, Curtin University, Perth, Australia
Pamela Meredith	Discipline of Occupational Therapy, University of the Sunshine Coast, Sunshine Coast, Queensland, Australia
Patricia Tran	Faculty of Health Sciences, Curtin School of Allied Health, Curtin University, Perth, Australia
Phil Morgan	Therapies and Quality (Mental Health), Dorset Healthcare University NHS Foundation Trust, Poole, Dorset, United Kingdom
Robert Pereira	Department of Occupational Therapy, University of Canberra, Canberra, ACT, Australia
Roshan Galvaan	Department of Occupational Therapy, University of Cape Town, Cape Town, South Africa
Rachel Oliver	Faculty of Health Sciences, Curtin School of Allied Health, Curtin University, Perth, Australia
Sam Thew	Department of Occupational Therapy, Child Development Centre, Prince George, British Columbia, Canada
Stewart Alford	School of Health Sciences, University of Southern Queensland, Occupational Therapy Program Ipswich, Queensland, Australia
Shalini Quadros	Department of Occupational Therapy, Manipal University, Manipal, Karnataka, India

Smrithi Natanasubramanian　　Department of Occupational Therapy, Manipal University, Manipal, Karnataka, India

Sonya Girdler　　Faculty of Health Sciences, Curtin School of Allied Health, Curtin University, Perth, Australia

Tawanda Machingura　　Head of Discipline Occupational Therapy Program, University of Notre Dame Australia, Sydney, Australia

Tongai F. Chichaya　　Department of Occupational Therapy, Coventry University, Coventry, England, United Kingdom

Zonia Weideman　　Department of Allied Health and Therapies, Metro North Hospital and Health Service, Brisbane, Queensland, Australia

Part 1
Occupational Therapy Models in Mental Health Practice

• Summary of the common occupational therapy models used in mental health practice.

• Summary of theoretical constructs and historical evolution of each model.

• Case and practice examples of how occupational therapists can use models in various practice contexts.

Models provide a structure to guide practice. Models help to delineate our key values and beliefs as occupational therapists and help articulate our understanding of occupational performance as a transaction between the person, the environment, and the occupation. However, many experienced occupational therapists have traditionally not seen themselves as using any model but rather relying on their professional reasoning.

The issue at hand is that the profession is ever-changing and exists in an ever-changing environment requiring occupational therapy practitioners to continuously adapt and respond to current and future client needs. Theoretical models help occupational therapists to be able to respond to current and future needs.

The purpose of this section is not to recommend any specific model but to summarise theoretical models commonly used by mental health occupational therapists so that the reader is able to choose an appropriate model to use for their clients in their contexts. When it comes to theoretical models, there is no one-siz--fits-all. This section will summarise the Model of Human Occupation (MoHO), the Person, Occupation, and Environment (PEO) model, the Canadian Model of Occupational Performance and Engagement (CMOP-E), and the Kawa model.

CHAPTER 1

The Model of Human Occupation (MOHO)

Tawanda Machingura[1,*], Edwin Mavindidze[2] and Clement Nhunzvi[3]

[1] *Head of Discipline Occupational Therapy Program, University of Notre Dame Australia, Sydney, Australia*

[2] *Department of Occupational Therapy, University of Zimbabwe, Harare, Zimbabwe*

[3] *Occupational Therapy Program, Bond University, Gold Coast, Australia*

Abstract: In this chapter, the Model of Human Occupation (MOHO) and its concepts are introduced to the reader. More specifically, each of the four components of the MOHO is defined and described, and examples from everyday practise are provided.

Keywords: Assessment , Model , Mental health , Occupational therapy , Occupation , Occupational behaviour , Occupational performance , Occupational therapy , Participation .

INTRODUCTION

Occupational therapists rely on occupation-based models of practice when working with their clients to enable them to do the things they want to, need to, or are expected to do. Occupation-based models are premised on the ontological stance in the philosophy of occupational therapy that "ever-changing humans, interconnected with everchanging environments, occupy time with ever-changing occupations and thereby transform – and are transformed by- their actions, environments and states of health" (Hooper & Wood, 2014, p.38). As such, occupation-based models focus on three interconnected elements that make up the occupational experience: person, environment, and occupation. Occupation-based models are built on the foundations laid by earlier frames of reference in occupational therapy, refocusing beyond just dysfunction and providing a more holistic outlook on occupation, even in those without impairments. A frame of reference or practice model is "a set of interrelated, internally consistent concepts, definitions, and postulates derived from or compatible with empirical data, providing a systematic description of or prescription for particular designs of the

---
* **Corresponding author Tawanda Machingura:** Head of Discipline Occupational Therapy Program, University of Notre Dame Australia, Sydney, Australia; E-mail: tawanda.machingura@nd.edu.au

environment for the purpose of facilitating evaluation an effecting change "(Mosey, 1986, p.5). It is a body of knowledge generated through research and practice used to develop a theory that is used by occupational therapists to inform them in a particular area of practice (Kielhofner, 2009a). Therefore, each model presents a unique perspective on the person, environment, and occupation illuminating the characteristics of each element that contributes to occupational being and ultimately supporting well-being. The occupational therapist uses occupation-based models as a magnifying glass, focusing on specific aspects of the occupational experience, gaining a deeper understanding, and targeting them. Mosey (1986), however, warns that practice models are "not a formula for action; but rather only a guide" (p.5).

This chapter focuses on one of the most popular occupation-based models of practice used in mental health practice, the Model of Human Occupation (MOHO) (Kielhofner, 2008). The MOHO was first published in 1980 as a series of four articles in the American Journal of Occupational Therapy (Kielhofner & Burke, 1980; Kielhofner, 1980a, 1980b; Kielhofner *et al.*, 1980). Since then, it has been the most extensively evidenced and most used occupation-based model, with about 80-92.1% of occupational therapists around the world now using this model (Cheung & Fung, 2020; J. Lee, 2010; S. W. Lee *et al.*, 2008, 2012). The MOHO is presented here, starting with a brief history of its foundations followed by an extensive discussion following the seven elements of an occupational therapy practice model: *the theoretical base, function-dysfunction continuum, the behaviours indicative of function and dysfunction, postulates regarding change, the primary assumptions, goals for intervention, and occupational therapy assessment and intervention techniques* (Creek, 2014; Hagedorn, 1992; Hinojosa & Kramer, 1993; Mosey, 1986).

The functions of MOHO as a conceptual model can be classified into four domains: Descriptive, Delimiting, Generative, and Integrative.

Descriptive – The MOHO can be used to describe the occupational phenomenon and provide operational definitions to aid the application of occupation to practice. Relevant variables are described, and the variations between them are also explained.

Delimiting – Just as lenses work, MOHO can be used to identify and filter in and out certain information about phenomena, helping to focus and organise data into meaningful units. This function is expanded on in assessments and evaluations supported by the model.

Integrative – True to its theoretical influences, the MOHO facilitates the systematic bringing together of other theoretical constructs and data into a consistent, meaningful, and unified whole.

Generative – The model continues to be a utility in research, innovation, and development. MOHO can be used as a conceptual framework in testing hypotheses and generation of new ideas.

A BRIEF HISTORY

MOHO evolved from the work of Mary Reilly during the 1960s and 1970s, who, at the time, was working on the Model of Occupational Behaviour (Fig. 1). Like many in occupational therapy, Reilly believed that humans transform their health and well-being through the use of their hands and minds. In the 1961 Eleanor Clarke Slagle Lecture, she famously said, 'Man, through the use of his hands as they are energised by mind and will, can influence the state of his own health' (Reilly, 1962, p.6, 1963). Mary Reilly opposed the medical model and felt that occupational therapists did not simply aim to reduce their clients' illness but their incapacity. Reilly defined occupational behaviour as activities that occupy time, involve achievement, and address the economic realities of life (Reilly, 1962). In her model, the goal of occupational behaviour is to reduce the disruptions and incapacities in occupational behaviour. Some of the basic assumptions at the time were that humans have an intrinsic need to master, occupation is intrinsically motivated, humans need occupation, and health is a balance of rest, work, and leisure. Reilly's work became the basis for MOHO, occupational science, and a new paradigm in occupational therapy where, once again, occupation was regarded as front and centre in occupational therapy practice.

Gary Kielhofner, Mary Reilly's student, was the architect of MOHO. In 1975, Kielhofner wrote an unpublished master's thesis on the model that formed the basis of the MOHO first published in 1980 (Kielhofner & Burke, 1980). Kielhofner believed that routines, habits, and motivation are part of a dynamic system influenced by the social and physical environment (Kielhofner & Burke, 1980). The diagrammatic representation of the original model is shown in Fig. (1) below.

When using MOHO, the routine and habits of the person are key to adaptation, and so are the motivation and meaning of the activity to the person. The MOHO underwent progressive development over the years to incorporate new knowledge and progressive changes in the profession's philosophy and domain of practice. After Gary Kielhofner's untimely death in 2010 (Braveman *et al.*, 2010), colleagues across the world have continued to develop the MOHO and research its applications across the occupational therapy domain and in various contexts

(Bowyer *et al.*, 2019, 2020; Cezar da Cruz *et al.*, 2019; Lin & Fisher, 2020; Parkinson, 2014; Parkinson & Brooks, 2020; Prior *et al.*, 2020; Taylor, 2017).

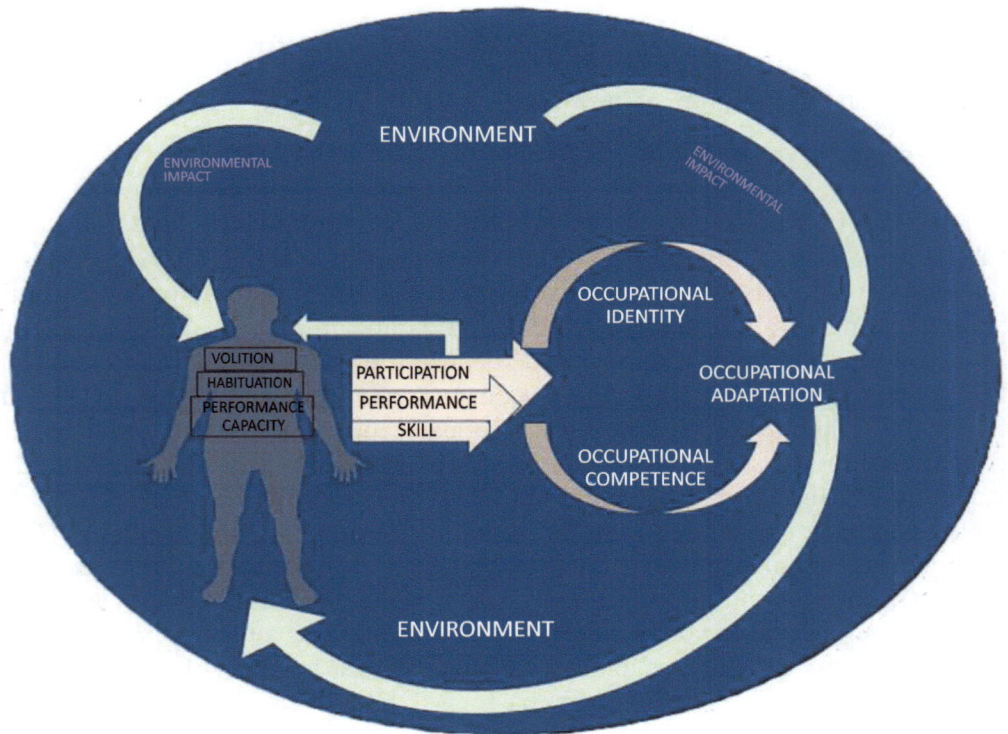

Fig. (1). Adapted from R. Taylor (Ed.) (2017), Kielhofner's Model of Human Occupation: Theory and application (5th ed.).

THEORETICAL BASE OF THE MODEL OF HUMAN OCCUPATION

Kielhofner, like Reilly, based his model of human occupation on dynamic systems theory. It suggests that there is an input, throughput, output, and feedback process in which individuals are linked to their environments as a dynamic system, and their occupations are shaped by both the individual's internal state and the external environment (Kielhofner, 2009b), The MOHO explains how the human system functions to perform occupations and how continued successful engagement shapes the sense of who individuals are or want to be (Kielhofner, 2009b). MOHO explains how people are motivated (also called *volition*) to perform occupations, how they repeat their behaviour over time (also called *habituation*), how the individual's inherent abilities support, how they perform occupations (also called *performance capacity)*, and how the entire process unfolds within a social and physical *environment*. The model's focus is on:

- Occupational performance rather than performance components
- The motivation for occupation
- The influence of the environment on occupational performance
- The nature of skilled performance
- The patterning of occupational behaviour/performance into routines and lifestyles

In a nutshell, MOHO conceptualises humans as being made up of three heterarchical interrelated components or subsystems:

- **Volition**: the motivation for engaging in an occupation.
- **Habituation:** the process by which behaviour is repeated and organised into patterns or routines.
- **Performance capacity**: the physical and mental abilities or skills that underlie occupational performance.

According to MOHO, human occupational performance is the result of an interaction between the person (volition, habituation, and performance capacity) and the environment (physical, social, or cultural) (Kielhofner, 2008). A dynamic and complementary relationship exists between the subsystems, which together influence occupational behaviour (Haglund & Kjellberg, 1999). No one component is more important than the other, but it is a complementary mix of factors from all the subsystems that result in specific occupational behaviors. Therefore, a disruption in one subsystem has a cascading effect on all other subsystems, resulting in occupational dysfunction. Furthermore, the environment can shape the human subsystems impacting occupational performance, or the person may select the best environment to perform specific tasks and occupations (Kielhofner, 2009b).

The model's focus is on:

- Occupational performance rather than performance components
- The motivation for occupation
- The influence of the environment on occupational performance
- The nature of skilled performance
- The patterning of occupational behaviour/performance into routines and lifestyles

Concepts of the MOHO

MOHO explains how a person becomes motivated to engage in an occupation, for example:

Tamaki was a 35-year-old woman and basketball Paralympian. She grew up in a school and social system where her goals of playing basketball were not always supported. Tamaki, however, always went to watch school basketball games in her school years and played basketball with her friends at home. With the help of her occupational therapist, she joined a professional basketball team in her teenage years and became a professional wheelchair basketball player by the time she was twenty. MOHO can explain how habits and routines are formed to support the chosen occupation. For example, Tamaki needed to develop certain habits; those habits involved things like regularly waking up in the morning to train, warming up, and eating healthy foods at specified times so that she could engage successfully in playing basketball. Such habits support successful engagement in occupations. Also important is the individual's perception of their own abilities and capacities. This perception changes and develops over time.

MOHO is evidence-based, holistic, and occupation-focused and complements other models. Each of these aspects is further described below.

MOHO is evidence-based. MOHO is an evidence-based conceptual practice model that explains how people adapt to severe disability and rediscover satisfying and meaningful ways to live their lives (Taylor, 2017). MOHO is supported by a substantial body of research conducted over the past four decades. Consequently, MOHO has a wide range of assessment tools designed to seek out information on the various elements of the model across various occupations and clients. Collectively, there is evidence that supports the validity of the concepts described by the model and confirms the validity and reliability of the model assessments. An evidence-based search engine can be found at www.MoHO.uic.edu.

MOHO is practice-based and holistic. MOHO assists in explaining how people can adapt to severe disability and rediscover satisfying, meaningful ways to live their lives. It provides a range of assessment tools, case studies, protocols, and programs. It involves practitioners and consumers in research and is grounded in the real world.

MOHO is client-centred. Practitioners observe and ask questions that facilitate an understanding of the client's immediate needs and perspectives. They incorporate the client's perspectives and desires in shaping therapy. They support and respect the client's values, sense of capacity and efficacy, roles, habits, performance experience, and environment. The client's choice, action, and experience are central to the therapy process. MOHO conceptualises the client's own doing, thinking, and feeling as central to the therapy process. Disability occurs as a result of a misfit between the environment and the person.

MOHO compliments other models. The model was developed at a time when most models in occupational therapy were impairment-focused. MOHO considers impairment alongside the client's motivation and lifestyle, as well as their environment The model components are detailed in Table **1**. The model was always intended to be used alongside other occupational therapy models and interdisciplinary concepts. In an eclectic combination of practice frameworks (Ikiugu & Smallfield, 2011), the MOHO is a versatile organising model of practice that can be combined with a wide range of other practice models across different practice contexts.

Table 1. A model of human occupation (Kielhofner, 2008).

Volition • Personal causation • Values • Interests	Performance Capacity • Motor skills • Processing • Communication and interaction skills	Dimensions of doing • Occupational participation • Occupational performance • Occupational skill
Habituation • Roles • Routines	Environment • Space • Social • Cultural • Political	Occupational adaptation • Occupational identity • Occupational competence

The versatility of the model is as a result of MOHO being based on assumptions that are common in other occupational therapy models. This assumptions are detailed in Table **2**.

Table 2. MOHO assumptions and their practice applications (adapted from B. Boyt Schell, G. Gillen, & M. Scaffa (Eds.), Willard and Spackman's Occupational Therapy (13th ed.). Lippincott Williams & Wilkins)

Assumptions	Practice Application
Humans are biologically mandated to be active.	People have a fundamental neurologically- based need for action and doing. The innate need is a dominant source of motivation for participation in occupation.
Thinking, feeling, and doing are influenced by a dynamic interaction between one's internal components and the environment.	Systems theory helps the practitioner to understand that there are multiple factors within the person and the environment that influence each other.
Humans are an open system that can change and develop through interaction with the environment. Parts of the open cycle include input, throughput, output, and feedback.	Clients learn about themselves by experimenting with behaviours and receiving feedback about behaviour (output).
Context demands will determine how human variables organise themselves to achieve a sense of order.	The client's environment influences how personal variables interrelate.

(Table 2) cont.....

Assumptions	Practice Application
Occupational competence (the degree to which one sustains a pattern of occupational participation that represents one's occupational identity).	Clients demonstrate competency when they organise their lives to meet their basic responsibilities to themselves and the role obligations of society in satisfying and meaningful ways.
Occupational adaptation (the outcome of a positive occupational identity and achievement of occupational competence).	Occupational therapy acts as a form of feedback that can impact how one changes and alters behaviours
Humans are a dynamic system.	Occupational behaviour is explored and understood from a systems theory perspective. Elements of the system work together to produce behaviour, which is dynamic and context-dependent.
Occupations are central to human experience, survival, and satisfaction.	Therapy enables people to reshape their occupational abilities and identities, therefore becoming more adaptive.

FUNCTION/ DYSFUNCTION CONTINUUM: MOHO CONCEPTS

Operationalizing the client's innate capacities along a function/ dysfunction continuum enables the occupational therapist to observe and measure changes in occupational functioning (Gutman *et al.*, 2007). A clear conceptualisation of such innate capacities makes it easier for the occupational therapist to identify changes in these capacities and functions. Function/ dysfunction continua define the extremes of dysfunction (need for occupational therapy intervention) and function (goal of occupational therapy intervention). Each function/ dysfunction continuum should be accompanied by observable and measurable (quantifiable or qualifiable) behaviours indicative of function/ dysfunction.

MOHO conceptualises humans as being made up of three interrelated heterarchical concepts or subsystems, each with a number of elements: Volition-values, interests, and personal causation; Habituation- habits and roles; and Performance Capacity- the mental and physical attributes and lived experiences. These elements are internal to humans but influence the behaviours that we then observe. These actions are described as dimensions of doing, which are the three levels of occupational participation, occupational performance, and occupational skills (Kielhofner, 2008). Each dimension of doing builds from the level that precedes it. The MOHO also links the internal self and the dimensions of doing to development and sustaining occupational identity, competence, and adaptation. MOHO defines function/dysfunction continua across the internal subsystems, dimensions of doing, and occupational adaptation. However, it should be noted that behaviours indicative of function and dysfunction relate only to dimensions of doing, even for the internal subsystems or occupational adaptation. For example, for a function/dysfunction continuum such as 'Role competence-Role dysfunction' within an internal subsystem of habituation, behaviours indicative of function/ dysfunction can only be observed within dimensions of doing like participation of the role within the context of relationships or performance of tasks culturally expected for the role. These MOHO concepts associated with the person and occupation are considered in more detail below, following which attention is turned to the last MOHO concept, Environment.

Volition

Volition is the motivation for engaging in occupations. Humans have a biological, neurologically-based mandate to be active, which is a product of an evolutionary process. This provides a foundation for motivation towards occupation. Volition is mediated through other physical phenomena such as mood, energy level, and fatigue (Kielhofner, 2002). Thoughts and feelings are also essential to volition. Volition is reflected in the wide range of thoughts and feelings people have about the things they have done, are doing, or might do (Kielhofner, 2002). Volition is conceptualised as being made up of personal causation, values, and interests. *Personal causation* refers to one's sense of competence and effectiveness. *Values* refer to what one finds important and meaningful. *Interests* refer to what one finds enjoyable or satisfying to do.

Habituation

Habituation is the process by which occupation is organised into patterns or routines. "The world around us, our habitat, has a certain stability; we, in return, also have a tendency to act in consistent, patterned ways" (Keilhofner, 2002). Habituation is the semi-autonomous patterning of behaviour in the form of habits and roles. Habituation is defined as an "internalised readiness to exhibit consistent patterns of behaviour guided by our habits and roles and fitted to the characteristics of routine temporal, physical, and social environments" (Kielhofner, 2002).

Performance Capacity

Performance capacity is the physical and mental abilities and lived experiences that underlie occupational performance. Emphasis is on subjective experience and its role in shaping how people perform. Occupational performance is also considered objectively (a person's musculoskeletal, neurologic, cardiopulmonary, and other bodily systems, mental an cognitive abilities). Performance capacity can be described as the ability to receive, plan, and program plans of action and effect action through the body. Performance components are important for performance but do not cause or produce behaviour directly.

Dimensions of doing: Behaviours Indicative of Function/ Dysfunction

Occupational Participation

Occupational participation is the engagement in a repertoire of tasks within work, play, or activities of daily living that are part of the social context, expected of an individual based on their gender, age, and culture, and contribute to their well-being (Kielhofner, 2009b). It is not just performance – it is doing things of personal and social significance (*e.g.*, volunteering, working part-time, maintaining one's living space, or attending college).

Occupational Performance

"Occupational performance is the doing, the action, the active behavior, or the active responses exhibited within the context of an occupational form" (Nelson, 1988. 634). Occupational performance describes the act of executing tasks that act as the foundation of occupational participation (Kielhofner, 2009b).

Performance Skills

All performance requires numerous skills, defined as purposeful, observable actions that are used while performing. Performance skills differ from performance capacity in that performance capacity is an underlying potential or preparedness for performance, while performance skills are actions towards a desired end. In other words, performance skills are an enactment of the performance capacity. There are three main types of skills: motor, process, and communication and interaction skills. These are influenced by both environmental and personal factors. Various body structures, personal factors, and environmental contexts converge to shape performance skills. In addition, body functions, such as mental, sensory, neuromuscular, and movement-related functions, are identified as the capacities that reside within the person and also converge with structures and environmental contexts to emerge as performance skills.

Occupational Identity, competence, and adaptation

Charles Christiansen, in his 1999 Eleanor Clarke Slagle Lecture, proposed that our identities are shaped by what we do and how we view that doing in the context of others (Christiansen, 1999).

Occupations are more than movements strung together, more than simply doing something. They are opportunities to express the self, to create an identity. (Christiansen, 1999, p.552)

MOHO acknowledges this assertion, conceptualising that the enactment of the dimensions of doing overtime develops the individual's occupational identity. Occupational identity is an individual's sense of self and the possible selves as occupational beings (Kielhofner, 2009b). Occupational identities are better understood in the context of occupational narratives, which are live stories being told and enacted based on an individual's volition, habituation and performance capacities under the influence of the environment (Kielhofner, 2009b). When occupational identities are enacted and sustained overtime, they result in occupational competence. MOHO conceptualises occupational adaptation as the positive experience of occupational identity.

Environment

The environment provides opportunities for performance and pressors for certain behaviour. It provides press and, concurrently, synergy of influences to channel behaviour. The environment is comprised of physical, social, cultural, economic, and political aspects. It impacts how occupations are motivated, organised, and performed. People seek to explore and master their environments. It contains objects, spaces, occupational tasks and culture, and economic and political influences. The temporal nature of human performance is key to understanding the influence of the environment. MOHO also accommodates the diversity and continuum of effects of the environment as occupational beings act on it through the plethora of their occupations.

Strengths of MOHO

MOHO is a particularly popular model in mental health practice. The strengths of MOHO are that:

- It reorients practice to be more occupation-based.
- It is a highly researched model.
- It is amenable to use in a variety of settings.
- It provides a framework for addressing difficulties of coping with roles and developing desired habits/Behaviour.
- It has clearly defined theoretical constructs.
- It has led to the development of many assessment instruments, which have been validated and are frequently used in research and practice.
- It uses a client-centred approach.
- It is applicable to all ages.

Weaknesses of MOHO

The weaknesses of MOHO are that:

- It offers limited intervention guidance.
- Its application of prevention vs intervention is unclear.
- The terms used can be confusing and are not intuitive. People may define or interpret terms differently, leading to confusion.
- It is rarely sufficient to identify all of the client's issues on its own.

Professional Reasoning and MOHO

Understanding the client's needs and current level of function requires the occupational therapist to think critically through the client's circumstances, existing knowledge on how to achieve change, and the possible action to achieve this change. Therefore, to achieve the best outcomes, the occupational therapist requires a guiding framework (Mosey, 1986) to guide their professional reasoning.

Professional reasoning denotes the occupational therapist's critical thinking about the client throughout the occupational therapy process (Unsworth & Baker, 2016). Professional reasoning allows the occupational therapist to think through the various elements that surround the case and may influence the outcome of the case. These elements of professional reasoning include scientific, diagnostic, procedural, pragmatic, narrative, conditional, interactive, and ethical reasoning. The foundations of professional reasoning in occupational therapy are rooted in the profession's philosophy and refined by the therapists' understanding of their practice context as well as the practice model they use.

The MOHO guides the following elements of professional reasoning:

Scientific reasoning: MOHO provides an evidence-based framework to think through the case, leading to a diagnosis of the occupational problems faced by the client, and offers procedures for evaluation and suggested interventions.

Diagnostic reasoning: MOHO defines occupational problems within the sub-systems of the human. It also provides the rationale of how these then affect occupational participation and performance.

Procedural reasoning: MOHO provides a wide range of assessment tools with clear procedures and manuals to follow

Narrative reasoning: MOHO highlights the client's occupational narratives, which may predict the client's adaptation. Occupational narratives may be better understood through case formulation.

MOHO Case Study

John, a 30-year-old Māori Indigenous male, was admitted to an acute inpatient unit on the Gold Coast in Australia with a diagnosis of schizophrenia. Physically, he was tall and overweight, with visible cultural tattoos covering his entire body, including face, head, and neck. This was John's third presentation to the acute inpatient unit in the last 12 months. He had presented with marked delusions and hallucinations following a period of not taking his medications. In the ward, he kept to himself. Most staff left him to himself, only talking to him when needed, such as during medication time and mealtimes. He had been secluded once when he had pushed a fellow patient to the follow following an incident where this other patient had made some negative comments about his tattoos.

John was seen for an initial assessment by his OT.

Reflection Questions

1. Is the structure of the routine in the ward helping John to engage in meaningful occupations whilst in the hospital?

2. In what way is it helping or not helping?

Information Gathered using MoHO

Volition: John valued his culture (*values*) and enjoyed listening and playing music (*interests*). He used to play in a band that played in pubs in New Zealand, where he was born. He believed he was a very good guitar player (*personal causation*).

Habituation: When not in the hospital, John spent most weekends going to pubs to listen to music (*habits*). This seemed to take precedence over things like self-care or home maintenance activities such as mowing the lawns. His neighbours had complained, and he had been given the notice to vacate his unit by the landlord. He no longer played in a band and, instead, hung out with members of a local biker gang renowned for selling drugs and violence. He saw himself as a gang member (*roles*).

Environment: John lived alone in a privately rented unit in the Upper Coomera suburb of the Gold Coast (physical environment). He had no friends, just acquaintances who all happened to be gang members or drug dealers (social environment). He had lost touch with family members who had remained in New Zealand when he emigrated to Australia 10 years ago.

Performance Capacity: John struggled to maintain his unit and had been issued with a notice to vacate the property. He did not pay rent on time and often ran out of money for groceries. He was not on any pension and survived by selling drugs or doing odd jobs for the gang, including being a debt collector. Physically he was overweight but mobile and active. He was disorganised and did not plan his days at all, rather "going with the flow".

Reflection Questions

1. What do we know about John's occupational identity?

2. Is John appropriately appraising his own abilities in terms of self-care, leisure, or productivity? Can John organise himself within his self-care, productivity, and leisure (process skills)? Does John have a supportive social and physical environment to allow for meaningful self-care, productivity, and leisure? How is John motivated for self-care, productivity, and leisure?

3. What could interventions focus on from a MoHO perspective?

Possible Answers to Reflection Questions

*1. **Occupational identity**: John identified as a gang member. He was also a proud Māori man and a musician.*

*2. **Appraisal of abilities**: He does not seem to be appropriately appraising his abilities. Appraisal of abilities reflects motivation for occupation. John does not seem to engage in self-care, leisure, and productive occupations on a consistent basis.*

*3. **Intervention:** The intervention was centred around constructing a positive occupational identity and achieving occupational competence over time in the context of his environment.*

MOHO Assessments

MOHO has a range of standardised and non-standardised assessment tools to aid practice. To access assessment forms and manuals, please visit www.moho.uic.edu. Some of these are overviewed here.

The Model of Human Occupation Screening Tool (MOHOST) aims to give a broad overview of occupational participation. It consists of 24 items, four for each of the following sections: Volition (or 'motivation for occupation'); Habituation (or 'pattern of occupation'); Communication and Interaction skills; Process skills; Motor skills; and the Environment. This tool is used *in situ*ations where accurate self-assessment may not be possible and lengthy interviews may not be appropriate (*e.g.*, a person lacks insight).

Occupational Performance History Interview-Second Version (OPHI-II) gathers information about a client's past and present occupational adaptation using three steps:

1. A semi-structured interview exploring the client's occupational life history
2. Rating scales measuring occupational identity, occupational competence, and the impact of the client's occupational behaviour, and
3. A life history narrative designed to capture the salient qualitative features of the occupational life history.

Occupational Self Assessment (OSA) gathers the clients' perceptions of their own occupational competence. It also allows clients to indicate personal values and to set priorities for change.

Occupational Circumstances Assessment Interview and Rating Scale (OCAIRS) is a semi-structured interview that provides a structure for gathering, analysing, and reporting data on the extent and nature of an individual's occupational participation.

Assessment of Communication and Interaction Skills (ACIS) is a formal observational tool designed to measure an individual's performance in an occupational form and/or within a social group of which the person is a part.

The Occupational Questionnaire (OQ) is a pen and paper, self-report instrument that asks the individual to provide a description of typical use of time and utilises Likert-type ratings of competence, importance, and enjoyment during activities.

The Role Checklist is a self-report checklist that can be used to obtain information about the types of roles people engage in, which organise their daily lives.

The Worker Role Interview (WRI) is a semi-structured interview designed to be used as the psychosocial/environmental component of the initial rehabilitation assessment process for the injured worker.

The Work Environment Impact Scale (WEIS) is a semi-structured interview designed to gather information about how individuals with disabilities experience and perceive their work settings.

Despite there being a wide range of MoHO Assessments, the user of these tools need to be aware of administration procedures and client requirements. These procedures and requirements are detailed in Table **3** below.

Table 3. Therapist and Client Requirements for commonly used MoHO Assessments (adapted from B. Boyt Schell, G. Gillen, & M. Scaffa (Eds.), Willard and Spackman's Occupational Therapy (13th ed.). Lippincott Williams & Wilkins)).

Assessment	Therapists' Requirements for Administration	Client Requirements to Participate	Estimated Total Therapist Time [Removed Hyperlink Field]
Assessment of Communication and Interaction Skills	Observe the client in a goal-oriented activity that involves social interaction, complete scale[b]	Engage in some social interaction	20-60 minutes
Assessment of Occupational Functioning	Administer interview or explain the self-report format to the client	Answer interview questions (interview format). Read and write (self-report format)	20-30 minutes as an interview and 12 minutes as self-report
Model of Human Occupational Screening Tool	Collect information *via* chart review, interview, observation from surrogates, and complete scale[c]	Minimally interact with the environment	10-40 minutes
Occupational Circumstances Assessment—Interview and Rating Scale	Conduct semi-structured interviews, and complete scale	Answer questions	25-50 minutes
Occupational Performance History Interview—II	Conduct a semi-structured interview; complete three scales and complete the life history narrative slope	Answer questions	45 minutes-1 hour

(Table 3) cont.....

Assessment	Therapists' Requirements for Administration	Client Requirements to Participate	Estimated Total Therapist Time [Removed Hyperlink Field]
Occupational Questionnaire	Explain instructions, discuss client responses	Concentrate, read, write	15-30 minutes
Occupational Self Assessment	Explain instructions and discuss client responses	Concentrate, read, write	15-35 minutes
Role Checklist	Explain instructions, discuss client responses	Concentrate, read, write	10-15 minutes
Volitional Questionnaire	Observe client across 1 or 2 settings: complete scale	Minimally interact with the environment	15-30 minutes each observation 5-10 minutes for the rating scale
Worker Role Interview	Conduct semi-structured interviews, complete scale[c]	Answer questions	30 minutes-1 hour
Work Environment Impact Scale	Conduct semi-structured interviews and complete scale	Answer questions	30 minutes-1 hour

[a] Does not include time for clients to complete self-administered assessments.
[b] Completing MoHO instrument scales ordinarily involves using a 4-point rating scale and entering clarifying/qualifying comments.
[c] There are interview formats available that allow the MOHOST or WRI to be combined with the OCAIRS, saving administration time.

Reflection Questions (Refer to Case Study)

1. What do we know about John's communication and interaction skills?

2. What do we know about John's patterns of doing?

3. What are John's strengths and limitations?

4. What assessment tools and outcome measures do you think you might use?

5. Would MOHOST be an appropriate assessment tool? Why? Or why not?

6. If using the MOHOST, what ratings would you give John for environment occupational demands in the hospital (e.g., Facilitates/ Allows/ Inhibits/ Restricts)?

MOHO Case Formulation

The MOHO case formulation is a process of applying occupational therapy clinical and occupational reasoning to re-assemble the occupational information about the person to understand and make sense of their situation in moving from assessment to intervention. Forsyth (2017) makes reference to an occupational formulation, which they posit as a process or stage within the occupational therapy process (Brooks & Parkinson, 2018), specifically created after informal or formal assessment and leading to identifying and setting measurable goals (Forsyth, 2017).

Parkinson and Brooks (2020) suggest a guide in case formulation, framing it as occupational formulation. They frame it as a process involving five self-explanatory iterative stages, that is:

1. Structuring the occupational identity section
2. Structuring the occupational competence section
3. Determining the key occupational adaptation issues
4. Wrapping up formulation
5. Determining and negotiating measurable occupational goals

Three basic questions to answer in case formulation (Table **4**) include Who is the person? What are the occupational issues?, and Why are they having those challenges? A narrative approach is recommended for formulation as it aligns well with the concept of occupational narrative already established in occupational therapy practice. Emphasis should be placed on making the process collaborative, thereby strengthening the shared decision-making, rapport, and client-therapist relationship.

Table 4. Case Formulation Quick Questions

Question	Occupational Formulation Concept	Focus
Who is the person?	Occupational influences	The occupational profile The occupational identity (principal role, values, beliefs, and goals)
What are the occupational issues?	Occupational presentation	Occupational competence issues, including challenges in fulfilling principal roles and responsibilities

(Table 4) cont.....

Question	Occupational Formulation Concept	Focus
Why is the person having challenges in their occupations?	Occupational focus	Occupational adaptation in relation to other components. A critical analysis of the factors influencing doing drawn from volition, habituation, or the environment

In summary, a well-articulated occupational formulation should allow readers to picture and engage with the person's identity and competence whilst scoping the way forward. It reads like a hybrid narrative, relying on the person's subjective statements describing their occupational influences and a more objective description of their occupational presentation to inform the occupational focus (Brooks & Parkinson, 2018).

MOHO-based Interventions

MOHO-based therapeutic reasoning is client-centred. Therapists must understand and consider all domains of the model including their client's values, sense of performance capacity, and personal environment. Assessments gather information, and interventions provide opportunities for clients to improve their perspectives on these factors. MOHO conceptualises the client's own thinking, feeling, and doing as the important factors in realising change, and interventions need to be based on the client's choices, needs, and experiences.

Practitioners who use MoHO commonly use occupations as a method to achieve positive outcomes. The method of measuring intervention outcomes is increases or changes in engagement in desired occupations (Creek, 2002). It helps clinicians to be occupation-focused rather than generic (Bassett & Lloyd, 2001).

Commonly used interventions are listed in Table **5** below.

Table 5. Commonly used MOHO-based intervention strategies.

Commonly used MOHO-based interventions	Description
Advising	This is a process where the therapist recommends goals or interventions to the client using their professional expertise. This may involve the therapist providing information on a recommended option. When using this strategy, the client must still maintain autonomy and the right to choose their preferred option. It is also critical that all possible options are discussed with the client.

(Table 5) cont.....

Commonly used MOHO-based interventions	Description
Giving Feedback	This is a process of gathering and analysing information and then conceptualising the information as feedback to the client with the purpose of enhancing the skills and occupational performance of the client. This may involve sharing assessment results with clients, providing feedback on behaviour in group settings, or providing praise on choices or progress in therapy.
Negotiating	This is a process used to resolve differences or to compare and contrast different perspectives by using a give-and-take approach. The therapist may use this strategy to assist the client in choosing a less harmful behaviour or life choice.
Structuring	This is a process where the therapist establishes parameters for choice and performance by setting limits, offering clients alternatives, and establishing some ground rules. (Scott & Haggarty, 984)
Coaching	This strategy involves the therapist assisting a client to take responsibility for self-direction in naming priorities and goals that are most meaningful to them. The therapist collaboratively works with the client to identify challenges, set goals, and work towards achieving those goals. The therapist working in this way may offer feedback on occupational performance in order to support and enhance occupational behaviour and engagement in occupations. (Townsend & Polatajko, 2007). The therapist uses guiding, demonstrations, prompting, and instructing to enable the client to improve their skills and enhance occupational performance.
Encouraging	This is a process of providing positive feedback, emotional support, and reassurance to the client with the aim of promoting a particular desired behaviour, feeling, or thought. It is a feedback mechanism from therapist to client.
Validating	The therapist identifies and appropriately acknowledges the feelings, emotions, perspectives, and lived experiences of the client. The therapist demonstrates an active interest in the client's thoughts, feelings, and experiences and demonstrates empathy and understanding as well as monitors and responds to the client's responses. (Bailliard *et al.*, 2020)
Identifying	This is a process where the therapist engages with the client and structures tasks and activities for the client to actively participate in the process of identifying personal and environmental opportunities and resources.

Below is a template that could be used to plan MOHO-based interventions.

The form presented in Table **5** can be used as a guide to record client goals and planned interventions using MOHO concepts and intervention strategies. Using this form will give confidence to the practitioner that they are using an evidence-based approach to working with their client and may help improve communication and clarity on the OT role within a multi-disciplinary team environment. The below process is suggested when completing the form:

Table 6. MOHO-based Intervention Planning.

Client Demographic Details			
Client Name:	DoB:	Age:	Sex:
Address:			

Setting Details			
Name of Referrer:	Designation:	Ward/ Team:	OT Name:

Presenting occupational issues	
Self-care:	Productivity:
Leisure:	Social Participation and Inclusion:

Interventions Plan			
MoHO Domain	Goals (Identify SMART occupational goals)	Therapeutic Strategies* (choose appropriate strategies in collaboration with the client)	Session Outline (Detail your first 3 treatment sessions)
Volition • Values • Interests • Personal causation	……..(Brooks & Parkinson) will be able to identify ……..occupations that are significant to them and are consistent with their current skills and abilities within ….(time frame)		
Habituation • roles • routines • habits	……..{client} will be able to…….(identify/ practice/ develop) a habit pattern that will support achievement of ………….(desired occupations) within ……(time frame).		
Performance Capacity • motor skills • communication and interaction skills • abilities	……..{client} will be able to perform in ……..{occupation} using…………{skills/ adapted techniques} …………{independently/ with assistance} at/ in …..{setting} within …..(time frame).		
Environment • social • physical • cultural • digital	……..{client} will be able to live in ……..{type of dwelling} with …………{supports} …………{independently/ with assistance} within…..{time frame}.		

1. The practitioner is encouraged to complete the client demographic details and setting details first.
2. The practitioner then collaborates with the client to devise priority areas of

primary concern to the client.

3. The practitioner and the client then collaborate to devise SMART occupation focused goals in each identified priority MOHO domain area.
4. The practitioner and the client then collaborate to devise appropriate MOHO-based intervention strategies to assist the client in achieving desired goals.
5. The practitioner utilises their knowledge of occupation, health, and well-being as well as the therapeutic use of self throughout the process.

*MOHO strategies include validating, identifying, advising, advocating, structuring, encouraging, giving feedback, physically supporting, and coaching.

CONCLUSION

This chapter has described the theoretical origins of MOHO and discussed the seven elements of an occupational therapy practice model: the theoretical base, function-dysfunction continuum, the behaviours indicative of function and dysfunction, postulates regarding change, the primary assumptions, goals for intervention, and occupational therapy assessment and intervention techniques (Creek, 2014; Hagedorn, 1992; Hinojosa & Kramer, 1993; Mosey, 1986). This chapter has presented case studies to assist the reader in understanding and applying the model in practice. MOHO is dynamic and will continue to evolve and change over time. It is a model based on evidence, is holistic, and complements other models.

Key Points

- MOHO is evidence-based, holistic, occupation-focused, and complements other models.
- MOHO has a range of standardised and non-standardised assessment tools to aid practice.
- MOHO uses occupations as the method to achieve positive outcomes.

REFERENCES

Bassett, H., Lloyd, C. (2001). Occupational Therapy in Mental Health: Managing Stress and Burnout. *Br. J. Occup. Ther., 64*(8), 406-411.
[http://dx.doi.org/10.1177/030802260106400807]

Bailliard, A.L., Dallman, A.R., Carroll, A., Lee, B.D., Szendrey, S. (2020). Doing Occupational Justice: A Central Dimension of Everyday Occupational Therapy Practice. *Can. J. Occup. Ther., 87*(2), 144-152.
[http://dx.doi.org/10.1177/0008417419898930] [PMID: 31964168]

Bowyer, P., Muñoz, L., Tiongco, C.G., Tkach, M.M., Moore, C.C., Burton, B., Lim, D. (2020). Occupational therapy, cancer, and occupation-centred practice: impact of training in the model of human occupation. *Aust. Occup. Ther. J., 67*(6), 605-614.
[http://dx.doi.org/10.1111/1440-1630.12687] [PMID: 32820529]

Bowyer, P., Munoz, L., Tkach, M.M., Moore, C.C., Tiongco, C.G. (2019). Long-term impact of model of human occupation training on therapeutic reasoning. *J. Allied Health, 48*(3), 188-193.

[PMID: 31487357]

Braveman, B., Fisher, G., Suarez-Balcazar, Y. (2010). Achieving the ordinary things: a tribute to Gary Kielhofner. *Am. J. Occup. Ther., 64*(6), 828-831.
[http://dx.doi.org/10.5014/ajot.2010.64605] [PMID: 21218672]

Brooks, R., Parkinson, S. (2018). Occupational formulation: A three-part structure. *Br. J. Occup. Ther., 81*(3), 177-179.
[http://dx.doi.org/10.1177/0308022617745015]

Bryant, W., Fieldhouse, J., & Plastow, N. (Eds.). (2022). Creek's Occupational Therapy and Mental Health E-Book: Creek's Occupational Therapy and Mental Health E-Book. Elsevier Health Sciences.

Boyt, Schell, Gillen, G., Scaffa, M. *Willard and Spackman's Occupational Therapy (12th ed.).*. (Lippincott Williams & Wilkins).

Cruz, D.M.C., Parkinson, S., Rodrigues, D.S., Carrijo, D.C.M., Costa, J.D., Fachin-Martins, E., Pfeifer, L.I. (2019). Cross-cultural adaptation, face validity and reliability of the Model of Human Occupation Screening Tool to Brazilian Portuguese. *Cadernos Brasileiros de Terapia Ocupacional, 27*(4), 691-702.
[http://dx.doi.org/10.4322/2526-8910.ctoAO2007]

Cheung, P., Fung, X.C.C. (2020). Review Article A Review on the Case Studies of Using the Model of Human Occupation. *Social Health and Behavior, 3*, 3-9.
[http://dx.doi.org/10.4103/SHB.SHB]

Christiansen, C.H. (1999). Defining Lives: Occupation as Identity: An Essay on Competence, Coherence, and the Creation of Meaning. *Am. J. Occup. Ther., 53*(6), 547-558.
[http://dx.doi.org/10.5014/ajot.53.6.547] [PMID: 10578432]

Creek, J., Bannigan, K. (2002). Occupation and activity – a discussion. *Mentalhealth OT, 7*(1), 4-6.

Forsyth, K. (2017). Therapeutic reasoning: Planning, implementing, and evaluating the outcomes of therapy. *Kielhofner's Model of Human Occupation: Theory and Application* In T. RR (Ed.), Williams and Wilkins.

Forsyth, K. (2017). Therapeutic reasoning: Planning, implementing, and evaluating the outcomes of therapy. In T. RR (Ed.), Williams and Wilkins.

Forsyth, K., Kielhofner, G. (2006). The Model of Human Occupation. *Foundations for practice in occupational therapy.*

Gutman, S.A., Mortera, M.H., Hinojosa, J., Kramer, P. (2007). Revision of the occupational therapy practice framework. *Am. J. Occup. Ther., 61*(1), 119-126.
[http://dx.doi.org/10.5014/ajot.61.1.119] [PMID: 17302113]

Haglund, L., Kjellberg, A. (1999). A Critical Analysis of the Model of Human Occupation. *Can. J. Occup. Ther., 66*(2), 102-108.
[http://dx.doi.org/10.1177/000841749906600206] [PMID: 10605160]

Haglund, L., Kjellberg, A. (1999). A Critical Analysis of the Model of Human Occupation. *Can. J. Occup. Ther., 66*(2), 102-108.
[http://dx.doi.org/10.1177/000841749906600206] [PMID: 10605160]

Hooper, B., Wood, W. (2014). The Philosophy of Occupational Therapy: A Framework for Practice. In: Boyt Schell, B., Gillen, G., Scaffa, M., (Eds.), *Willard and Spackman's Occupational Therapy.* Lippincott Williams & Wilkins.

Ikiugu, M.N., Smallfield, S. (2011). Ikiugu's eclectic method of combining theoretical conceptual practice models in occupational therapy. *Aust. Occup. Ther. J., 58*(6), 437-446.
[http://dx.doi.org/10.1111/j.1440-1630.2011.00968.x] [PMID: 22111646]

Kielhofner, G., Burke, J.P. (1980). A model of human occupation, part 1. Conceptual framework and content. *Am. J. Occup. Ther., 34*(9), 572-581.
[http://dx.doi.org/10.5014/ajot.34.9.572] [PMID: 7457553]

Kielhofner, G. (1980). A model of human occupation, part 2. Ontogenesis from the perspective of temporal adaptation. *Am. J. Occup. Ther., 34*(10), 657-663. a
[http://dx.doi.org/10.5014/ajot.34.10.657] [PMID: 7425070]

Kielhofner, G. (1980). A model of human occupation, Part 3, benign and vicious cycles. *Am. J. Occup. Ther., 34*(11), 731-737. b
[http://dx.doi.org/10.5014/ajot.34.11.731] [PMID: 7212009]

Kielhofner, G. (2008). *Model of Human Occupation: Theory and application.* Lippincott Williams & Wilkins.

Kielhofner, G. (2009). Conceptual Foundations of Occupational Therapy Practice. *Conceptual Foundations of Occupational Therapy Practice.* Kielhofner, G. (2009). Conceptual foundations of occupational therapy practice. FA Davis.

Kielhofner, G. (2009). Model of Human Occupation *In Conceptual Foundations of Occupational Therapy Practice.*

Kielhofner, G., Burke, J.P. (1980). A model of human occupation, part 1. Conceptual framework and content. *Am. J. Occup. Ther., 34*(9), 572-581.
[http://dx.doi.org/10.5014/ajot.34.9.572] [PMID: 7457553]

Kielhofner, G., Burke, J.P., Igi, C.H. (1980). A model of human occupation, Part 4. Assessment and intervention. *Am. J. Occup. Ther., 34*(12), 777-788.
[http://dx.doi.org/10.5014/ajot.34.12.777] [PMID: 7282839]

Kirsh, B., Martin, L., Hultqvist, J., Eklund, M. (2019). Occupational therapy interventions in mental health: A literature review in search of evidence. *Occup. Ther. Ment. Health, 35*(2), 109-156.
[http://dx.doi.org/10.1080/0164212X.2019.1588832]

Lee, J. (2010). Achieving best practice: a review of evidence linked to occupation-focused practice models. *Occup. Ther. Health Care, 24*(3), 206-222.
[http://dx.doi.org/10.3109/07380577.2010.483270] [PMID: 23898928]

Lee, S.W., Kielhofner, G., Morley, M., Heasman, D., Garnham, M., Willis, S., Parkinson, S., Forsyth, K., Melton, J., Taylor, R.R. (2012). Impact of using the Model of Human Occupation: A survey of occupational therapy mental health practitioners' perceptions. *Scand. J. Occup. Ther., 19*(5), 450-456.
[http://dx.doi.org/10.3109/11038128.2011.645553] [PMID: 22214401]

Lee, S.W., Taylor, R., Kielhofner, G., Fisher, G. (2008). Theory use in practice: a national survey of therapists who use the Model of Human Occupation. *Am. J. Occup. Ther., 62*(1), 106-117.
[http://dx.doi.org/10.5014/ajot.62.1.106] [PMID: 18254437]

Lin, T.T., Fisher, G. (2020). Applying the Model of Human Occupation During the Pandemic Stay-at-Home Order. *Open J. Occup. Ther., 8*(4), 1-7.
[http://dx.doi.org/10.15453/2168-6408.1770]

Mosey, A. (1986). *Psychosocial components of occupational therapy.*

Muñoz, J.P., Lawlor, M., Kielhofner, G. (1993). Use of the model of human occupation: A survey of therapists in psychiatric practice. *Occup. Ther. J. Res., 13*(2), 117-139.
[http://dx.doi.org/10.1177/153944929301300204]

Nelson, D.L. (1988). Occupation: Form and Performance. *Am. J. Occup. Ther., 42*(10), 633-641.
[http://dx.doi.org/10.5014/ajot.42.10.633] [PMID: 3059801]

O'Brien, J. C., Hinojosa, J., Kramer, P., Royeen, C. B. (2017). Model of human occupation. *Perspectives on human occupation: Theories underlying practice,* 93-136.

Pan, A.W., Fan, C.W., Chung, L., Chen, T.J., Kielhofner, G., Wu, M.Y., Chen, Y.L. (2011). Examining the validity of the Model of Human Occupation Screening Tool: using classical test theory and item response theory. *Br. J. Occup. Ther., 74*(1), 34-40.

[http://dx.doi.org/10.4276/030802211X12947686093648]

Park, J., Gross, D.P., Rayani, F., Norris, C.M., Roberts, M.R., James, C., Guptill, C., Esmail, S. (2019). Model of Human Occupation as a framework for implementation of Motivational Interviewing in occupational rehabilitation. *Work, 62*(4), 629-641.
[http://dx.doi.org/10.3233/WOR-192895] [PMID: 31104046]

Parkinson, S. (2014). Programme design: Applying the Model of Human Occupation. *In Recovery Through Activity Routledge.*

Parkinson, S., Brooks, R. (2020). A Guide to the Formulation of Plans and Goals in Occupational Therapy. *A Guide to the Formulation of Plans and Goals in Occupational Therapy..* Issue February.
[http://dx.doi.org/10.4324/9781003046301]

Prior, S., Maciver, D., Aas, R.W., Kirsh, B., Lexen, A., van Niekerk, L., Irvine Fitzpatrick, L., Forsyth, K. (2020). An enhanced individual placement and support (IPS) intervention based on the Model of Human Occupation (MOHO); a prospective cohort study. *BMC Psychiatry, 20*(1), 361.
[http://dx.doi.org/10.1186/s12888-020-02745-3] [PMID: 32641009]

Reilly, M. (1962). Occupational therapy can be one of the great ideas of 20th century medicine. *Am. J. Occup. Ther., 16*(1), 1-9.
[PMID: 14491211]

Reilly, M. (1963). The Eleanor Clarke Slagle: Occupational Therapy can be one of the great ideas of 20th century medicine. *Can. J. Occup. Ther., 30*(1), 5-19.
[http://dx.doi.org/10.1177/000841746303000102]

Scott, A.H., Haggarty, E.J. (1984). Structuring Goals *via* Goal Attainment Scaling in Occupational Therapy Groups in a Partial Hospitalization Setting. *Occup. Ther. Ment. Health, 4*(2), 39-58.
[http://dx.doi.org/10.1300/J004v04n02_04]

Taylor, R., Bowyer, P., & Fisher, G. (2023). Kielhofner's model of human occupation. *Lippincott Williams & Wilkins.*

Unsworth, C., Baker, A. (2016). A systematic review of professional reasoning literature in occupational therapy. *Br. J. Occup. Ther., 79*(1), 5-16.
[http://dx.doi.org/10.1177/0308022615599994]

CHAPTER 2

Canadian Model of Occupational Performance and Engagement

Tawanda Machingura[1,*] and **Sam Thew**[2]

[1] *Head of Discipline Occupational Therapy Program, University of Notre Dame Australia, Sydney, Australia*

[2] *Department of Occupational Therapy, Child Development Centre, Prince George, British Columbia, Canada*

Abstract: This chapter describes the key aspects of the CMOP-E model and how occupational performance and engagement are understood through the lens of the CMOP-E model. The chapter ends with a case study illustrating the application of the model in practice.

Keywords: Case study, Client-centred practice, Canadian Model of Occupational Performance and Engagement, Engagement, Occupation, Occupational performance, Person-environment-occupation transactions.

INTRODUCTION

The Canadian Model of Occupational Performance and Engagement (CMOP-E) is a key model that helps practitioners understand how individuals engage in occupations within their unique social, physical, cultural, personal, political, and economic contexts. The model particularly emphasises the importance of spirituality, which is at the core of the person, and the fact that occupation is the bridge that connects the person and their environment. CMOP-E is a comprehensive and commonly used model of practice in occupational therapy mental health practice.

In this chapter, we will explore the origins of the model, the core components of the model, including the person, occupation, and environment components, and how these transact to enhance or hinder occupational performance. The chapter will end by utilising a case study to illustrate how this model can be used in practice.

---

* **Corresponding authors Tawanda Machingura:** Head of Discipline Occupational Therapy Program, University of Notre Dame Australia, Sydney, Australia; E-mail: tawanda.machingura@nd.edu.au

The CMOP-E theory

CAOT has been working together with members to provide a vision for the conceptual grounding, processes, and outcomes of occupational therapy in Canada for many years. This vision was first articulated in the Guidelines for Client-Centred Practice published in 1983, 1986, and1987 and consolidated in 1991, followed by the OT guidelines for client-centred mental health practice in 1993.

Enabling Occupation: An Occupational Therapy Perspective was re-printed with an updated preface in 2002. These publications have been integral to guide Canadian occupational therapy practice and are now used in many countries around the world. The 2007 publication entitled Enabling Occupation II: Advancing an Occupational Therapy Vision for Health, Well-being, and Justice through Occupation was launched in July 2007 in St John's, Newfoundland.

Here are some key historical facts:

- The Canadian Model of Occupational Performance (CMOP)- Townsend *et al.* (1997; 2002)
- 1980s-early 1990s: Canadian occupational therapists and medical representatives developed guidelines to facilitate an occupationally focused, client-centred practice of occupational therapy (Townsend *et al.* 1997, 2002).
- A key driver for the work was to demonstrate the effectiveness of interventions, justify actions, and promote the profession of occupational therapy.
- Emphasis was placed upon ensuring that occupation was recognised as a core concept of occupational therapy practice.
- The original model was based upon the work of Reed and Sanderson (1999) and called the Occupational Performance Model (OPM) (1982, 1983, and 1991), with occupation divided into self-care, productivity, and leisure.

As the name suggests, the Canadian Model of 'Occupational Performance and Engagement' is the result of this vision of CAOT. The change from CMOP to CMOPE was made because the authors felt that occupational performance alone was limiting and did not capture the full scope of OT practice. OTs are involved in not just enabling people to 'do' occupations but to be engaged in 'doing'. Polatajko *et al.* defined occupational performance as the dynamic interaction of a person, occupation, and environment. It does not have a specific depiction of the model but is encompassed within the whole model. A pictorial representation of the model is in Fig. (**1**) below.

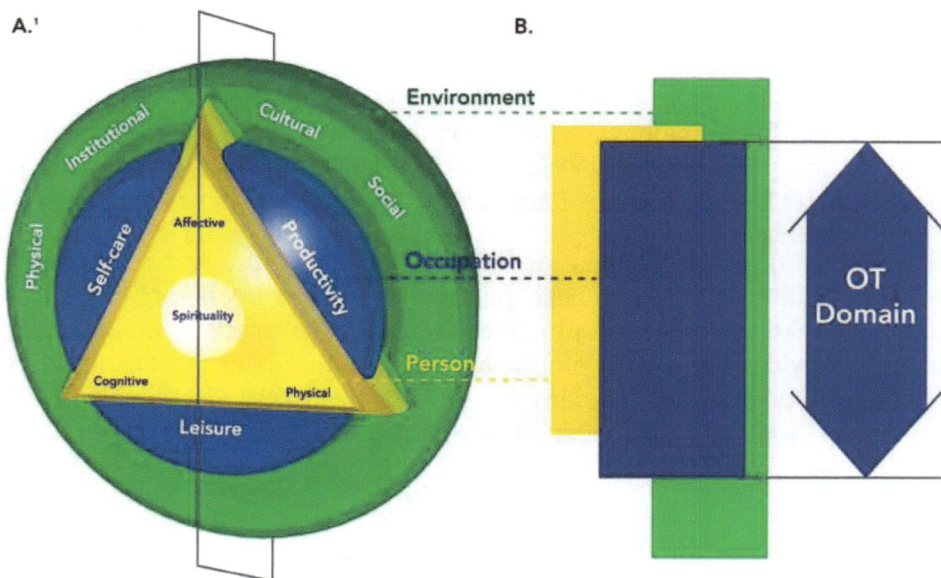

A.' Referred to as the CMOP in *Enabling Occupation* (1997a, 2002) and CMOP-E as of this edition
B. Trans-sectional view

Polatajko, H. J., Townsend, E. A., Craik, J. (2007). *Canadian Model of Occupational Performance and Engagement (CMOP-E)*. In E. A. Townsend and H. J. Polatajko, *Enabling Occupation II: Advancing an Occupational Therapy Vision of Health, Well-being, & Justice through Occupation*. p.23 Ottawa, ON: CAOT Publications ACE.

Fig. (1). The Canadian Model of Occupational Performance and Engagement (Polatajko *et al.*, 2007)

Occupational enablement means enabling people to choose, organize, and perform those occupations they find useful and meaningful in their environment. The CMOP-E can be used with individuals, families, groups, communities, organisations, and populations.

Person

Spirituality: Spirituality can be described as a life force that gives a sense of a higher self, acts as a source of will and self-determination, and gives a sense of meaning, purpose, and connectedness (Duncan, 2020).

Cognitive (thinking): Memory, orientation, concentration, intellect, insight, judgement, general knowledge.

Affective (feeling): Emotions, mood, affect, volition, self-esteem, coping skills, and ability to adapt to changing circumstances.

Physical (doing): Movement, strength, coordination, balance, endurance, sensation, pain, appearance, physical health of body systems and structures.

Environment

Physical Environment: All built and natural aspects.

Social environment: The people a person interacts with

Cultural: Sets of values, conventions, or social practices that guide how we perform or engage with certain occupations.

Institutional: The practices, relationships or organisations within society, culture, or organisation.

Occupation

Groups of activities and tasks of everyday life that are named and organised and have value and meaning.

Self-care: Any aspect of personal care/looking after themselves

Leisure: Recreation, rest, rejuvenation

Productivity: Contributing to the social and economic fabric of their communities

Fig. (**2**) below summarises the model, process and practice framework of the Canadian Model of Occupational Performance and Engagement.

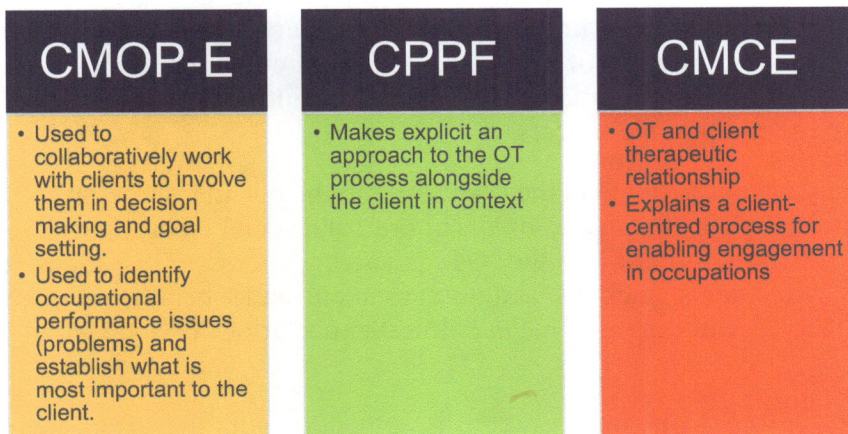

CMOP-E	CPPF	CMCE
• Used to collaboratively work with clients to involve them in decision making and goal setting. • Used to identify occupational performance issues (problems) and establish what is most important to the client.	• Makes explicit an approach to the OT process alongside the client in context	• OT and client therapeutic relationship • Explains a client-centred process for enabling engagement in occupations

Fig. (2). Model, Practice Framework and Process.

CMOP-E in Practice

Both the CPPF and the Model of Client-Centred Enablement (CMCE) are processes that provide additional guidance to OT practice when using the CMOP-E. However, they are not processes that need to be exclusively used with the CMOP-E. The CPPF details the action points that occur in collaboration with the client throughout OT practice. This approach to the process of OT practice explains that practice is also influenced by the broader societal and practice context.

There are other practice process frameworks; however, these are the two we are primarily going to explore this teaching period.

The Canadian Practice Process Framework (CPPF)

The CPPF has its origins in the Canadian Association of OT and the CMOP-E. The CPPF is appropriate to use with individuals, groups, communities, organisations, or populations. The CPPF guides OTs through a process that is occupation-based, evidence-based, and client-centred to enable change in occupational performance and engagement.

Within the CPPF, four primary elements of the OT practice process are illustrated. There is the societal context (outer box), the practice context (inner box), the frames of reference (large circle), and the action points (smaller circles). The diagram demonstrates the potential pathways of action in the OT and client relationship. This is shown by the solid and dotted arrows, as in Fig. (**3**) below.

The circle represents the frames of reference, which are embedded in the practice context and inform the 8 action points of the OT process. In this case, 'Frames of Reference' more broadly encompasses any of the paradigms, conceptual practice models, and specific frames of reference that might guide the OT's practice. The CPPF highlights the importance of OT theory to guide the therapist's reasoning throughout each step of the process.

The societal context outlined in the CMOP-E, on the outside, shows aspects of the broader societal physical, institutional, cultural, and social environments that have an influence on all parts of the OT practice process. This might include institutional elements such as state government-wide healthcare policies or funding policies. Cultural may mean cultural expectations or societal values and expectations.

The practice context (the inner square) is embedded within the societal context. The same environmental components of physical, institutional, cultural, and social are considered; however, it refers to the specific personal and practice contexts of the therapist and client. This might include the physical space where therapy or assessment occurs (*i.e.*, Home visit versus clinic setting). The social elements might include what other team members are involved or significant others supporting the client, is there a specific institutional culture in the workplace or a model of service delivery that the clinician has to operate within? Furthermore, both the OT and the client bring their own personal factors that influence the process and OT/client relationship. The OT has specific knowledge, skills, and attitudes they bring, and the client also has knowledge, skills, and abilities about their conditions, experiences, and occupations to share.

There is a dotted line between these two contexts because they have a mutual influence on each other. The institutional contexts determined by society, such as governmental policies, will influence the specific practice context (such as the resources, funding, supports, or limitations available to the client).

Actions

Actions are completed by OTs to ensure that their practice is centered on the client and their occupational goals. Shading of the circles demonstrates that the client and the therapist are collaboratively engaged in each action point. The practice process needs to be flexible. Some clients will progress in a linear pathway (solid arrows), and others may require an alternate route. Looking at the legend, the client is represented by yellow, and OT is represented by blue. Shading of the circles between 'set the stage' and 'evaluate outcome' demonstrates that the client and the therapist are collaboratively engaged in each action point. This is to emphasise the importance of being client-centered and power sharing as much as possible to empower the client to pursue their occupational performance or engagement goals.

Actions in the process are flexible. Not every client will seamlessly move through every action point – this is influenced by societal and practice contexts such as client needs or service models. This flexibility is represented by the solid and dotted lines demonstrating the range of pathways the process might take.

We have identified that the pathways and action points can be influenced by the contexts. Similarly, it is important to note that some of these action points may happen at different points of contact with the client, and some may occur simultaneously. The process begins when the occupational therapists receives a referral or when the client contacts the therapist as in self referrals. The process that ensures is detailed in Fig. (**3**) below.

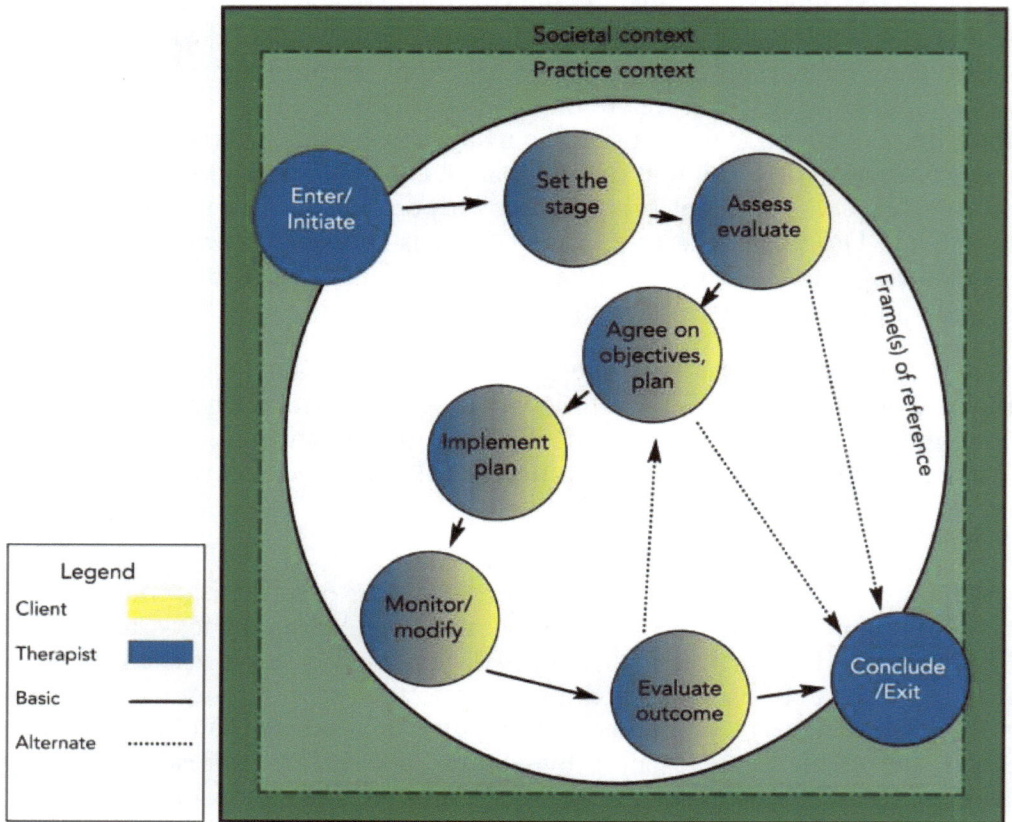

Polatajko, H. J., Craik, J., Davis, J., & Townsend,E. A. (2007). Canadian Practice Process Framework. In E. A. Townsend and H. J. Polatajko, *Enabling occupation II: Advancing an occupational therapy vision for health, well-being, & justice through occupation.* p. 233 Ottawa, ON: CAOT Publications ACE.

Fig. (3). The Canadian Practice Process Framework (Polatajko *et al.*, 2007)

Enter/initiate

The type of client is identified, and the OT may consider if the referral is appropriate. This is the first point of contact. This stage can happen with or without the client, *e.g.*, when the OT receives the referral and reviews other available documentation. OTs use this information to start to think about how this information will be used in initial interaction with the client and finding out about their occupational challenges. Consent for OT input is identified at this stage. This leads to setting the stage for future action.

- Who is the client?
- Who else is involved?
- Reviewing referral
- Obtaining consent
- Initiating a partnership with the client
- Beginning to identify occupational challenges

Setting the stage

Setting the stage: This is where the strengths and resources of the client may be identified as the occupational performance issues. It involves building rapport, setting ground rules, and clarifying expectations. Doing an occupational profile and gathering an occupational history might be relevant to understanding the client's past experiences and finding the meaning attributed to occupational performance, engagement, roles, identities, *etc*. The overarching conceptual practice model being used by the therapist should influence the structure of how information is gathered. For example, if applying the CMOP-E, the OT might consider using the COPM. This is where the OT might start to select other frames of reference in addition to OT models that will help guide the strategies.

- Identifying occupational performance issues
- Building rapport
- Setting ground rules and expectations for the therapeutic relationship and scope of the OT's practice within the service, *etc.*

Assess/Evaluate

Further in-depth assessment of factors influencing occupational performance is important. It helps to further identify potential breakdowns in occupational performance or the client's strengths. Clinical reasoning and OT theory will help to inform what assessment methods are chosen. Assessment methods may be informal or standardized. They might occur in the context of the occupations – however, if this is not made possible by the practice context, it may be simulated or observed in some other way. It is important for the assessment to be occupation-based or focused where possible. Analysis of information gathered throughout the previous three steps then informs the next.

- Further in-depth assessment of factors influencing occupational performance.
- Sometimes the context will influence the assessment tools utilized.
- Clinical reasoning and OT theory will help to inform assessment methods.

Agree on the Objectives and Plan

Engaging the client collaboratively is vital in this step. This means we do not just ask for their agreement or consent to proceed with the objective identified by the OT – it means we allow the client to express their priorities, needs, and approach to address goals. Negotiating an agreement requires a collaborative decision-making process and involves "reflecting upon the client's occupational challenges, the priority ¬ occupational issues, and assessment/evaluation findings, including data on occupations and the personal and environmental factors influencing occupational engagement."

Goals may be negotiated or clarified. The OT and client can decide together the steps (objectives) to reach the client's goals. Frames of reference or service-specific resources may also inform this process. These key points should be clearly documented. *e.g.* GARSS uses a client treatment agreement form.

- Ensure that the client is at the center of this process
- Goals may be negotiated or clarified
- Decide on an approach and the steps needed to achieve goals together.
- Steps to achieve client goals (the objectives and plan) should be documented.

Implement Plan

In this stage, the OT implements the plan identified and agreed with the client, using approaches and techniques informed by selected frames of reference. OTs employ tools to engage the client in intervention (this is one point where the CMCE can be brought in). Practice contexts may also influence implementation, *e.g.*, are there boundaries to how often you can visit a client's home for therapy? Or maybe there are appropriate therapy groups being offered within your particular service that might not be available in others.

This is where it is important to maintain an occupation-based or focused approach in order to promote progress towards the client's occupational goals whilst balancing this with the boundaries of the practice context or the protocols associated with the chosen approaches.

- Implement the plan identified in action point 4.
- Approaches and techniques are informed by the frames of reference.
- OT employs tools to engage the client in intervention.
- Practice contexts may also inform implementation.

Monitor and Modify

It involves ensuring that the plan continues to be appropriate and is supporting the client towards their goals. It may include communication with other stakeholders or intermittent assessment. It is essential to negotiate any modifications to the plan with the client. People's needs, circumstances, or priorities may change over time; this may mean progressing earlier than expected to the next step in order to re-establish the objectives and plan or an early conclusion to therapy. OTs engage in reflective practice to monitor their approach or the impact of external influences to identify enablers and barriers to progression towards client goals.

- Involves ensuring that the plan continues to be appropriate and is supporting the client towards their goals.
- May include communication with other stakeholders or intermittent assessment
- Essential to negotiate any modifications to the plan with the client

Evaluate Outcome

It is more of a summative evaluation to determine if occupational goals were achieved. When we place clients at the centre of care, this action point primarily hinges on the client's perceptions of their goals and their satisfaction with their occupational performance or engagement. Evaluation of goals and re-assessment of measures previously completed inform next steps – this could mean a new plan, goals, and transition into re-commencing parts of the OT process or transition towards the conclusion of the relationship.

- What is the outcome of the implemented plan/treatment?
- How does the client perceive they have progressed towards or achieved their goals?
- Evaluation of goals and re-assessment of measures previously completed inform next steps – either a new plan, goals, or transition towards the conclusion of the relationship.

Conclude/Exit

At this stage, a mutual decision between the therapist and client is made to conclude occupational therapy input. This may be because the client has achieved their goals or identified a level of satisfaction with their occupational performance to continue independently. There may be personal factors impacting the client determining the conclusion of therapy prior to completing their agreed plan or reaching their goals. There may be practice/service influences (such as length of stay or having reached the limitations of funding) influencing the OT's capacity to continue service delivery. Final documentation and summaries of care are completed, and transition to alternate appropriate services may be coordinated and agreed upon.

- A mutual decision between the therapist and client to conclude occupational therapy.
- Requires further planning or transition and documentation.

In summary, the CPPF guides the OT to support clients in achieving their occupational performance and engagement goals. The CPPF highlights how the societal and practice contexts influence all aspects of the client's journey and need to be considered by the OT in planning their approach with the client to the ground. In the first few actions of the CPPF, practice models and frames of reference are vital in supporting gathering a holistic view of the person, their occupations, environments, and personal goals and determining the best approach to therapy.

The Canadian Model of Client-Centred Enablement (CMCE)

CMCE provides a visual metaphor for client-centred enablement in order to promote health, well-being, and justice through occupation. It relates to the CMOP-E where foundational concepts of enablement and engagement. This model depicts the enablement skills therapists employ that are essential for improving occupational engagement and performance in a client-centred and collaborative way.

The relationship between the client and the professional is represented by the two asymmetrical curved lines. Where they intersect shows the entry and exit points of the OT process – like that outlined in the CPPF. These lines also emphasise that the sharing of power throughout the whole process is central to a client-centred approach. There are 10 enablement skills that are used throughout the OT process. If you were using this alongside the CPPF, you would employ these enablement skills throughout the 8 action points of the practice process framework.

CMOP-E can help us understand barriers and enablers to occupational performance and engagement. The CMCE complements this by giving OTs a framework for how to engage with clients in a therapeutic relationship.

There are 6 foundations that help us to enable clients in a client-centered, occupation-based way. These 6 foundations describe the values, beliefs, or perspectives that can shape our thinking when we are focussed on enabling. These are not seen in the model but are underlying concepts that inform our approach to being client-centred and enabling our clients as shown in Fig. (**4**) below.

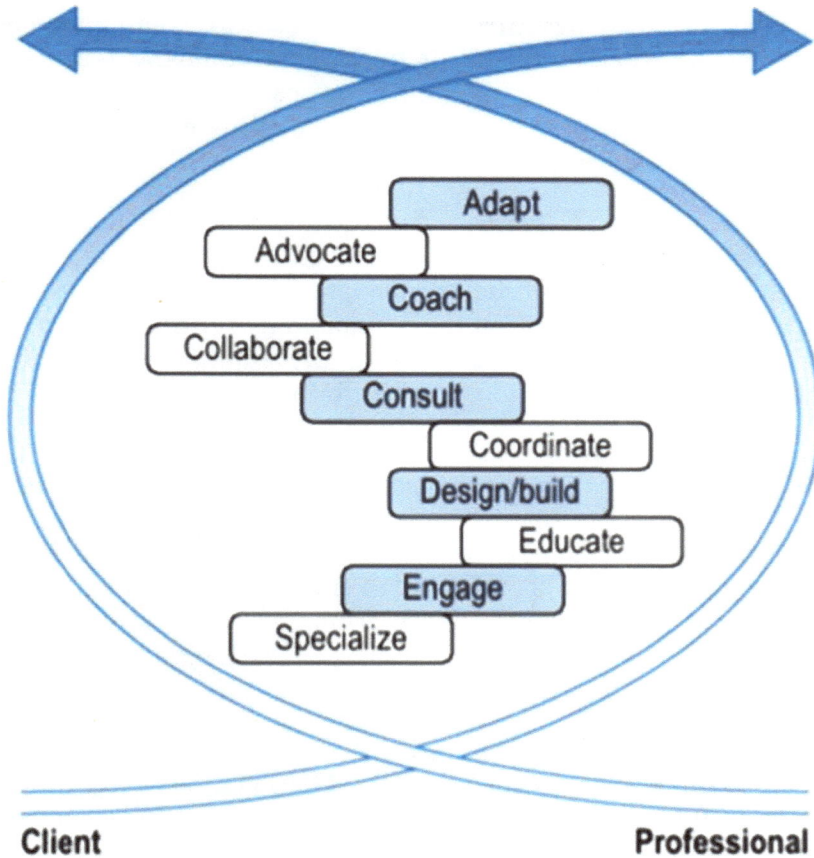

Fig. (4). The Canadian model of client-centred enablement.

Empower clients to make decisions: Occupational therapists have an ethical obligation to respect client views, experiences, interests, and safety by respecting their client's right to make choices and live with risk. This is a core principle of client-centred practice not just in the context of this model. If clients are not involved in making decisions about their own healthcare, values, lifestyle, *etc.*, then we are either making assumptions about what people want, making decisions for them, and then doing therapy for them – not empowering them to have an active role in their journey.

Client participation: There is so much evidence out there to say that when clients are actively involved and participating in their care, they are more likely to engage in therapy/occupation/maintaining the progress made, *etc.*

Visions of possibilities: Clients must be encouraged to imagine the possibilities and to think about what might be or even what could be rather than being constrained by how things are at the time (Townsend *et al.*, 2007). Occupational therapists must encourage their clients to imagine a life that may not be expected of them and that they may not have expected themselves.

Enabling change: The OT's role when enabling clients might include (a) developing transitions across the life course, (b) maintaining occupational engagement, health, and well-being 'or preventing change' (think of the prevention priority/goal prompt on the occupational profile form), (c) restoring occupational potential and performance, or (d) preventing occupational losses and deprivation, occupational alienation, or other forms of occupational injustice.

Occupational justice: Townsend *et al*. identified four aspects of a "justice" perspective on enabling. These are related to recognizing injustices that are encountered by various groups in society and the systems we all engage in, accepting people as they are, advocating for people and their rights to participate equally in society to access occupations of meaning, and noticing when we or others assume that people need to change or improve some aspect of themselves to be more acceptable (as distinct from when a client might identify the goal to change).

Power sharing: The authors identified that power-sharing is central to client-centred collaboration, and this requires an explicit and conscious process. They stated, "Successful, collaborative power-sharing involves genuine interest, acknowledgement, empathy, altruism, trust, and creative communication" and demonstrated the 10 enablement skills depicted in the model.

CMCE provides a visual representation of client-centred enablement in order to promote health, well-being, and justice through occupation. This model depicts the enablement skills therapists employ that are essential for improving occupational engagement and performance in a client-centred and collaborative way. The relationship between the client and the professional is represented by the two asymmetrical curved lines. Where they intersect shows the entry and exit points of the OT process – like that outlined in the CPPF. These lines also demonstrate that the authors felt it important to emphasise that the sharing of power throughout the whole process is central to a client-centred approach. There are 10 enablement skills in the space between the two lines that are used throughout the whole OT process.

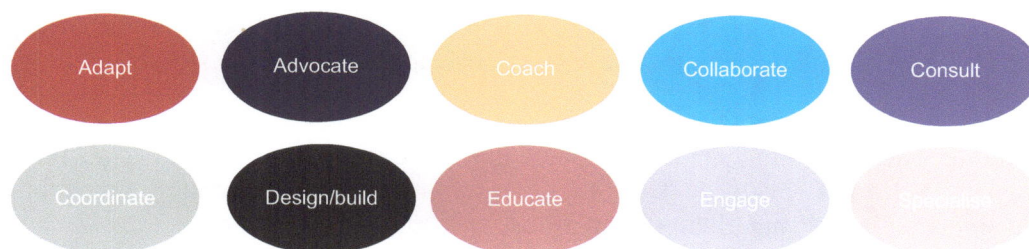

Fig. (5). Enabling Strategies.

Advocate: It means raising awareness in others of issues and promoting the need for change amongst those with appropriate power or resources, or challenging others to think differently about an issue. Give an IPE example.

Coach: Coaching is a skill that requires practice. As OTs, when we use 'coaching', we are trying to encourage clients to reflect and discover their own motivations in desired occupations. For example, having conversations with clients about their occupations may facilitate occupational engagement when they have been coached to self-identify their strengths, resources, challenges, and desired goals.

Collaborate: This is a key skill for power-sharing and being client-centred. It means to work with people rather than doing things to them or for them.

Consult: It requires occupational therapists to gather information, synthesize it into an in-depth understanding of the situation or issue, and involve actions such as giving advice, making recommendations, and advocating for change. It can be relevant to contexts outside of direct service provision, such as management, education, and research (*e.g.*, OT director role in QH) – or when working with groups, communities, or populations rather than individuals.

Coordinate: They coordinate information, people, services, and organizations and may be acting in direct service and case coordination roles, as well as management roles. It may require occupational therapists to "educate those involved, and to facilitate, mediate, or actively negotiate networking, links, and resolutions."

Design/build: It might relate to designing and building AT or orthotics, making splints, designing environmental modifications, and designing programs and services. Potentially, one of the skills OTs are most associated with for our skills in creating, designing, and fabricating products or environmental adaptations, however is broader than that, as it refers to the ability to enable clients through the design of new therapeutic strategies or intervention approaches, adapting environments, advocating for social change and inclusive design in communities, and enabling clients to participate in all of these activities.

Educate: OTs use occupations to promote learning through doing, being able to simulate, and practicing skills outside of the contextual environment (*e.g.*, rehab ward with limited resources). It provides clients with information to support decision-making, about their occupations, treatment, health, *etc.*

Engage: Engaging clients in occupation actively as a means or an end. It is often combined with other enablement skills.

Specialise: OTs develop a range of skills in specific techniques or approaches. *e.g.*, the use of sensory modulation in mental health, UL rehabilitation techniques, and extensive knowledge of available AT solutions. It is important to remain client-centred; however, when applying specialised knowledge, make sure that clients understand, agree, consent to, and actively participate in the specialised approaches.

If you are using CMCE alongside the CPPF, you will employ these enablement skills throughout the 8 action points of the practice process framework.

Reflection

How can the CMOP-E frame your practice beyond performance to include modes of occupational interaction and engagement such as occupational development, capacity, and repertoire?

CONCLUSION

- CMOP-E is a client-centred model that seeks to enable occupational performance and engagement.
- People can engage in occupations without necessarily performing them.
- Person, occupation, and environment are the three layers, with the person at the centre.
- Spirituality is at the core of the person and the model.
- Occupation is the bridge between the person and their environment.

REFERENCES

Craik, J., Townsend, E., Polatajko, H. (2008). Introducing the new guidelines-enabling occupation II: Advancing an occupational therapy vision for health, well-being, & justice through occupation. *Occupational Therapy Now, 10*(1), 3-5.

Fazio, K., Hicks, E., Kuzma, C., Leung, P., Schwartz, A., Stergiou-Kita, M. (2008). The Canadian Practice

Process Framework: Using a conscious approach to occupational therapy practice. *OT Now, 10*(4), 6-9.

Gibson, J. (1986). *The ecological approach to visual perception.*. Hillsdale, N.J.: Erlbaum.

Lawton, M.P., Nahemow, L. (1973). Ecology and the aging process. In: Eisdorfer, C., Lawton, M.P., (Eds.), *Psychology of Adult Development and Aging.*. Washington, DC: American Psychological Association. [http://dx.doi.org/10.1037/10044-020]

 Polatajko, H. J., Townsend, E. A., & Craik, J. (2007). Canadian model of occupational performance and engagement (CMOP-E). Enabling occupation II: Advancing an occupational therapy vision of health, well-being & justice through occupation, 23.

Stadnyk, R., Phillips, J., Sapeta, S., MacAulay, A., Champion, M., Tam, L., Craik, J. (2009). The Canadian Model of Client-Centred Enablement: Reflections from diverse occupational therapy practitioners. *OT Now, 11*(3), 26-28.

Zhang, C., McCarthy, C., Craik, J. (2008). Students as translators for the Canadian Model of Occupational Performance and Engagement. *OT Now, 10*(2), 3-5.

CHAPTER 3

Kawa Model

Tawanda Machingura[1,*]

[1] *Head of Discipline Occupational Therapy Program, University of Notre Dame Australia, Sydney, Australia*

Abstract: This chapter overviews the Kawa Model as developed by Michael Iwama and colleagues. It starts off with some insights into a conversation with Dr Iwama following a chance meeting with the author in 2006. This chapter then explores model concepts and ends with an exploration of how the Kawa Model may be utilized in practice.

Keywords: Collectivist cultures, Life flow, Occupational therapy, Kawa model.

INTRODUCTION

The Kawa model was developed by Michael Iwama. I had the pleasure of having a conversation with Dr. Michael Iwama in 2006 in New Zealand when he came to the National Occupational Therapy Conference to present the Kawa Model. I will share what he said and what I got out of our conversation.

According to Dr. Iwama, the word Kawa means 'River' in Japanese (Iwama, 2006). Dr. Iwama told me that he was originally from Japan; however, he was educated in the USA and Canada and worked in Canada at the time. He stated that he regarded himself as a Japanese Canadian occupational therapist and social scientist. He stated that the humble beginnings of the Kawa model were the time he travelled back to Japan and realised that Japanese Occupational Therapists and, indeed, the Japanese people, in general, had a different view of what occupation was. Occupation, as perceived and described in the West, meant something completely different to Japanese people. In Japanese, he advised that occupation meant 'boring, laborious work'. This did not sit well with him, so he collaborated with a group of Japanese occupational therapists to design a model of occupational therapy practice that would resonate with the Japanese people, people from the East, and indeed many people around the world. The model was

---

[*] **Corresponding author Tawanda Machingura:** Head of Discipline Occupational Therapy Program, University of Notre Dame Australia, Sydney, Australia; E-mail: tawanda.machingura@nd.edu.au

subsequently published in 2006 and is one of the newest models in occupational therapy practice even today.

To understand this model, it is important to place it in the sociocultural and geopolitical context in which it was developed. The model was originally developed in response to a perceived need for an occupational therapy model that was relevant to non-western contexts, initially, which was the Japanese occupational therapy practice context. The authors sought a way to challenge the Western dominance in the field of occupational therapy that did not seem to value the collectivist view of many people from non-Western backgrounds. OT as a profession originated in Western culture in the USA. Dr Iwama and many occupational therapists from non-western backgrounds, myself included, are of the view that many of the assumptions that the profession was founded on differ from our own experiences of occupation and understanding of life and the nature of humans. Collectivist cultures such as Japanese/Asian or African or indigenous people in many countries, including New Zealand, Australia, Canada, and the USA, view the individual or the 'self' differently. In fact, in many non-western cultures, the concept of a self is not completely separate from the other people, plants, animals, and inanimate structures that surround them.

The question might be so how is the Kawa Model different? Dr. Iwama and the group he was working with found out that what resonates with Japanese people are metaphors. The Kawa model was built on the foundation of a metaphor of a river flowing from the mountains where it originates, probably from the melting of ice and flowing all the way to the sea where it ends and empties all its contents, *i.e.*, the water. The river may also start due to rainwater. Depending on the environment, water will start to flow and form a river (Fig. **1**). Sometimes, they flow into lakes or the sea. The twists and turns in life will always be unique. The breadth, depth, and flow of the river will vary and change throughout the journey. The river is taken to be all its elements, which include the riverbed and the river walls that shape the river, the water that flows in the river, the rocks that impede the water flow, and the driftwood that either impedes the water flow when it gets logged between the rocks or enhances water flow when it knocks off some rocks to increase water flow.

Concepts and Components of the Model

The model is a metaphor for a river that symbolises 'life flow' or 'life energy'. The elements of the model include the water, rocks, driftwood, and river floor and walls. Rivers start due to rain and flow from up high in the mountains towards a low point in the land. In the application of the model to humans, the river is a metaphor for life as a journey beginning when one is born (origins of the river), and as one goes through life, there are ups and downs and twists and turns just like a river (Fig. (2); as we know, life will end at some point when one dies just as a river ends when it flows into a dam, sea, or ocean.

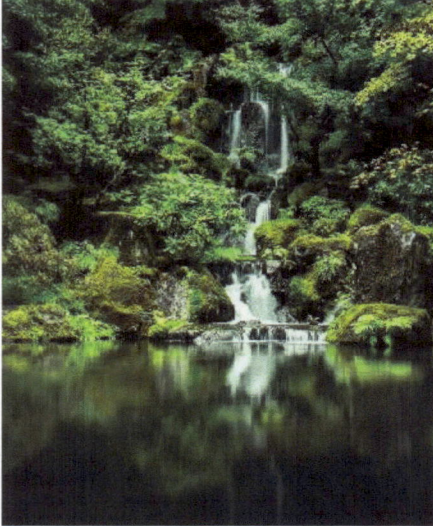

Beginning of the river in the mountains.

Symbolises beginning of life's journey.

Fig. (1). The beginning of river or life.

Photo by Anders Ipsen on Unsplash

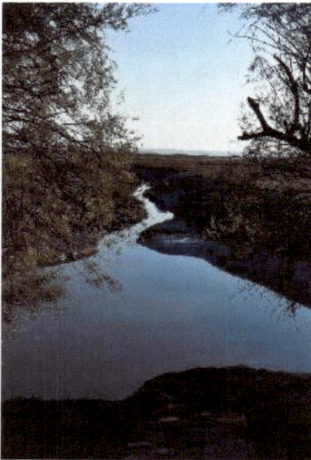

Twists and turns symbolize the ups and downs in life

Fig. (2). Twists and turns in a river.

Photo by Pauline on Unsplash.

The spaces (Sukima)

Sukima (Japanese word) are the spaces between the rocks, driftwood, river walls, and riverbed. These spaces are the gaps through which the client's life energy or flow is channelled through and flows. In the context of Kawa, the channels through which water flows offer opportunities for growth and enhanced occupational performance and engagement. Occupational therapists look for these channels to enable clients to achieve their occupational performance goals. The role of OT is to facilitate life flow and balance between all aspects/elements of the river. The whole river depicts the whole life of a person, and cross sections can be taken at different points in a person's life to reveal elements acting within their life at that time. Each cross-section of the river will look different depending on their life circumstances at the time. An optimal state of well-being in one's life or river can be portrayed by an image of a strong, deep, unimpeded flow, such as in Fig. (**3**) below.

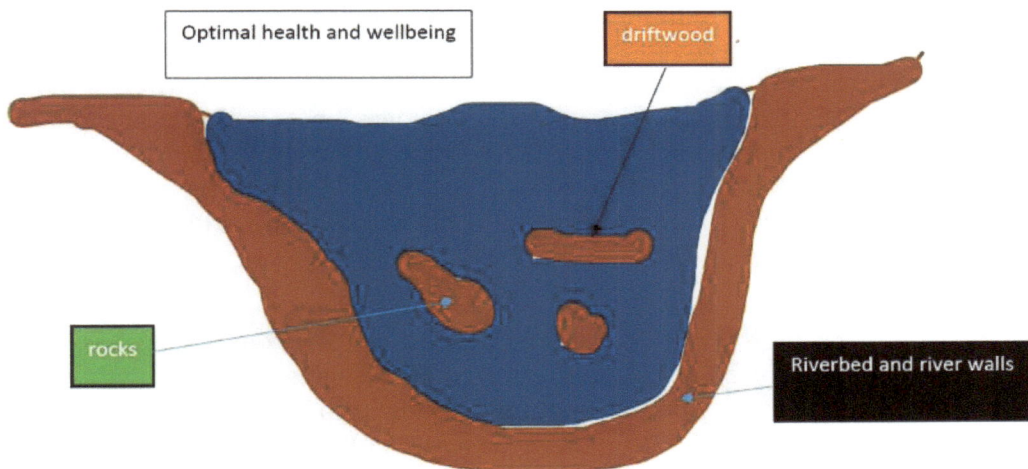

Optimal health and wellbeing

driftwood

rocks

Riverbed and river walls

Fig. (3). Optimal Health and Well-being.

The riverbed and river walls (kawa no soku-heki and kawa no zoko)

Kawa no soku-heki and kawa no zoko are Japanese terms for riverbed and riverwalls (Iwama, 2006). The reader is reminded that since this model is about a person's journey told by the person themselves, this model relies heavily on narrative reasoning. Another thing to note is that all components of this model are transactive in nature, which means they are all interrelated and affect overall health and well-being without any element being more important than the other. The riverbed and river walls represent environmental factors, the context in which the occupation occurs, or the context in which the person lives, works, or plays. It must be noted that occupation cannot be separated from life flow within the person's context (Iwama, 2007). Some examples of context are:

- *Physical*- buildings, structures, buildings
- *Social*- family, friends, groups, networks
- *Cultural*- cultural norms, protocols, and values
- *Technological*-mobile technologies, online platforms, internet, web technologies
- *Institutional*- rules, laws, policies, procedures

All these elements are interrelated and can affect occupational performance and engagement.

The river will take shape depending on the river walls and riverbed in the Kawa Model. The depth of the river or the size of the walls represent the environment, including the social and physical environments that may impact someone's ability to perform their occupations. In discussing the river walls and riverbed in the context of collectivist cultures, the influence of the social environment is particularly significant (Iwama, 2007). The social environment refers to those people with which clients have direct relationships with, such as friends, family, neighbours, distant relatives, workmates, classmates, pets, cultural and religious leaders, customs, and so forth. There is no 'optimal' shape for the river floor and walls; what matters is the amount of water that is still able to flow, depending on the interaction between the river floor and walls and elements within the river.

Water (Mizu)

Mizu is the Japanese word for water (Iwama, 2006). Water appears to mean different things in different cultures, but in most cultures, it appears to represent life, life flow, or life energy. Occupational therapy aims to enable and maximise life flow (Iwama, 2006, 2007). In many different cultures, water has been used to symbolise life. Water may symbolise different meanings for life and spirituality in different cultures – and understanding this meaning for the cultures we engage in may be relevant. Because water is fluid, it has the ability to flow over and around through obstacles and challenges. Water is considered cleansing, pure, and renewing. Water can help push obstacles downstream. It has the power to change the shape or flow. Water can be contained in things or impeded by these obstacles. It can also shape the things around it. Similarly, collectively oriented people place greater value on belonging. They are influenced by their sociocultural context, which emphasises and places more worth in belonging over individual wants or needs.

Rocks (Iwa)

The Japanese word for rocks is Iwa (Iwama, 2006). This is used to represent life circumstances that impede life flow and are regarded by the client as problematic and are considered by the client as difficult to move or remove. Rocks are barriers to function and impact life flow. In a river there are rocks that are difficult to move depending on the size. The size and shape of the rock represent how big the barrier is to life flow. Examples of rocks may be injury, sickness, poor mental health, or any injury or illness that impacts someone's ability to engage in desired occupations. Rocks may significantly impede the life flow, and in other circumstances, they might be sitting on the edges but do not significantly limit the water flow. The rocks, in relation to the river walls and floor, determine how much influence they have on the life flow. It is important when using the Kawa model that the occupational therapist discusses with the client the extent to which their potential rocks (difficult-to-move problems) and obstacles to life flow are perceived by them as impacting their life. Examples of rocks may be injury, sickness, low motivation, poor mental health, difficulties with activities of daily living, or money. It is any injury or illness that impacts someone's ability to perform ADLs. If a problem is temporary and can be easily addressed to enhance occupational performance, then it is likely to be driftwood rather than a rock.

The driftwood (Ryuboku)

Ryuboku is Japanese for driftwood (Iwama, 2006). Driftwood is less permanent than rocks. Driftwood can be carried along with the river and can be used positively to push rocks downstream. Sometimes, they can get caught on the rocks. Driftwood represents the attributes and resources of the client. They are neither positive nor negative; their effect is dependent on whether they act to enhance occupational performance or to inhibit occupational performance for the individual. A value such as 'hard working' may help the person if they are having poor performance issues at work but may hinder them if they are having mental health issues exacerbated by stress. Other examples of driftwood include:

- personal attributes *e.g.*, a person's values, personality, character, or special skills
- Resources *e.g.*, finances, equipment, assets, and other material things the person may have.

Attributes and resources are described as assets and liabilities based on the impact that they have on the life flow, which can be positive or negative. Driftwood is designed to push rocks down the stream and expand the life flow or positively affect life flow.

Case Example

Farayi is a lecturer in occupational therapy who has recently moved to work for a new university in Sydney. He is originally from Africa. His family lives in Zimbabwe, and some of his siblings live in South Africa. His friends still live in Queensland, a state he has lived in since coming to Australia in 2009. He feels isolated from his friends. At work, he has been given a very lucrative role he has always wanted; however, there is plenty to do and very little time to do it. He is finding this job very stressful and affecting his mental health.

Farayi went to see a psychiatrist, and he has been referred to you as the community occupational therapist. As a culturally sensitive OT, you have engaged with him and determined that the Kawa Model will be the best model to use to understand your client's circumstances. You have asked him to draw his Kawa as it is right now, and he has drawn Fig. (**4**) below:

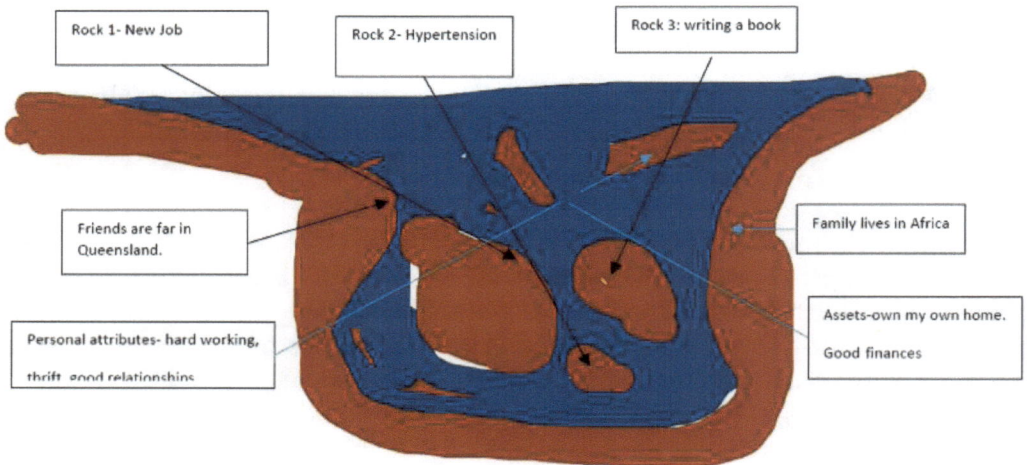

Fig. (4). Farayi's Kawa.

Reflection Questions

- Describe the client's context
- What environmental factors are impacting occupational performance?
- What would be the focus of OT Interventions?

Occupational therapy practice using the Kawa Model

When a person's life flow is impeded, the role of the OT is to understand all of the elements in the river in context and help facilitate better life flow. As described above, the spaces are the entry points for occupational therapy interventions. It is important that each problem is understood within the broader context of the person, which includes the personal and environmental contexts. Occupational therapists enable occupational performance and engagement by considering all components of the person's Kawa. The aim is to facilitate the life flow of the client's river in the context of their environment. OTs aim to enhance harmony between the person and their environment. The OT's role is to look at the person's current occupations and aim to facilitate better life flow.

When practicing using the Kawa Model, occupational therapists must adopt a strength-based approach. The aim is to maximise life flow using the person's driftwood, river wall, and riverbed in the process rather than just focusing on reducing the size of the rocks. The Kawa model suggests that occupational therapists must focus on spaces between rocks, driftwood, and riverbed or river walls rather than the objects themselves (Iwama, 2006, 2007, 2009). Other areas to focus on could be:

- Reducing the size and shape of rocks (problems),
- Making channels in or changing the shape of the riverbed (environment)
- Maximising the person's strengths and resources

Kawa model appears to differ from many other occupational therapy models is its use in practice. The majority of occupational therapy models have been developed as theoretical perspectives that are used to guide occupational therapists in their conceptualization of humans and human occupation and performance and are used by OTs to guide how we collect, organize, and integrate information (Tupe, 2014; Turpin, 2011; Supyk-Mellson & McKenna, 2010). In contrast, the Kawa model was designed to be used as a basis for discussion with clients. It can be a way for clients to tell and understand their own stories – which could be empowering. However, we also need to be aware that the river metaphor may not always be the best metaphor to use with a client, and in this case, one needs to consider modifying the metaphor or deciding that it may not be appropriate. Overall, when selecting this model, we might find it relevant for clients who come from a cultural background that has more collectivist rather than individualistic perspectives or for clients where it may be relevant and helpful to use the metaphor as a tool to collaboratively understand their journey, their current circumstances, and the tools/strategies, which may increase their life flow.

CONCLUSION

In the Kawa Model, water represents 'life energy' or 'life flow'. The river floor and walls represent the physical and societal context. The driftwood is the personal attributes and resources. Rocks represent life circumstances that are perceived to be problematic. The spaces between these elements are opportunities to create flow.

REFERENCES

Iwama, M.K. (2006). *The Kawa model: Culturally relevant occupational therapy.*. Philadelphia: Churchill Livingstone Elsevier.

Iwama, M. (2007). Culture and occupational therapy: meeting the challenge of relevance in a global world. *Occup. Ther. Int., 14*(4), 183-187.
[http://dx.doi.org/10.1002/oti.234] [PMID: 17966112]

Iwama, M.K., Thomson, N.A., Macdonald, R.M., Iwama, M.K., Thomson, N.A., Macdonald, R.M. (2009). The Kawa model: The power of culturally responsive occupational therapy. *Disabil. Rehabil., 31*(14), 1125-1135.
[http://dx.doi.org/10.1080/09638280902773711] [PMID: 19479503]

Supyk-Mellson, J., McKenna, J. (2010). Understanding models of practice. In: Curtin, M., Molineux, M., Supyk-Mellson, J., (Eds.), *Occupational therapy and physical dysfunction: Enabling occupation.* (6th ed., pp. 67-79). London, UK: Elsevier.

Tupe, D. (2014). Emerging theories. In: Boyt Schell, B.A., Gillen, G., Scaffa, M.E., (Eds.), *Willard & Spackman's occupational therapy.* (12th ed., pp. 553-562). Philadelphia: Wolters Kluwer Health/Lippincott Williams & Wilkins.

Turpin, M., Iwama, M.K. (2011). *Using occupational therapy models in practice: A field guide.*. London, UK: Elsevier.

CHAPTER 4

Person-Environment-Occupation Model and its Derivatives

Tawanda Machingura[1,*] and **Michelle Fair[2]**

[1] Head of Discipline Occupational Therapy Program, University of Notre Dame Australia, Sydney, Australia

[2] Department of Occupational Therapy, University of Tasmania, Tasmania, Australia

Abstract: This chapter will provide an overview of the Person-Environmen-
-Occupation (PEO) and the Person-Environment Occupation Performance (PEOP)
Models. The PEO model emphasises the importance of congruence between person,
environment, and occupation (PEO fit) and the subsequent occupational performance
within an event. Another ecological model, PEOP, focuses on the client and relevant
intrinsic (person) and extrinsic (environment) influences on the performance of
everyday occupations. The chapter discusses how these models can be applied to
individuals, groups (or organizations), and populations.

Keywords: Environment, Models, Occupation, Person.

INTRODUCTION

One way that can help us to understand complex ideas is to represent them as a
model. When we talk about a model, we are simply referring to a visual
representation of a concept or system. These visual images can help us to better
understand complex concepts as they aim to convey large amounts of information
in a simple and clear way.

OT theory has moved from a biomedical model, which was more popular pre
1990s, to a transactive model, which is based on the systems theory. In a
transactive model of occupational performance (OP), the word 'transactive' is
used to denote the product of a dynamic interwoven relationship between the
person (P), the environment (E), and the occupation (O) and where behaviour
cannot be separated from contextual influences.

---

* **Corresponding author Tawanda Machingura:** Head of Discipline Occupational Therapy Program, University of
Notre Dame Australia, Sydney, Australia; E-mail: tawanda.machingura@nd.edu.au

The PEO Model

The PEO model was founded by Law *et al.* (1996) in response to an identified need articulated through occupational therapy literature. This model was based on knowledge from person-environment models and client-centred practice, which was an emerging framework in Canada at the time (Strong *et al.*, 2010). The purpose of this model was to supplement existing models and provide occupational therapists with a framework to assess clients, provide interventions, and articulate their practice to others, including clients, other professionals, and funders (Strong *et al.*, 2010). The key concept of this model is the interconnectedness between the person, the environment, and the occupation (Fig. 1). The PEO model (Law et, 1996) is a framework that guides clinical reasoning through the analysis of interdependent transactions. It is used by many occupational therapists as a framework that they apply when working with their clients and guides their practice. The transactional approach in this model emphasises the interdependence between the environment and the person and enables users to explain occupational performance. It is a very simple model to explain a very complex phenomenon. Indeed, the very simplicity of the model is deceptive, given how complex occupational performance is.

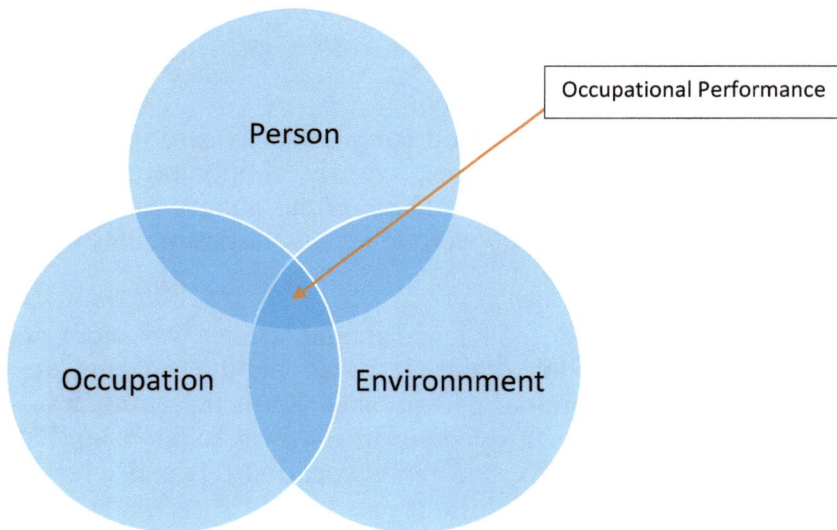

Fig. (1). PEO.

Visually, the model consists of three overlapping circles with an occupational performance at the centre where all three circles overlap. Each circle represents one aspect: the person, the environment, and the occupation. It must be emphasised that the relationship between the P, E, and O is dynamic and changes over time (Law *et al.*, 1996). The following is a description of the components of the model.

Person

The person is a unique being who assumes multiple roles and cannot be separated from contextual influences. The person should be considered from a biopsychosocial perspective, and they bring to the context a set of attributes, skills, knowledge, and experience. The person will have an influence on the environment around them, just as their environment will influence them.

Environment

The environment is defined as the context within which occupational performance takes place, and it is categorised into cultural, socioeconomic, institutional, physical, and social (Turpin *et al.*, 2024). All the environmental categories are equally important to consider according to the model. We consider the environment from the unique perspective of the person, household, neighbourhood, and/or community. It is clear here that ecological systems theory forms a foundation for this model. The person's cultural environment is typically made up of the shared values, beliefs, and attitudes of the relevant community. Whether a person connects with their cultural environment or not will influence their occupational performance (MacRae & Boggis, 2019). The socioeconomic aspect of the environment considers a person's social and economic position in society and how it influences their behaviour. At an institutional level, we consider concepts such as governance, regulations, laws, and policies that influence society. The physical aspects of the environment have tended to be more recognisable, and historically, a central consideration for occupational therapists. Over time, as we moved away from the medical model and towards the social model of disability, the other aspects of the environment have become equally important. The social model of disability suggests that it is not a person's impairments that disable them; instead, it is due to the barriers that exist in their broader environment (Oliver, 2013). Finally, when considering the social aspects of the environment, we can consider a person's intimate social environment, their community, and broader society. To enable us to unpack the social environment even further, using other relevant models, such as Bronfenbrenner's ecological systems theory (Bronfenbrenner, 1974) can be valuable. Bronfenbrenner considers five different systems: the microsystem, the mesosystem, the exosystem, the macrosystem, and the chronosystem, which can all influence a child's behaviour and growth. They highlight the complex dynamic systems that exist whereby a person is influenced by their environment, and, in turn, they influence the world around them (Bronfenbrenner, 1979).

Occupation

Occupations are the things that people do everyday and throughout their lives, either alone or with others, that give meaning and purpose to their life. The PEO model identifies the areas of occupation as self-care, productivity, and leisure (Law *et al.*, 1996). Occupations are pursued to fulfil the inherent desire for self-care, self-expression, and overall life pleasure. These tasks are performed in various settings to meet the demands of appropriate roles at different stages of development. It is crucial to take into account the temporal dimensions of the person's occupational habits over time. This includes the timing, sequence, and length of routines and habits and how these may change over time given how a person's roles will vary across their lifespan. When analysing occupations, it is important to consider the attributes of each task, such as their structure, duration, complexity, and demands.

Occupational Performance

Occupational performance is the outcome of the transactions between the person, the environment, and the occupation. We often describe this as the 'PEO fit'. When there is good alignment between all domains, occupational performance is enhanced (Fig. **2**). Alternatively, when alignment is poor, occupational performance is diminished (Fig. **3**). To understand this further, we look at the transactions between the P and E, the E and O, and the O and P. Effectively, we look at the barriers and enablers to an occupational performance that exist in these transactions and recognise that this is dynamic and changes over time.

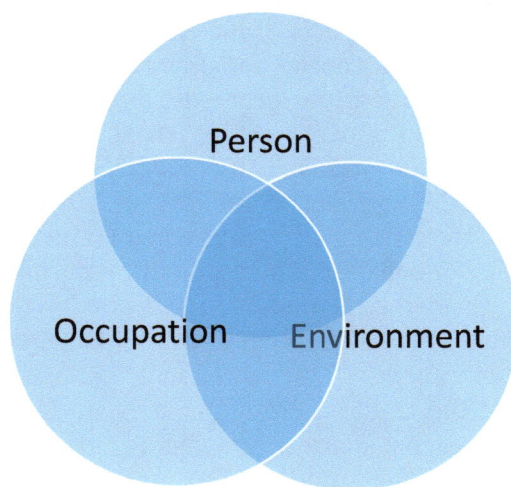

Fig. (2). PEO- Good alignment.

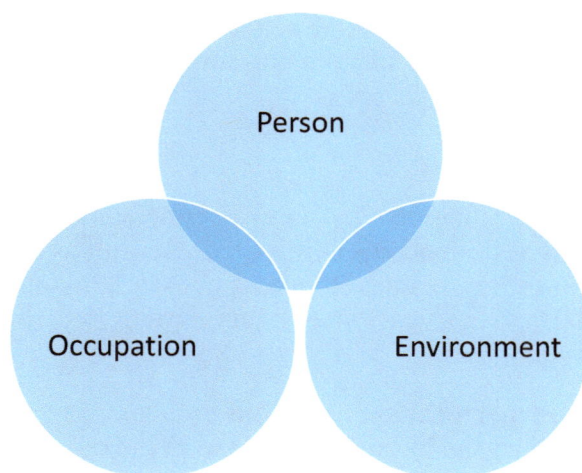

Fig. (3). PEO – Poor alignment.

Case Study

Let's explore this using a case study.

Meet Mary. Mary is a 40-year-old Australian woman living in Darwin and is married with two children. She is outgoing and enjoys socialising with friends and family on a regular basis. Mary attends her local church, and her faith plays an important role in her life. Fifteen years ago, Mary was diagnosed with relapsing-remitting multiple sclerosis. Her flare ups have been infrequent, and up until recently, Mary has continued to work full-time as an accountant and play netball in the local competition. Over the last year, Mary has noticed her symptoms have become more severe and are impacting her ability to complete her daily occupations. Specifically, she has reported issues with balance, mobility, anxiety, continence, and visual disturbances such as double vision, fatigue, and sensitivity to heat. Subsequently, Mary has noticed she lacks motivation, her sleep is impaired, and she can no longer concentrate and make decisions. Her general practitioner has now diagnosed her with depression (MS Australia, 2024).

Person-Environment Transactions

Barrier: Given where Mary lives and the exercise she participates in, her symptoms are likely to flare up, even if only temporarily. This is because Darwin has a tropical climate where temperatures can reach up to 38 degrees Celsius and typically reach a maximum of over 30 degrees Celsius every month of the year (Bureau of Meteorology, 2024). With multiple sclerosis, a person's symptoms can flare when they are exposed to heat, such as from the weather or exercise.

Enabler: Mary has a supportive social network and enjoys interacting with her friends and family. A supportive social environment can enable Mary and foster a sense of connectedness and inclusion.

Person – Occupation Transactions

Barrier: Mary reports that she is now feeling more fatigued and lacks concentration, and her vision has been impacted. Her job as an accountant can be demanding and requires her to spend much of her workday on a computer. There are also peak periods of the year when Mary is required to work overtime to manage the business demands.

Barrier: Mary values her occupational role as a mother; however, given the increase in her symptoms, she has been unable to participate in family activities in the usual way and can no longer prepare fresh meals every night for the family.

Occupation-Environment Transactions

Barrier: Mary historically attended church every weekend,; however, her local church is at a long distance from the car parking facility and has two flights of stairs to access the building. Given Mary's current issues with balance and mobility, she is unable to independently attend church. Furthermore, this has escalated Mary's anxiety, and she is worried she will not be able to access the toilet quickly if needed.

A visual depiction of Mary's current occupational performance can be seen in Fig. (**4**).

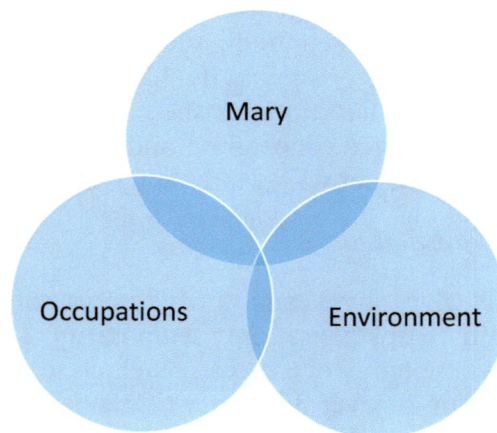

Fig. (4). Mary's poor PEO fit.

By considering Mary's needs holistically using the ecological approach of the PEO model, we can identify barriers and enablers to performance and, as a result, identify interventions to promote occupational performance. By addressing the barriers and creating more congruence between each domain, Mary's occupational performance can be improved. For example, by encouraging Mary to identify an indoor sporting activity where the temperature is lower and controlled using air conditioning, she can still participate but has less chance of her symptoms flaring up. In addition, staying well hydrated and taking regular breaks will allow her body temperature to be more stable (MS Australia, 2024). Another example could be assessing options for equipment and support within the workplace. Using text to speech software may be of benefit to allow Mary a visual break from reading information on her computer. Negotiating reduced hours at work when her symptoms have flared up could assist her in managing her symptoms and enable her to continue completing her other daily activities. Additionally, scheduling appointments with her healthcare team, for example, to assess if adaptations to her glasses, such as prisms to realign the two images (MS Australia, 2024), and meeting with a mental health occupational therapist to investigate solutions for improving motivation and managing symptoms associated with anxiety and depression can be helpful. By considering the context in which Mary lives her life and fully analysing the transactions that occur between her, the environment, and her chosen occupations, we are well placed to then recommend interventions that can enhance her occupational performance (Fig. **5**).

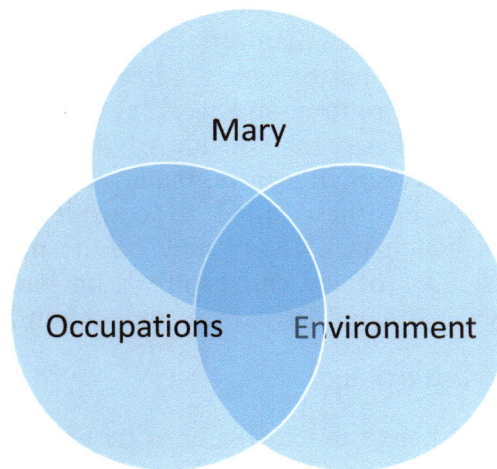

Fig. (5). Mary's good PEO fit.

We have applied the model for Mary as an individual, but now let's explore how we can apply PEO to groups of people or an organisation. In this example, we will explore the impact in the context of a workplace.

We can adapt our visual representation slightly to reflect the workplace. Fig. (**6**) depicts the 'person' as workers, the 'occupation' as work tasks, and the 'environment' as the workplace.

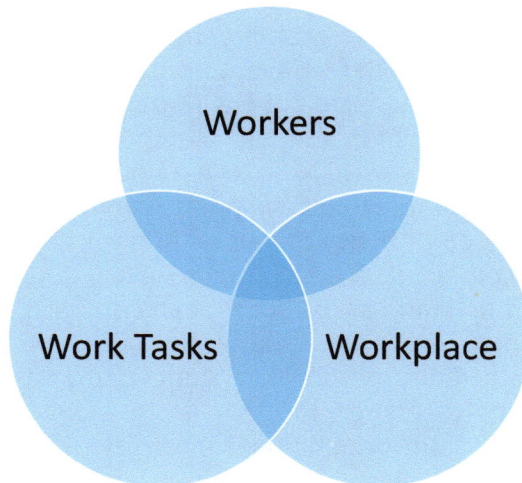

Fig. (6). Adapted PEO for Workplace.

In our scenario, the business is an insurance provider, and the workers are claims officers who work in a call centre. The call centre is located in the central business district of a major city, in an office building that is air-conditioned and has good accessibility. Staff work in an open plan office set up and have daily targets they must meet as part of their key performance indicators. They have low levels of control regarding their work routine and work content. Their break times are scheduled, and if they need a break outside of these times, they must seek permission from their supervisor. Recently, management has rolled out all new office task chairs; however, they failed to consult with workers or seek professional advice on which task chairs may be the most suitable. Within a period of three weeks, 80% of the call centre team had lodged a workplace incident related to back and shoulder pain when performing their work duties.

Worker – Workplace Transactions

Barrier: Organisational change is less likely to be effective if workers are not consulted and engaged during the process. The management team did not engage with the end users of the office task chairs and, as such, failed to understand their needs. Furthermore, by not utilizing a professional to assist with assessing which chairs would be most appropriate or conducting a risk assessment before introducing a new piece of equipment, they failed to identify any hazards associated with this rollout of furniture.

Enabler: The physical workplace enables workers by offering a thermostatically controlled environment and accessibility for all workers.

Worker-Work Tasks Transactions

Barrier: Psychosocial hazards can negatively impact worker health and workplace productivity. Having low levels of job control has been identified as one key psychosocial hazard experienced in workplaces (Safe Work Australia, n.d). As the workers were very restricted over an extended period of time in regard to the tasks they perform, when they perform them, and when they can take breaks, their health and wellbeing can be negatively affected.

This poor 'PEO fit' can result in both human and financial costs associated with the business (Fig. **7**).

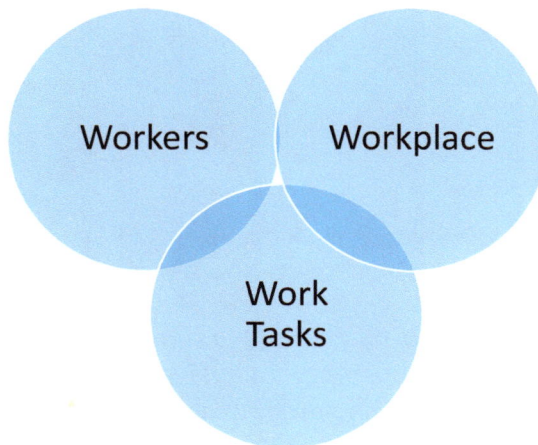

Fig. (7). Poor PEO Fit.

Through analysis using the PEO model, we can identify the relevant barriers and seek to address the impaired occupational performance. In this scenario, examples of solutions may include:

- Ergonomic workplace assessment to review the needs of the workers
- Improvements to processes surrounding change management and ensuring workers are consulted in the future
- Brainstorming session with staff about ways to improve levels of job control within a call centre operation.

Once effective solutions have been implemented, we are likely to have more alignment between the domains and improved occupational performance (Fig. **8**).

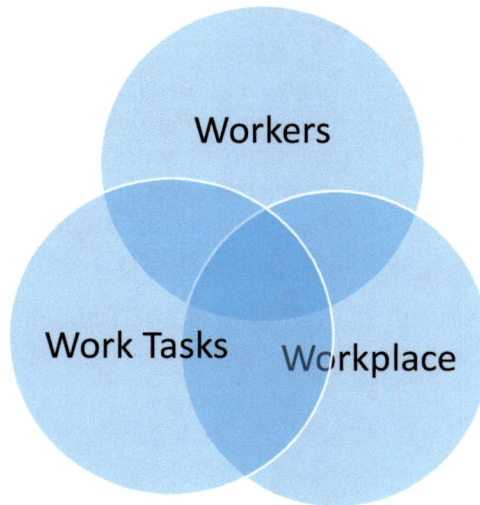

Fig. (8). Good PEO Fit.

PEO Summary

In summary, the Person-Environment-Occupation (PEO) model highlights how occupational performance is influenced by the interplay between an individual, their surroundings, and their chosen activities. The person domain encompasses various factors such as role, self-perception, cultural heritage, personality traits, physical well-being, cognitive ability, physical capabilities, and sensory capacities. The environmental domain encompasses the physical, cultural, institutional, social, and socio-economic aspects of the environment. Occupations are the various activities that an individual (or group of people) undertakes to fulfil their personal needs, express themselves, and achieve personal satisfaction. The three areas are interdependent and mutually influenced in this transactive and dynamic system. When the congruence between domains is high, occupational performance is improved. Alternatively, when there is a lack of congruence or alignment between these domains, occupational performance is diminished. Furthermore, the PEO model adopts a comprehensive viewpoint that considers the entire lifespan, resulting in changes in all three domains and occupational performance throughout one's life. Thus, this model can be used as an evaluative instrument for comprehending and examining problematic areas that impact clients' occupational performance. Alternatively, it can be utilised as an intervention tool to enhance clients' occupational performance by addressing barriers and improving the alignment of the three domains.

Person-Environment Occupation Performance (PEOP) Model

The PEOP model is an ecological systems model that was originally developed with the intention to be suitable across all areas of occupational therapy and to be used with diverse clients across their lifespan (Baum, Bass, and Christiansen, 2015). Like PEO, it focuses on the person, their environment, and the occupations that are being performed. In addition, it has a fourth component – the narrative. The narrative can be seen as a starting point to understand the needs and goals from the individual, community, or population perspective and contributes to the development of an occupational profile. Baum, Bass, and Christiansen (2015, p.40) refer to occupational performance in this model as "the doing of meaningful activities, tasks, and roles through complex interactions between the person and environment". It is a person, community, and population-centred model of occupational performance. First published in 1991, the PEOP model has undergone a number of iterations, with updates published in 1997, 2005, and 2015 (Turpin, Garcia, and Iwama, 2024). Fig. (**9**) summarises the development of the model over time. For the purposes of this chapter, we will focus on the current iteration. The key underpinnings of this model are that it is focused on occupational performance, it emphasizes a systems perspective, it is collaborative, and it supports client-centered practice. Let's explore what each of these means.

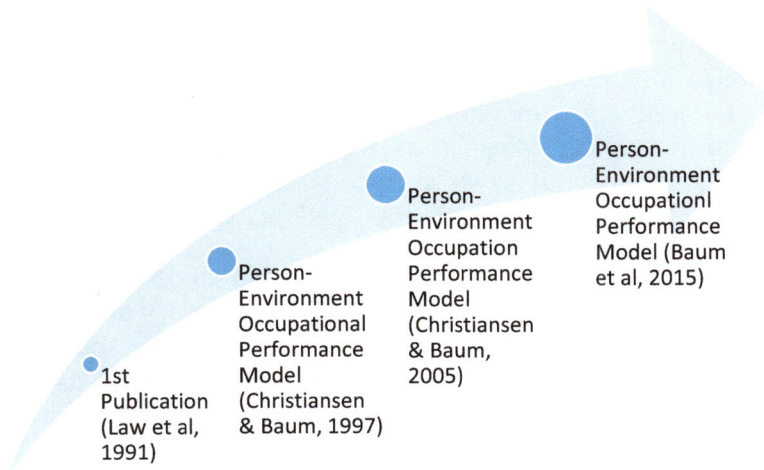

Fig. (9). Development of the PEOP model.

Occupational Performance

The concept of occupational performance is central to the profession of occupational therapy. It is the intersection between the person's capacities, the environment in which they live, work, and play, and the activities or tasks that are meaningful to them. Positive occupational performance supports the participation and well-being of people (Baum, Christiansen, and Bass, 2015).

Systems Approach

Systems theory recognises that each element of the system can impact another and, subsequently, the overall functioning of the system. It is a dynamic process where these transactions will shape a person, the environment, and how occupations are performed.

Collaborative

At the core, this model values clients and requires their active participation. It sees this as a positive way to influence your own life situation. This collaborative approach is designed to facilitate the development of an intervention plan with the client.

Client-Centred Practice

This model places the client (person, organisation, population) front and centre, ensuring we consider the past, current, and future perceptions, choices, interests, goals, and needs that are unique to them (the narrative). This enables the development of tailored goals specific to that person and encourages the client to be an active participant in the collaborative process. Ultimately, the goal is to support participation, performance, and well-being (Baum, Christiansen, and Bass, 2015). To do this, the model recognises the impairments of the person that limit participation and performance as well as the abilities and strengths that enable their performance. It gives due consideration to the environment and context in which the person lives, works, and plays.

The person factors consider all aspects of the individual, including their cognitive capacity, psychological status, physiological status, sensory and perceptive skills, motor functioning, and spirituality. Environmental factors span culture, social factors, policy and societal resources, and physical features such as the natural and built environment, including assistive technology. The model is transactive and acknowledges how the doing of the occupations (activities, tasks, and roles) is either supported by or impaired by personal and environmental factors (Baum, Christiansen, and Bass, 2015). Occupation is described in terms of participation, performance, and well-being. Fig. (**10**) depicts the PEOP model.

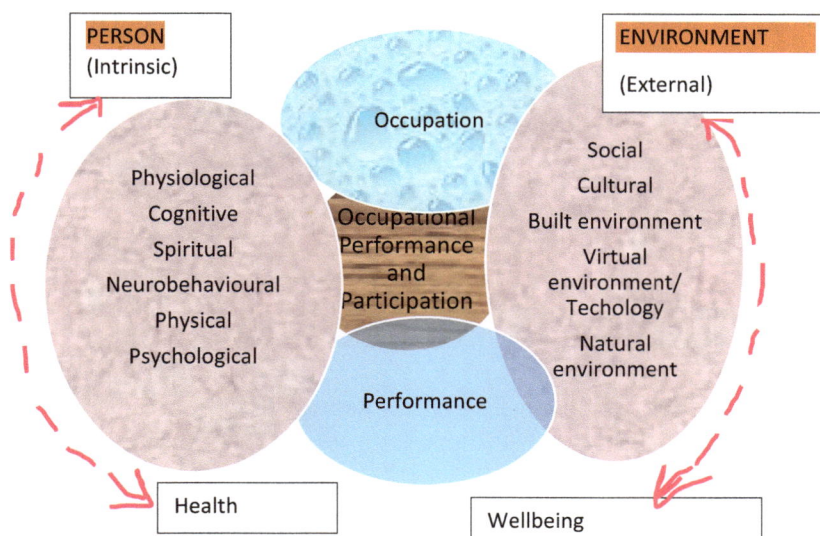

Fig. (10). PEOP Model (Adapted from Baum *et al*. 2015).

Application of PEOP

Below are some key steps to consider when using the PEOP in practice.

- Collaborate with the client throughout the occupational therapy process to improve occupational performance and participation.
- Develop an occupational profile of the client – interview the client/ gather information to develop an in-depth understanding of the person's past, current, and future perceptions, choices, interests, goals, and needs.
- Use a top-down approach to problem identification and decision-making, starting with the client's well-being, performance, and participation goals (highest-order factors).
- Provide interventions to enable the client to participate in desired social, cultural, socioeconomic, or political goals.
- Measure occupational performance by evaluating the person's ability to perform (do) desired occupations for the purposes of engagement in daily life and well-being.

PEOP SUMMARY

In summary, the PEOP Model is a framework that emphasizes the importance of occupational performance, participation, and well-being in everyday life. It focuses on the relationships between person, environment, and occupation factors that support these factors. The model is a bridge between biomedical and sociocultural approaches and is aligned with the Occupational Therapy Practice Framework and the International Classification of Function, Disability, and Health. It is suitable for various clients and practice settings, including individuals, groups, organizations, and populations. The PEOP can be used for providing occupational therapy to individuals, organizations, and populations.

Think of this model as consisting of layers.

- **First layer:** Foundation is the person (abilities) and environment.
- **Second layer:** Occupation (roles, occupations, and tasks) and performance (actions)
- **Third layer:** Occupational performance (actions that are meaningful) and participation (context of meaningful and purposeful participation).

SUMMARY

This chapter has provided an overview of the PEO and PEOP Models. The PEO model focuses on the fit or congruence between the person, environment, and occupation (PEO fit). The PEOP model focuses on the client and relevant intrinsic (person) and extrinsic (environment) influences on the performance of everyday occupations. Both models can be applied to individuals, groups (or organizations), and populations.

REFERENCES

Baum, C.M., Bass, J.D., Christiansen, C.H. (2015). Theory, models. Frameworks, and classifications. *Occupational Therapy Performance, Participation, and Well-Being (4th ed)* Christiansen, Baum and Bass (Eds.) SLACK, Incorporated.

Bureau of Meteorology. (2024). Northern Territory Weather and Warning Summaries. Australian Government. Available from: http://www.bom.gov.au/nt/?ref=hdr.

Bronfenbrenner, U. (1974). Developmental research, public policy, and the ecology of childhood. *Child Dev., 45*(1), 1-5.
[http://dx.doi.org/10.2307/1127743]

Bronfenbrenner, U. (1979). *The ecology of human development: Experiments by nature and design..* Harvard University Press.
[http://dx.doi.org/10.4159/9780674028845]

MacRae, A., Boggis, T. (2019). Cultural Identity and Context. *Psychosocial Occupational Therapy: An evolving practice (4th ed)* Cara and MacRae's (Eds.) SLACK, Incorporated.

MS Australia. (2024). *MS Symptoms*. Available from: https://www.msaustralia.org.au/what-is-multip-e-sclerosis-ms/symptoms/.

Oliver, M. (2013). The social model of disability: thirty years on. *Disabil. Soc., 28*(7), 1024-1026.
[http://dx.doi.org/10.1080/09687599.2013.818773]

Safe Work Australia. (n.d.). Psychosocial Hazards. Available from: https://www.safeworkaustralia.gov.au/safety-topic/managing-health-and-safety/mental-health/ psychosocial-hazards.

Strong, S., Rigby, P., Stewart, D., Law, M., Letts, L., Cooper, B. (1999). Application of the Person-Environment-Occupation Model: a practical tool. *Can. J. Occup. Ther., 66*(3), 122-133. [http://dx.doi.org/10.1177/000841749906600304] [PMID: 10462885]

Turpin, M.J., Garcia, J., Iwama, M.K. (2024). *Using Occupational Therapy Models in Practice.* Elsevier.

Part 2
Conditions in Mental Health Practice

• Summary of the common occupational therapy models used in mental health practice.

• Summary of theoretical constructs and historical evolution of each model.

• Case and practice examples of how occupational therapists can use models in various practice contexts.

This section builds on the understanding of theoretical models in occupational therapy practice. The models provide occupational therapists with an explanation and understanding of human behaviour, function, and dysfunction. Leading on from models, key considerations in occupational therapy theory and practice are the person components as these transact with the environment and the occupation and either facilitate or inhibit occupational performance.

The purpose of this section is to provide practitioners with an understanding of the person components through an introductory understanding of common mental health conditions encountered in practice. This section contains chapters on conditions such as eating disorders, personality disorders, mood disorders, and psychotic disorders. The intention was never to cover all conditions but to introduce occupational therapists to some common mental health conditions and explain how occupational therapists can provide evidence-based interventions when working with people experiencing those particular conditions.

CHAPTER 5

Psychotic Disorders

Tawanda Machingura[1,*]

[1] *Head of Discipline Occupational Therapy Program, University of Notre Dame Australia, Sydney, Australia*

Abstract: Psychosis is a debilitating group of symptoms that affects an individual at the same time and occurs over a period of time. These symptoms often include disturbances in behaviour, the thinking process, thought content, perception, affect, and mood. This chapter with briefly explore what psychosis is and then focus on one of the most debilitating psychotic disorders known to mankind, schizophrenia.

Note

This chapter is meant to be introductory, and the reader is encouraged to seek further information from comprehensive psychiatric texts. This chapter can also be used as a quick revision chapter for students and clinicians.

Keywords: Bipolar, Delusional disorder, Psychotic disorders, Schizophrenia, Schizoaffective disorder, Schizophreniform disorder, Substance-induced psychotic disorder.

INTRODUCTION

It is important to first acknowledge that there is debate in the field of psychiatry around what is a mental disorder, with some pointing out past turnarounds and failures; for example, homosexuality used to be regarded as a mental disorder (Stein *et al.*, 2021). Recently, the DSM-5 definition has refered to dysfunction in 'psychological, biological, or developmental processes' (American Psychiatric Association, 2013). In writing this chapter on psychosis, the DSM-5 definition of mental disorder is assumed.

The term 'psychosis' was derived from the Greek word 'psyche', meaning 'mind', and the Latin word 'osis', meaning abnormal condition. The literal translation of the word psychosis is, therefore, 'abnormal condition of the mind'. A key feature of psychosis is that the person is affected by a collection of symptoms that occur

---

* **Corresponding author Tawanda Machingura:** Head of Discipline Occupational Therapy Program, University of Notre Dame Australia, Sydney, Australia; E-mail: tawanda.machingura@nd.edu.au

at the same time and do so over a period of time ranging from one week to several months or even years. The most commonly described symptoms of psychosis include a deterioration in social and occupational functioning (behaviour), a loss of mental functioning (thinking processes), a loss of ability to distinguish fantasy from reality (perception), and changes in mood and affect [emotions or feelings; Howes *et al.*, 2012]. Psychosis affects the way a person thinks, feels, and behaves. Psychosis tends to occur in a spectrum ranging from subclinical symptoms to severe psychosis, such as in schizophrenia (Mennigen & Bearden, 2020). Fig. (**1**) below shows the spectrum of common psychotic disorders.

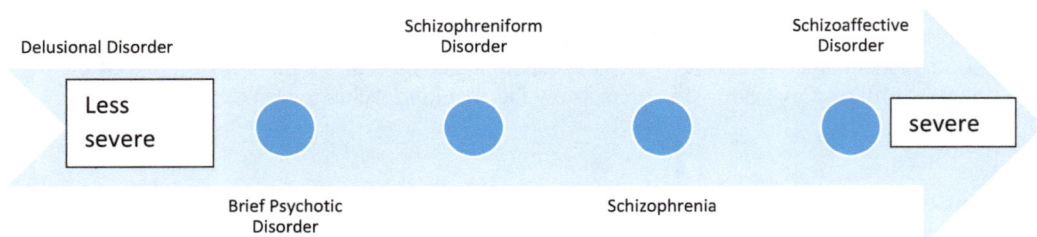

Fig. (1). Spectrum of psychotic disorders.

A large part of the population with subclinical symptoms does not seek help (Mennigen & Bearden, 2020).

Onset

The first onset of psychotic disorders is usually in adolescence or young adulthood. Recent research, however, indicates that nearly a quarter of first onsets occur after the age of 40 when looking at population data obtained from the World Health Organization (McGrath *et al.*, 2015; McGrath *et al.*, 2016). This implies that psychotic symptoms in childhood and adolescence do not always predict the onset of a major mental illness later on in life (Mennigen & Bearden, 2020).

Types

The different types of psychotic disorders are determined by the spectrum of symptoms that one presents with and also how long those symptoms last. The symptoms can be for short periods of time, lasting a few days or weeks, and others can take much longer, lasting a month or more (Bhati, 2013). Table **1** provides more details on specific types.

Table 1. Types of Psychotic Disorders[1]

Type	Brief description / Duration
Brief Psychotic Disorder	Duration of an episode of the disturbance is at least 1 day to 1 month with eventual full return to premorbid level of functioning.
Schizophreniform Disorder	Two of the following symptomsmust be present for a significant portion of time during a 1-month period (or less if successfully treated): delusions, hallucinations, disorganized speech, disorganized behaviour, and negative symptoms. At least one of the following must be present: delusions, hallucinations, or disorganized speech.
Substance-Induced Psychotic Disorder	Prominent hallucinations or delusions developed within a month of substance intoxication or withdrawal that cannot be better accounted for by a psychotic disorder that is not substance induced.
Schizoaffective disorder	2 weeks of delusions and hallucinations alone, periods where hallucinations and delusions are accompanied by major depression or mania, and the mood symptoms are present for a significant period of the total duration of the illness.
Schizophrenia	Two of the following must be present for a significant portion of time during a 1-month period (or less if successfully treated): delusions, hallucinations, disorganized speech, disorganized behaviour, and negative symptoms. At least one of the following must be present: delusions, hallucinations, or disorganized speech. Continuous signs of the disturbance persist for at least 6 months. This 6-month period must include at least 1 month of symptoms (or less if successfully treated) that meet Criterion A (*i.e.*, active-phase symptoms) and may include periods of prodromal or residual symptoms.
Delusional Disorder	Duration is 1 month or longer. Functioning is not markedly impaired, and behaviour is not obviously odd or bizarre. If mood episodes are present, their total duration is brief relative to the duration of the delusional periods.

Etiology

The causes of psychosis are not fully understood. What is known is that psychosis is often associated with early life adversities, and these manifest as childhood emotional and behavioural problems (Menningen & Bearden, 2020). There are other known risk factors for developing overt psychotic symptoms later on in life, and these include:

- Genetic risk- such as a family history of psychosis,
- Early exposure to drugs -such as cannabis,
- Early neurodevelopmental problems- such as autism spectrum symptoms, lower IQ, and delayed early motor development,
- Early life stress and childhood trauma -such as complications in eutero or during birth, *e.g.*, birth asphyxia, and socioeconomic difficulties (Menningen & Bearden, 2020).

The importance of understanding risk factors is that most of these upstream determinants of health can be mitigated.

Incidence

Psychotic symptoms are a strong indicator of the future development of severe mental illnesses (Fusar-Poli *et al.*, 2017). McGrath (2004) defines incidence as the number of new cases that occur in a population over a given period of observation. The prevalence of psychotic symptoms in the general population is 5.8%, with these symptoms being reported to be often accompanied by cognitive difficulties, poor quality of life, increased substance use, poor social and occupational functioning, and suicidality (McGrath *et al.*, 2015; McGrath *et al.*, 2016).

Treatment

Medical treatment of psychosis includes mainly the use of atypical antipsychotic drugs. Interestingly, the term 'atypical' was first used to describe clozapine, which had been found to have very different properties from the traditionally used and older typical neuroleptics (Siegfried *et al.*, 2001). Other examples of atypical antipsychotics include risperidone, olanzapine, quetiapine, sertindole, ziprasidone, aripiprazole, and amisulpride (Siegfried *et al.*, 2001). These drugs, however, are of major concern because of their tendency to induce weight gain and alter glucose and lipid metabolism (De Oliveira & Juruena, 2006).

Psychosocial interventions for psychosis also have mixed efficacy. The most common evidence-based psychosocial interventions include:

- Regular exercise (Mittal *et al.*, 2017)
- Yoga (Mittal *et al.*, 2017)
- Virtual reality-assisted therapies for psychosis (Rus-Calafell *et al.*, 2018)
- Individual cognitive and behavioral therapies (Rus-Calafell *et al.*, 2018)
- Family interventions for psychosis (Haddock & Spaulding, 2010)
- Neuropsychological and cognitive remediation approaches (Haddock & Spaulding, 2010)
- Social skills training and other skills training approaches (Rus-Calafell *et al.*, 2018)
- Contingency management approaches (Haddock & Spaulding, 2010).

Schizophrenia

Schizophrenia is a major psychotic disorder that is characterised by symptoms such as hallucinations, delusions, disorganized speech, poor planning, reduced motivation, blunted affect, and reduced interpersonal and occupational functioning (APA, 2015). Arguably, schizophrenia is one of the most stigmatised and ill-treated conditions in the world today. 'Schizo' is a Greek word that means 'split', and 'phrenia' is a Greek word for 'mind', so the literal translation of the word schizophrenia is 'split mind' (Bhati, 2013). We, however, now know that this is not an accurate description of the condition. We now know that schizophrenia is an illness affecting how a person thinks, acts, and feels, leaving them with an altered perception of reality, and consists of positive, negative, and cognitive symptoms, which in combination, significantly impair the person's ability to live, work, study, and socialize in the community of their choice.

There is ongoing philosophical debate in the field of psychiatry and mental health and in the general population on the accuracy of diagnostic labels, particularly in differentiating what is culturally appropriate versus abnormal behaviour (Bathi, 2013; Stein *et al.*, 2021). There is, however, very little to no debate among clinicians about the clinical application and usefulness of those labels. Clinicians use provisional and arbitrary constructs such as ICD 10 and DSM V to facilitate international communication and guide treatment and research (Bathi, 2013). According to DSM IV, schizophrenia is "a disturbance that lasts for at least 6 months and includes at least 1 month of active-phase symptoms (*i.e.*, two [or more] of the following: delusions, hallucinations, disorganized speech, grossly disorganized or catatonic behaviour, negative symptoms)" (DSM IV p.273). DSM 5 further details the diagnosis in Table **2** below.

Adapted from DSM 5: Diagnostic and Statistical Manual of Mental Disorders, Fifth Edition (APA)

To be diagnosed with schizophrenia, one must have marked social and occupational dysfunction with symptoms for more than 6 months, as in Table 2 above.

The reason why schizophrenia is a major problem is that it causes significant impairment in an individual's social and occupational functioning and is a known major contributor to the burden of disease worldwide (APA, 2015). Furthermore, people with schizophrenia have high rates of comorbidities, which further complicates their recovery and contributes to their significantly reduced life expectancy (APA, 2015).

Prevalence

Schizophrenia is of low prevalence (McGrath, 2004). The prevalence and incidence rates of schizophrenia tend to be similar across populations; however, deviations from this trend have also between found within and between populations (McGrath, 2004). In the general population, lifetime risk is approximately 1%. However, the risk is greatly increased in families, pointing to a genetic correlation. As an example, a child born to one schizophrenic parent has a 14% risk of developing schizophrenia. The risk increases to 25% if both parents have schizophrenia. In a non-twin sibling, the risk is lower: 8%. In non-identical twins (dizygotic), there is a 10% risk for the other twin to develop schizophrenia. The risk rises to 40-50% in identical, monozygotic twins (McGrath, 2004).

Table 2. Summary of symptoms and diagnosis of schizophrenia

Criteria	Description
A	Two (or more) of the following, each present for a significant portion of time during a 1-month period (or less if successfully treated). At least one of these must be present (1, 2, or 3): 1. Delusions 2. Hallucinations 3. Disorganized speech or Disorganised thinking 4. Grossly disorganized or catatonic behaviour 5. Negative symptoms.
B	For a significant portion of the time since the onset of the disturbance, the level of functioning in one or more major areas is markedly below the level achieved prior to the onset (or when the onset is in childhood or adolescence, there is failure to achieve the expected level of interpersonal, academic, or occupational functioning).
C	Continuous signs of the disturbance persist for at least 6 months. This 6-month period must include at least 1 month of symptoms (or less if successfully treated) that meet Criterion A (*i.e.,* active-phase symptoms) and may include periods of prodromal or residual symptoms.
D	Schizoaffective disorder and depressive or bipolar disorder with psychotic features have been ruled out.
E	The disturbance is not attributable to the physiological effects of a substance (*e.g.*, a drug of abuse, a medication) or another medical condition.
F	If there is a history of autism spectrum disorder or a communication disorder of childhood onset, the additional diagnosis of schizophrenia is made only if prominent delusions or hallucinations, in addition to the other required symptoms of schizophrenia, are also present for at least 1 month (or less if successfully treated).

Onset

The disorder usually starts in young adulthood. Despite optimal treatment, approximately two-thirds of affected individuals have persisting or fluctuating symptoms (APA, 1994). In the Australian population, two-thirds of people with schizophrenia experienced their initial episode before age 25, and many of them had experienced disabling, unremitting symptoms since the onset of their illness (Morgan *et al.*, 2011). Life expectancy is also reduced by death from suicide and other causes. Approximately 40% of patients with schizophrenia attempt suicide at some point in their lifetime, and 15 – 20% succeed. Lifetime risk among people with schizophrenia is approximately 10% (Sher & Kahn, 2019)

Management

The general management of schizophrenia is similar to what has been discussed under the management of psychotic conditions. This section will, therefore, focus on the role of occupational therapy and other interventions not already discussed.

Occupational therapists are concerned with how people interact with their environment and their chosen occupation, the product of which is regarded as occupational performance (Chapparo & Ranka, 1997). Many people with schizophrenia will have difficulties in a number of life domains, including:

- Basic activities of daily living, such as personal care, and instrumental activities of daily living, such as home maintenance (Aubin *et al.*, 2009).
- Work and employment skills (Waghorn *et al.*, 2009)
- Social skills and use of leisure time (Waghorn *et al.*, 2009).

These are the very domains of the profession of occupational therapy. An occupational therapist may provide the following interventions:

- Facilitating social connections and support- includes building social connections with friends, family, neighbours, and carers and engaging in social activities in the community.
- Providing case management -this is professional help in the coordination and navigation of services the person needs, as well as the provision of supportive therapy and assistance with problem solving.
- Assisting with hospital admission -this includes inpatient/ outpatient clinic and hospital services when the person needs it and for as long as the person needs it.
- Providing social skills training – this is skills training from a health professional to enable the person to relearn interpersonal skills.
- Providing crisis intervention/early intervention services- this is a crisis service provided to the person when they need it and where they need it which is usually at home or in the community. It also includes education concerning early warning signs and practising and planning for crisis management before one is in a crisis.
- Returning a person to person to more productive roles in society
- Enabling access to supported employment- helps a person return to work.
- Providing other psychosocial interventions- to help the person break unhelpful thinking patterns and manage distress.

- Enabling access to housing and financial support- helps people with basic human needs such as food and shelter needs and forms a starting point for health and well-being.
- Enabling a person to access peer support – includes opportunities to learn from peers who have a lived experience.
- Encouraging and facilitating medication compliance- Medications -including neuroleptics (oral/ depot)

CONCLUSION

Below are some key facts about psychosis:

- The lifetime incidence of 1:300 people worldwide,
- Associated with alcohol, tobacco, or other drug use,
- The causes of psychosis are not fully understood
- Risk factors include genetics, early childhood experiences, early exposure to alcohol or other drugs
- Treatment involves the use of atypical antipsychotics.
- Management involves evidence-based psychosocial interventions.

REFERENCES

American Psychiatric Association, D. S. M. T. F., & American Psychiatric Association. *Diagnostic and statistical manual of mental disorders: DSM-5* Washington, DC: American psychiatric association.(5)

American Psychiatric Association. (2000). Diagnostic and statistical manual of mental disorders. *Text revision.*

Bhati, M.T. (2013). Defining psychosis: the evolution of DSM-5 schizophrenia spectrum disorders. *Curr. Psychiatry Rep., 15*(11), 409.
[http://dx.doi.org/10.1007/s11920-013-0409-9] [PMID: 24057160]

Chapparo, C., Ranka, J. (1997). Towards a model of occupational performance: Model development. *Occupational performance model (Australia)*

De Oliveira, I.R., Juruena, M.F. (2006). Treatment of psychosis: 30 years of progress. *J. Clin. Pharm. Ther., 31*(6), 523-534.
[http://dx.doi.org/10.1111/j.1365-2710.2006.00784.x] [PMID: 17176358]

Fusar-Poli, P., Rutigliano, G., Stahl, D., Davies, C., De Micheli, A., Ramella-Cravaro, V., Bonoldi, I., McGuire, P. (2017). Long-term validity of the At Risk Mental State (ARMS) for predicting psychotic and non-psychotic mental disorders. *Eur. Psychiatry, 42*, 49-54.
[http://dx.doi.org/10.1016/j.eurpsy.2016.11.010] [PMID: 28212505]

Haddock, G., Spaulding, W. (2010). Psychological treatment of psychosis. *Schizophrenia,* 666-686.

Howes, O.D., Fusar-Poli, P., Bloomfield, M., Selvaraj, S., McGuire, P. (2012). From the prodrome to chronic schizophrenia: the neurobiology underlying psychotic symptoms and cognitive impairments. *Curr. Pharm. Des., 18*(4), 459-465.
[http://dx.doi.org/10.2174/138161212799316217] [PMID: 22239576]

McGrath, J.J., Saha, S., Al-Hamzawi, A.O., Alonso, J., Andrade, L., Borges, G., Bromet, E.J., Oakley Browne, M., Bruffaerts, R., Caldas de Almeida, J.M., Fayyad, J., Florescu, S., de Girolamo, G., Gureje, O.,

Hu, C., de Jonge, P., Kovess-Masfety, V., Lepine, J.P., Lim, C.C.W., Navarro-Mateu, F., Piazza, M., Sampson, N., Posada-Villa, J., Kendler, K.S., Kessler, R.C. (2016). Age of onset and lifetime projected risk of psychotic experiences: cross-national data from the World Mental Health Survey. *Schizophr. Bull., 42*(4), 933-941.
[http://dx.doi.org/10.1093/schbul/sbw011] [PMID: 27038468]

McGrath, J.J., Saha, S., Al-Hamzawi, A., Alonso, J., Bromet, E.J., Bruffaerts, R., Caldas-de-Almeida, J.M., Chiu, W.T., de Jonge, P., Fayyad, J., Florescu, S., Gureje, O., Haro, J.M., Hu, C., Kovess-Masfety, V., Lepine, J.P., Lim, C.C.W., Mora, M.E.M., Navarro-Mateu, F., Ochoa, S., Sampson, N., Scott, K., Viana, M.C., Kessler, R.C. (2015). Psychotic experiences in the general population: a cross-national analysis based on 31 261 respondents from 18 countries. *JAMA Psychiatry, 72*(7), 697-705.
[http://dx.doi.org/10.1001/jamapsychiatry.2015.0575] [PMID: 26018466]

Mennigen, E., Bearden, C.E. (2020). Psychosis risk and development: what do we know from population-based studies? *Biol. Psychiatry, 88*(4), 315-325.
[http://dx.doi.org/10.1016/j.biopsych.2019.12.014] [PMID: 32061373]

McGrath, J., Saha, S., Welham, J., El Saadi, O., MacCauley, C., Chant, D. (2004). A systematic review of the incidence of schizophrenia: the distribution of rates and the influence of sex, urbanicity, migrant status and methodology. *BMC Med., 2*(1), 13.
[http://dx.doi.org/10.1186/1741-7015-2-13] [PMID: 15115547]

Mittal, V.A., Vargas, T., Juston Osborne, K., Dean, D., Gupta, T., Ristanovic, I., Hooker, C.I., Shankman, S.A. (2017). Exercise treatments for psychosis: a review. *Curr. Treat. Options Psychiatry, 4*(2), 152-166.
[http://dx.doi.org/10.1007/s40501-017-0112-2] [PMID: 29034144]

Rus-Calafell, M., Garety, P., Sason, E., Craig, T.J.K., Valmaggia, L.R. (2018). Virtual reality in the assessment and treatment of psychosis: a systematic review of its utility, acceptability and effectiveness. *Psychol. Med., 48*(3), 362-391.
[http://dx.doi.org/10.1017/S0033291717001945] [PMID: 28735593]

Siegfried, S. L., Fleischhacker, W., Lieberman, J. A., Lieberman, J. A., Murray, R. M. (2001). *Comprehensive care of schizophrenia: a textbook of clinical management.*

Stein, D.J., Palk, A.C., Kendler, K.S. (2021). What is a mental disorder? An exemplar-focused approach. *Psychol. Med., 51*(6), 894-901.
[http://dx.doi.org/10.1017/S0033291721001185] [PMID: 33843505]

Sher, L., Kahn, R.S. (2019). Suicide in schizophrenia: an educational overview. *Medicina (Kaunas), 55*(7), 361.
[http://dx.doi.org/10.3390/medicina55070361] [PMID: 31295938]

CHAPTER 6

Anxiety and Mood Disorders

Tawanda Machingura[1,*] and **Catherine Hurley**[2]

[1] *Head of Discipline Occupational Therapy Program, University of Notre Dame Australia, Sydney, Australia*

[2] *Discipline of Occupational Therapy, University of Notre Dame Australia, Sydney, Australia*

Abstract: This chapter gives an overview of anxiety and mood disorders. Anxiety and mood disorders are arguably the most common mental illness worldwide. The purpose of this chapter is to introduce the reader to the pathophysiology, aetiology, and epidemiology of these conditions so the reader can develop an in-depth understanding of how to work with people with anxiety and mood disorders. The occupational therapy perspective is woven in throughout this chapter.

Keywords: Anxiety, Bipolar disorder, Depression, Generalized anxiety disorder, Manic episode, Mood disorders, Obsessive-compulsive disorder, Occupational therapy, Occupational therapy, Panic disorder, Phobia, Post-traumatic stress disorder.

INTRODUCTION

Anxiety and depression are arguably the most common mental health conditions known to affect people worldwide. This chapter introduces anxiety disorders first and then delves into mood disorders, including depression. These conditions are presented in one chapter as they often co-exist and complicate one another. In general, anxiety disorders are characterised by excessive worry or fear of something that might happen, whereas mood disorders often affect how one perceives themselves and their environment. People with depression, for example, may also excessively worry about something that has already happened.

In this chapter, we will explore these disorders in detail, including their signs and symptoms, as well as medical and occupational therapy management. This chapter aims to equip the readers with an introductory yet comprehensive understanding of anxiety and mood disorders so that they are well-positioned to recognize and manage these conditions within the bounds of their professions.

* **Corresponding author Tawanda Machingura:** Head of Discipline Occupational Therapy Program, University of Notre Dame Australia, Sydney, Australia; E-mail: tawanda.machingura@nd.edu.au

Anxiety

Anxiety is a distressing, unpleasant emotional state of nervousness and uneasiness (Akinsulore, Owojuyigbe, Faponle, & Fatoye, 2015). It can be anticipatory before a threat, persist after a threat has passed, or occur without an identifiable threat (Craske & Stein, 2016). Anxiety is often accompanied by physical changes and behaviours similar to those caused by fear and occurs in a wide range of physical and mental disorders (Kandola *et al.*, 2018; Perusini & Fanselow, 2015).

Causes of Anxiety

Causes are not fully known and are often a combination of factors, including: —

- Environmental. This includes a response to stressful life events *e.g.*, job loss/ pregnancy/ abuse and/or significant exposure to life-threatening disasters (Porter, 2011). Trauma is thought to be a significant factor in the development of anxiety disorders (Bridley & Daffin, 2018).
- Humanistic, existential, and sociocultural theories. This emanates from a loss of sense of self and/ or concerns about the meaningfulness of life and the need for self-actualisation.
- Psychodynamic theory. Anxiety is linked to unresolved, unconscious psychological conflict that originates in the ego as it tries to moderate intense challenges from the id and superego (Duncan, 2005).
- Culture bound. Ancestral communication, curses, or omens (Duncan, 2005)
- Physical health problems. Examples include diabetes, asthma, and heart disease (Niles *et al.*, 2015)
- Biological factors (Martin, Ressler, Binder, & Nemeroff, 2009)
- Family history (genetic transmission) (van Sprang *et al.*, 2022)
- Sodium lactate and caffeine stimulate anxiety (Hermann, Lay, Wahl, Roth, & Petrowski, 2019; Lara, 2010)
- Substance use, especially heavy or prolonged (Vorspan, Mehtelli, Dupuy, Bloch, & Lépine, 2015)
- Cognitive, learning, and behavioural theories (Chorpita & Barlow, 2018; Hallion & Ruscio, 2011; Rector, Bourdeau, Kitchen, Joseph-Massiah, & Laposa, 2016)
- Learned responses, contributing to a highly strung personality style (Kotov, Gamez, Schmidt, & Watson, 2010).

Panic Disorder

Panic disorder is characterised by short, sudden attacks of fear, fear of losing control, or terror (Bouton, Mineka, & Barlow, 2018). The onset is often late adolescence or early adulthood (Olaya, Moneta, Miret, Ayuso-Mateos, & Haro,

2018). Signs and symptoms include heart pounding, feeling short of breath, feeling as if choking will occur, chest tightness, pain, dizziness, and other physical symptoms that appear quickly and peak within 10 minutes (Meuret *et al.*, 2011). It can happen unexpectedly and can be situationally bound or situationally predisposed (Copeland, 2003)

Phobia

A phobia is defined as having an irrational fear that leads to avoidance of certain objects and specific situations (Garcia, 2017). Its onset is in childhood or early adolescence (American Psychiatric Association, 2022). Phobias are classified by specific fears, such as a fear of places or situations that might cause panic (agoraphobia) or a fear of blood (Hemophobia) (Eaton, Bienvenu, & Miloyan, 2018). Phobias present with associated physical symptoms, as is the case with panic disorder (Samra & Abdijadid, 2018).

Obsessive Compulsive Disorder (OCD)

In OCD, obsessions are repetitive thoughts, and compulsions are ritualistic behaviours. A person may present with obsessions, compulsions, or both that one realises are unreasonable, unnecessary, intrusive, and irresistible. The average age of onset is late adolescence (Brakoulias *et al.*, 2017). Common compulsive behaviours include hand washing, cleanliness of the skin, checking appliances, locking doors, and counting, hoarding, and arranging items in a specific order (Abramowitz & Jacoby, 2015).

Generalised Anxiety Disorder (GAD)

GAD is characterised by excessive worry or anxiety about a variety of life events or activities, such as school, work, or family concerns, that are difficult to control (Groves, Binasis, Wootton, & Moses, 2023). These worries happen most days for a period of at least 6 months (Stein & Sareen, 2015). The Australian lifetime prevalence for GAD has been found to be 8% (Ruscio *et al.*, 2017).

Post Traumatic Stress Disorder (PTSD)

PTSD is a psychological stress disorder from exposure to traumatic events such as natural disasters, violent crime, torture, accidents, or war (Benjet *et al.*, 2016). It is characterised by chronic anxiety, exaggerated startle response, difficulties with concentrating, nightmares, and insomnia (Bryant, 2019). PTSD can present with comorbid depression and or substance misuse (Angelakis & Nixon, 2015; Flanagan, Korte, Killeen, & Back, 2016).

Treatment of Anxiety

Treatment of anxiety includes medications, usually antidepressant medications and benzodiazepines (sedatives). Psychosocial interventions include anxiety management, problem-solving, relaxation, mindfulness techniques, a healthy lifestyle, exercise, reduction of alcohol and other drugs, engagement in meaningful occupation, self-help, family therapy, and psychoeducation and grading activities.

Occupational Therapy with People with Anxiety

Occupational Performance Assessment

The first step in the occupational therapy process is developing an understanding of the person in context. This includes developing an occupational profile of the person as well as an assessment of functioning. Occupational assessments are conducted in the following areas: —

- BADLs/IADLs: self-care, sleep, habits, routines, homemaking, child care.
- Education/ Work: Work habits and routines
- Play/Leisure: Leisure interests and activities.
- Social participation: Life roles and role performance
- Sensorimotor: Fatigue, pain
- Cognitive: Attention, concentration, memory, executive functions
- Psychosocial: Fears or phobias, self-control, coping skills, self-image.

Assessment Tools

Assessment tools commonly used to assess people with anxiety by occupational therapists include the following:

- ACLS: (Allen cognitive level screen)
- Brookvale Living Skills Assessment
- COPM: (Law *et al.*, 2004) Canadian occupational performance measure
- OPHI-II: (Kielhofner *et al.*, 2004) Occupational performance history interview
- Sensory Profile: Taste/smell processing/movement/visual/touch/activity level/auditory processing
- VISA: Vocational interest survey
- BAI (Beck Anxiety Inventory)
- Battery of Anxiety Questionnaire (Powell, 1991) — DASS 21 and DASS 42:
- Depression, anxiety, and stress (mild/moderate/severe/extremely severe)
- Depression & Anxiety in Youth Scale (DAYS) (Newcomer *et al.*, 1994)

- K10 (Checklist for anxiety and depression symptoms) Beyond Blue
- Revised Children's Manifest Anxiety Scale (RCMAS-2) (Reynolds & Richmond, 2008)

Intervention Goals

Following assessment, the occupational therapist would then work with the person to assist them to:

- — Organise routines.
- — Manage sleep patterns.
- — Manage time.
- — Return to work.
- — Engage in leisure.
- — Build supportive relationships.
- — Participate in social groups.
- — Use community resources.
- — Participate in valued occupations, tasks, and roles.
- — Engage in physical activities.
- — Understand anxiety.
- — Promote wellbeing and quality of life.
- — Use coping skills to manage anxiety.
- — Learn to counteract negative self-assessment.
- — Manage diet.
- — Build feelings of security, ability, and self-acceptance

■ --- **Grading activities:** The occupational therapist can work with the person to approach situations that cause high levels of anxiety by breaking down the approach to such tasks into smaller, more manageable steps.

Mood Disorders

Mood refers to a person's emotional state, such as feeling sad, happy, angry, or excited. Most people experience these emotions at different times (Luomala & Laaksonen, 2000). For some people, however, these emotions can be extreme or more long-lasting. Extreme moods can become a problem if they start to get in the way of daily life — that is, when they interfere with work, study, or responsibilities around the home, or when they have a negative impact on relationships with workmates, family, or friends (Gitlin & Miklowitz, 2017). If a person experiences extreme moods that are affecting their daily life, they may have a mood disorder (Birken & Harper, 2017).

Mood disorders are more common among people who have alcohol, tobacco, or other substance misuse issues (Tolliver & Anton, 2015). Over 17% of people who have a substance misuse disorder have depression, and over 4% have bipolar disorder (Mills *et al.*, 2011). There is no single cause of mood disorders. However, there are several factors that can contribute to the development of a mood disorder, such as:

- — A family history of depression or mood disorders
- — Chemical imbalances in the brain
- — Life experiences (*e.g.*, stress)
- — Significant life events (*e.g.*, childbirth, menopause, bereavement)
- — Alcohol or other drug use

(D'cruz & Chaturvedi, 2022; Remes, Mendes, & Templeton, 2021).

Types of Mood Disorders

There are two main types of mood disorders: Depression and Bipolar disorder.

Bipolar Disorders

Bipolar disorders are also known as Affective Disorders or Bipolar Affective Disorders, Manic Depressive Disorder, or Manic-Depressive Psychosis. Bipolar disorders are characterised by mania and depression, which usually alternate (Tondo, H Vazquez, & J Baldessarini, 2017). The age of onset is teens to early adulthood, with the average age of onset being 17.5 years (Keramatian, Morton, Levit, & Nunez, 2023). The first 2 years present a high risk of relapse, recurring episodes, and recycling of mood (Najafi-Vosough, Ghaleiha, Faradmal, & Mahjub, 2016). People with bipolar disorder have a higher risk of suicide than those with depression, *i.e.*, 4 times more and 15 times more than in the general public. 50% of people with bipolar disorder attempt suicide at some point in their lives, and 11% die as a result. Prevalence is 1% worldwide (equal for men and women) (Vieta *et al.*, 2018). The cause is unknown but the following play a role: heredity, stress, physical disorders, or as part of other mental illnesses.

Bipolar Disorder (BPD) Types

- BPD 1: manic or mixed episode (Alteration of manic and major depressive episodes)
- BPD II: hypomania plus depressive episodes
- Cyclothymia: chronic but less severe mood disturbance
- Bipolar Disorder not otherwise specified (NOS): bipolar features that do not meet specific criteria

(American Psychiatric Association, 2022).

Mania

Mania is when a person has **persistently elevated, expansive, or irritable mood plus 3 or more of:**

- inflated self-esteem
- persistent elevation of mood or grandiosity
- decreased need for sleep
- increased talkativeness than usual
- flight of ideas or racing thoughts
- distractibility or increased goal-directed activity

(Pacchiarotti, Anmella, Colomer, & Vieta, 2020).

Hypomania is a less severe variant of mania lasting 4 days or longer (Mitchell, 2012). Manic psychosis is characterised by extreme manic symptoms with psychotic features (Nehme *et al.*, 2018).

Bipolar Signs and Symptoms

- -Grandiosity
- -Minimal need for sleep
- -Excessively talkative or having pressured speech
- -Racing thoughts or flight of ideas
- - Distractibility
- - Excessive goal-directed activity or psychomotor agitation
- - Impulsivity or participation in dangerous or risky activities

(McIntyre *et al.*, 2020).

Bipolar Medical Management

Mood stabilisers such as lithium, valproic acid, anticonvulsants *e.g.*, lamotrigine, and combinations are usually given. Mood stabilisers, however, have side effects. Common side effects of mood stabilisers include sedation, weight gain, tremors, dry mouth, excessive thirst (polydipsia), restlessness, acne, gastric irritation, and kidney malfunction (Orsolini, Pompili, & Volpe, 2020). ECT Shock treatment is reserved for those who are treatment-resistant to pharmacology (Schoeyen *et al.*, 2015).

Occupational Therapy with People with Bipolar Disorder

The OT enables occupational performance through a number of interventions:

- Skills training *e.g.*, time management, money management, following a medication schedule, communication
- Return to school/ work plan, specific work skills *e.g.*, looking for a job, applying, interviewing, conflict resolution
- Engage in leisure activities
- Sensory processing program
- Assist with goal-setting
- Relaxation training
- Provide opportunities to practice problem-solving
- Psychoeducation, which includes developing the person's knowledge of the impact cycling moods have on their life and functioning. Also, to develop with the person a plan of action for when symptoms start to present

Common occupational performance instruments include the Occupational Performance Questionnaire (Kusznir *et al.*, 1996) and Performance Assessment of Self-care Skills (PASS) (Rogers *et al.*, 1989).

Depression

Everyone feels sad or depressed from time to time, especially when faced with stress, relationship breakdowns, or disappointment. Feeling sad or depressed in these circumstances is normal, and these feelings usually only last a short time, usually hours (Leventhal, 2008). Depression is when these feelings are experienced excessively (for most of the day) or for a long period of time (two weeks or more) (American Psychiatric Association, 2022). Depression is characterised by severe and persistent sadness that interferes with function (Kolovos, Kleiboer, & Cuijpers, 2016). The person is at risk of suicide and may present with significant suicidal ideation (Cummins *et al.*, 2015). They may require hospitalisation, particularly when family support is lacking. The average age of onset is 30 years (Harder *et al.*, 2022). In their study, Kasturi, Oguoma, Grant, Niyonsenga, and Mohanty (2023) found that the overall pooled prevalence of depression and anxiety for those aged 10 to 24 years in Australia was 25.3%, and in a subgroup analysis, depression was found to be 21.3% for this age group. The overall incidence of depression is higher in women than in men (Kuehner, 2017).

Symptoms of Depression

Depression can affect the way a person feels, thinks, and behaves. Generally, the person presents with depressed mood, anhedonia, weight loss, altered sleep, change in psychomotor behaviour, fatigue/ loss of energy, feelings of worthlessness or guilt, impaired cognition, and thoughts of death or suicide.

Emotions include feeling sad, upset, worthless, guilty, or numb, as well as feelings of hopelessness and despair and loss of interest in activities that used to be enjoyable (Dobson, 2024). Physical reactions include tiredness or lack of energy, restlessness or agitation, having trouble sleeping, changes in appetite and eating habits, weight loss, and loss of interest in sex (Arya & Kumar, 2011; Judd, Schettler, Coryell, Akiskal, & Fiedorowicz, 2013). A person with depression may have trouble remembering things or concentrating, difficulty making decisions, negative thoughts about themselves, others, and the future, and thoughts of suicide (Trivedi, Greer, & Mayes, 2019). A person with depression may behave as follows: Withdraw from friends or family, cry a lot or feel unable to cry, move or talk more slowly than usual, and may have outbursts of irritability or anger (Buyukdura, McClintock, & Croarkin, 2011; Derntl *et al.*, 2011; Liu & Cole, 2021; Rottenberg, Gross, Wilhelm, Najmi, & Gotlib, 2002; Steer, 2011).

Treatment of Depression

Mood disorders can be treated effectively. Both psychological therapy and medication can help people affected by mood disorders (Kamenov, Twomey, Cabello, Prina, & Ayuso-Mateos, 2017).

Medications

Medication may be helpful alongside psychological therapy. Anti-depressant medication can help depressive feelings, restore normal sleep patterns and appetite, and reduce anxiety (Hantsoo & Mathews, 2019; Wichniak, Wierzbicka, & Jernajczyk, 2012). Mood stabilisers can also help balance out the mood swings people experience with bipolar disorder (Preston, O'Neal, Talaga, & Moore, 2021).

- SSRIs (serotonin reuptake inhibitors); Common side effects include nausea and
- sedation.

SNRI (norepinephrine reuptake inhibitors); Common side effects include headache and sedation.

- MAOIs (Monoamine oxidase inhibitors) 1st generation; Common side effects include sexual dysfunction, dry mouth, constipation, blurred vision, and increased risk of stroke.
- Electroconvulsive therapy (ECT): — This is "Shock treatment" for those who are treatment resistant to pharmacology
- Transcranial Magnetic Stimulation (rTMS) — This is repetitive magnetic stimulation.

Psychological therapy

Psychological treatments usually involve therapy that is focused on changing unhelpful patterns of thinking, behaviours, and beliefs (Locher, Meier, & Gaab, 2019). Cognitive behaviour therapy (CBT) is commonly used in the treatment of depression and bipolar disorder and has the best evidence of improving these conditions (Costa *et al.*, 2010; López-López *et al.*, 2019).

Occupational therapy with people with depression

The OT enables occupational performance through a number of interventions: —

- Skills training *e.g.*, time management, money management, sleep routines/ balance, following a medication schedule, healthy eating/ meal preparation, self-care, and exercise
- Assist the person in the development of daily and weekly routines consisting of a balanced range of meaningful activities
- Pursuit of school/ vocational interests
- Engage in leisure activities
- Encourage physical fitness
- Assist with goal setting, including breaking down goals into smaller steps so that they feel more manageable for the person to achieve
- Relaxation training
- Provide opportunities to practice problem-solving and decision making
- Stress management and coping skills training
- Supporting the person to link with social and leisure groups, including support groups
- Activities to improve self-esteem, and for self-expression, self-exploration, self-management
- Psychoeducation

Assessment Tools

Common occupational performance assessment tools include:

- Allen Cognitive Level Screen (ACLS) (Allen, 2000)
- Assessment of Communication & Interaction Skills (ACIS) (Forsyth *et al.*, 1998)
- Assessment of Motor & Process Skills (AMPS) (Fisher 2006)
- BDI (Beck Depression Inventory)
- Brookvale Living Skills Assessment
- Canadian Occupational Performance Measure (COPM) (Law *et al.*, 2005)
- Kohlman Evaluation of Living Skills (KELS) (Thompson, 1992)
- Occupational Performance History Interview v2 (OPHI-II) (Keilhofner *et al* ., 2004)
- Occupational Self-Assessment (OSA) (Kielhofner *et al.*, 2006)
- Performance Assessment of Self-care Skills (PASS) (Rogers *et al.*, 1989)

Case Study: Manic Episode

Sarah is a 24-year-old woman with a history of depressive episodes, recently admitted to an acute psychiatric facility. Three months ago, Sarah's mother passed away. Since that time, Sarah reports that her need for sleep has been declining to the point where she sleeps 2 hours per night. She states that she stays up most nights writing as she has made profound philosophical insights that she "must share with the world". Sarah states that she "rarely" feels the need to eat, and her family reports that Sarah has recently lost a significant amount of weight. Sarah is enrolled in a Masters of Education, although she has not submitted recent assignments as she feels she must focus on her philosophies. As a result, her enrolment is in jeapordy. Sarah does not seem bothered by this fact and states that as she is a famous philosopher and will no longer need her Masters qualification.

Sarah's sister Jessica states that Sarah has become more irritable over the last month, especially when Jessica tries to discuss a topc with Sarah other than her philosophical ideas. Jessica reports that Sarah has been talking rapidly and is often difficult to interrupt. Jessica also states that Sarah has been bathing less frequently and often appears dishevelled. Jessica also reports that Sarah has been spending excessively on items such as philosophy textbooks, electronic equipment, and clothing. Although she is not aware of Sarah's exact income, she is aware that Sarah is on a fixed income, being a part-time university student.

Occupational Therapy Assessment

With pharmacological treatment, Sarah's mental state began to stabilise. She was able to engage with the OT in a range of assessments and was able to identify the following goals:

- Reestablish a daily and weekly routine of tasks, including self-care, stress management activities, regular meals, social activities, and exercise
- Develop further insight into her mental illness and control its management
- Rengage with her university studies
- Review her spending and develop a budget

Occupational Therapy Intervention

- Sarah began to develop a regular routine on the ward, incorporating the Occupational Therapy ward group program. She began to see the OT regularly and planned a routine that she could realistically put into place post-discharge.
- Sarah and the OT discussed stress management techniques, including mindfulness activities.
- Sarah and the OT engaged in psychoeducation discussions about her illness. Together, they developed a relapse prevention plan so that Sarah could be more aware of when her symptoms were starting and put in place a plan to prevent a full relapse.
- The OT and Sarah contacted the university support staff, and together, they developed a graded plan for the recommencement of her studies.
- Sarah and the OT reviewed her recent spending and developed a budget, incorporating repayments for outstanding debts.

CONCLUSION

This chapter has overviewed anxiety and mood disorders. Common anxiety disorders such as generalized anxiety, OCD, and PTSD were discussed in detail. Anxiety and mood disorders are arguably the most common mental illness worldwide. This chapter also discussed mood disorders, which included depressive disorders and bipolar disorder. Anxiety and mood disorders are long-term disturbances to emotional states, which affect a person's ability to live successfully and with satisfaction and do the things they want to, need to, or are expected to do. The role of occupational therapy when working with these individuals, including assessments and interventions, has been presented in this chapter.

REFERENCES

Abramowitz, J.S., Jacoby, R.J. (2015). *Obsessive-compulsive disorder in adults.* Hogrefe Publishing GmbH.

Akinsulore, A., Owojuyigbe, A.M., Faponle, A.F., Fatoye, F.O. (2015). Assessment of preoperative and postoperative anxiety among elective major surgery patients in a tertiary hospital in Nigeria. *Middle East J. Anaesthesiol., 23*(2), 235-240.
[PMID: 26442401]

American Psychiatric Association. (2022). *Diagnostic and statistical manual of mental disorders : DSM--TR.* (5th edition, text revision. ed.). Washington, DC: American Psychiatric Association Publishing..

Angelakis, S., Nixon, R.D.V. (2015). The comorbidity of PTSD and MDD: Implications for clinical practice and future research. *Behav. Change, 32*(1), 1-25.
[http://dx.doi.org/10.1017/bec.2014.26]

Arya, A., Kumar, T. (2011). Depression: A review. *J. Chem. Pharm. Res., 3*(2), 444-453.http://dx.doi.org/

Benjet, C., Bromet, E., Karam, e.g., Kessler, R.C., McLaughlin, K.A., Ruscio, A.M., Shahly, V., Stein, D.J., Petukhova, M., Hill, E., Alonso, J., Atwoli, L., Bunting, B., Bruffaerts, R., Caldas-de-Almeida, J.M., de Girolamo, G., Florescu, S., Gureje, O., Huang, Y., Lepine, J.P., Kawakami, N., Kovess-Masfety, V., Medina-Mora, M.E., Navarro-Mateu, F., Piazza, M., Posada-Villa, J., Scott, K.M., Shalev, A., Slade, T., ten Have, M., Torres, Y., Viana, M.C., Zarkov, Z., Koenen, K.C. (2016). The epidemiology of traumatic event exposure worldwide: results from the World Mental Health Survey Consortium. *Psychol. Med., 46*(2), 327-343.
[http://dx.doi.org/10.1017/S0033291715001981] [PMID: 26511595]

Birken, M., Harper, S. (2017). Experiences of people with a personality disorder or mood disorder regarding carrying out daily activities following discharge from hospital. *Br. J. Occup. Ther., 80*(7), 409-416.
[http://dx.doi.org/10.1177/0308022617697995]

Bouton, M.E., Mineka, S., Barlow, D.H. (2018). A modern learning theory perspective on the etiology of panic disorder. *Neurotic Paradox, 2*, 265-324.
[http://dx.doi.org/10.4324/9781315619996-3]

Brakoulias, V., Starcevic, V., Belloch, A., Brown, C., Ferrao, Y.A., Fontenelle, L.F., Lochner, C., Marazziti, D., Matsunaga, H., Miguel, E.C., Reddy, Y.C.J., do Rosario, M.C., Shavitt, R.G., Shyam Sundar, A., Stein, D.J., Torres, A.R., Viswasam, K. (2017). Comorbidity, age of onset and suicidality in obsessive–compulsive disorder (OCD): An international collaboration. *Compr. Psychiatry, 76*, 79-86.
[http://dx.doi.org/10.1016/j.comppsych.2017.04.002] [PMID: 28433854]

Bridley, A., Daffin, L.W. (2018). *Fundamentals of psychological disorders.* (3rd edition (5-TR) ed.). Washington, D.C: Washington State University.

Bryant, R.A. (2019). Post-traumatic stress disorder: a state-of-the-art review of evidence and challenges. *World Psychiatry, 18*(3), 259-269.
[http://dx.doi.org/10.1002/wps.20656] [PMID: 31496089]

Buyukdura, J.S., McClintock, S.M., Croarkin, P.E. (2011). Psychomotor retardation in depression: Biological underpinnings, measurement, and treatment. *Prog. Neuropsychopharmacol. Biol. Psychiatry, 35*(2), 395-409.
[http://dx.doi.org/10.1016/j.pnpbp.2010.10.019] [PMID: 21044654]

Chorpita, B.F., Barlow, D.H. (2018). The development of anxiety: The role of control in the early environment. *Neurotic Paradox, 2*, 227-264.
[http://dx.doi.org/10.4324/9781315619996-2]

Costa, R.T., Rangé, B.P., Malagris, L.E.N., Sardinha, A., Carvalho, M.R., Nardi, A.E. (2010). Cognitive–behavioral therapy for bipolar disorder. *Expert Rev. Neurother., 10*(7), 1089-1099.
[http://dx.doi.org/10.1586/ern.10.75] [PMID: 20586690]

Craske, M.G., Stein, M.B. (2016). Anxiety. *Lancet, 388*(10063), 3048-3059.
[http://dx.doi.org/10.1016/S0140-6736(16)30381-6] [PMID: 27349358]

Cummins, N., Scherer, S., Krajewski, J., Schnieder, S., Epps, J., Quatieri, T.F. (2015). A review of depression and suicide risk assessment using speech analysis. *Speech Commun., 71*, 10-49. [http://dx.doi.org/10.1016/j.specom.2015.03.004]

D'cruz, M.M., Chaturvedi, S.K. (2022). Sociodemographic and cultural determinants of mood disorders. *Curr. Opin. Psychiatry, 35*(1), 38-44. [http://dx.doi.org/10.1097/YCO.0000000000000766] [PMID: 34812742]

Derntl, B., Seidel, E.M., Eickhoff, S.B., Kellermann, T., Gur, R.C., Schneider, F., Habel, U. (2011). Neural correlates of social approach and withdrawal in patients with major depression. *Soc. Neurosci., 6*(5-6), 482-501. [http://dx.doi.org/10.1080/17470919.2011.579800] [PMID: 21777105]

Dobson, K.S. (2024). *Clinical depression: an individualized, biopsychosocial approach to assessment and treatment.* (1st ed.). Washington, D. C: American Psychological Association. [http://dx.doi.org/10.1037/0000398-000]

Eaton, W.W., Bienvenu, O.J., Miloyan, B. (2018). Specific phobias. *Lancet Psychiatry, 5*(8), 678-686. [http://dx.doi.org/10.1016/S2215-0366(18)30169-X] [PMID: 30060873]

Flanagan, J.C., Korte, K.J., Killeen, T.K., Back, S.E. (2016). Concurrent treatment of substance use and PTSD. *Curr. Psychiatry Rep., 18*(8), 70. [http://dx.doi.org/10.1007/s11920-016-0709-y] [PMID: 27278509]

Garcia, R. (2017). Neurobiology of fear and specific phobias. *Learn. Mem., 24*(9), 462-471. [http://dx.doi.org/10.1101/lm.044115.116] [PMID: 28814472]

Gitlin, M.J., Miklowitz, D.J. (2017). The difficult lives of individuals with bipolar disorder: A review of functional outcomes and their implications for treatment. *J. Affect. Disord., 209*, 147-154. [http://dx.doi.org/10.1016/j.jad.2016.11.021] [PMID: 27914248]

Groves, D., Binasis, T., Wootton, B., Moses, K. (2023). Psychometric properties of the Generalised Anxiety Disorder Dimensional Scale in an Australian sample. *PLoS One, 18*(6), e0286634. [http://dx.doi.org/10.1371/journal.pone.0286634] [PMID: 37279207]

Hallion, L.S., Ruscio, A.M. (2011). A meta-analysis of the effect of cognitive bias modification on anxiety and depression. *Psychol. Bull., 137*(6), 940-958. [http://dx.doi.org/10.1037/a0024355] [PMID: 21728399]

Hantsoo, L., Mathews, S. (2019). Pharmlogical Treatment of Depressive Disorders. In: Evans, S.M., Carpenter, K.M., (Eds.), *APA handbook of psychopharmacology.* American Psychological Association. [http://dx.doi.org/10.1037/0000133-007]

Harder, A., Nguyen, T.D., Pasman, J.A., Mosing, M.A., Hägg, S., Lu, Y. (2022). Genetics of age-at-onset in major depression. *Transl. Psychiatry, 12*(1), 124. [http://dx.doi.org/10.1038/s41398-022-01888-z] [PMID: 35347114]

Hermann, R., Lay, D., Wahl, P., Roth, W.T., Petrowski, K. (2019). Effects of psychosocial and physical stress on lactate and anxiety levels. *Stress, 22*(6), 664-669. [http://dx.doi.org/10.1080/10253890.2019.1610743] [PMID: 31062999]

Judd, L.L., Schettler, P.J., Coryell, W., Akiskal, H.S., Fiedorowicz, J.G. (2013). Overt irritability/anger in unipolar major depressive episodes: past and current characteristics and implications for long-term course. *JAMA Psychiatry, 70*(11), 1171-1180. [http://dx.doi.org/10.1001/jamapsychiatry.2013.1957] [PMID: 24026579]

Kamenov, K., Twomey, C., Cabello, M., Prina, A.M., Ayuso-Mateos, J.L. (2017). The efficacy of psychotherapy, pharmacotherapy and their combination on functioning and quality of life in depression: a meta-analysis. *Psychol. Med., 47*(3), 414-425. [http://dx.doi.org/10.1017/S0033291716002774] [PMID: 27780478]

Kandola, A., Vancampfort, D., Herring, M., Rebar, A., Hallgren, M., Firth, J., Stubbs, B. (2018). Moving to

beat anxiety: epidemiology and therapeutic issues with physical activity for anxiety. *Curr. Psychiatry Rep.,* *20*(8), 63.
[http://dx.doi.org/10.1007/s11920-018-0923-x] [PMID: 30043270]

Kasturi, S., Oguoma, V.M., Grant, J.B., Niyonsenga, T., Mohanty, I. (2023). Prevalence Rates of Depression and Anxiety among Young Rural and Urban Australians: A Systematic Review and Meta-Analysis. *Int. J. Environ. Res. Public Health,* *20*(1), 800.
[http://dx.doi.org/10.3390/ijerph20010800] [PMID: 36613122]

Keramatian, K., Morton, E., Levit, A., Nunez, J.J. (2023). Evidence of factors influencing delays in the diagnosis and treatment of bipolar disorder in adolescents and young adults. Protocol for a systematic scoping review. *PLoS One,* *18*(11), e0292923.
[http://dx.doi.org/10.1371/journal.pone.0292923] [PMID: 37976281]

Kolovos, S., Kleiboer, A., Cuijpers, P. (2016). Effect of psychotherapy for depression on quality of life: meta-analysis. *Br. J. Psychiatry,* *209*(6), 460-468.
[http://dx.doi.org/10.1192/bjp.bp.115.175059] [PMID: 27539296]

Kotov, R., Gamez, W., Schmidt, F., Watson, D. (2010). Linking "big" personality traits to anxiety, depressive, and substance use disorders: A meta-analysis. *Psychol. Bull.,* *136*(5), 768-821.
[http://dx.doi.org/10.1037/a0020327] [PMID: 20804236]

Kuehner, C. (2017). Why is depression more common among women than among men? *Lancet Psychiatry,* *4*(2), 146-158.
[http://dx.doi.org/10.1016/S2215-0366(16)30263-2] [PMID: 27856392]

Lara, D.R. (2010). Caffeine, mental health, and psychiatric disorders. *J. Alzheimers Dis.,* *20*(s1) (Suppl. 1), S239-S248.
[http://dx.doi.org/10.3233/JAD-2010-1378] [PMID: 20164571]

Leventhal, A.M. (2008). Sadness, depression, and avoidance behavior. *Behav. Modif.,* *32*(6), 759-779.
[http://dx.doi.org/10.1177/0145445508317167] [PMID: 18403316]

Liu, Q., Cole, D.A. (2021). The association of phasic irritability (aggressive outbursts) and tonic irritability (irritable mood) to depression occurrences, symptoms, and subtypes. *J. Affect. Disord.,* *293*, 9-18.
[http://dx.doi.org/10.1016/j.jad.2021.06.012] [PMID: 34157615]

Locher, C., Meier, S., Gaab, J. (2019). Psychotherapy: a world of meanings. *Front. Psychol.,* *10*, 460.
[http://dx.doi.org/10.3389/fpsyg.2019.00460] [PMID: 30984050]

López-López, J.A., Davies, S.R., Caldwell, D.M., Churchill, R., Peters, T.J., Tallon, D., Dawson, S., Wu, Q., Li, J., Taylor, A., Lewis, G., Kessler, D.S., Wiles, N., Welton, N.J. (2019). The process and delivery of CBT for depression in adults: a systematic review and network meta-analysis. *Psychol. Med.,* *49*(12), 1937-1947.
[http://dx.doi.org/10.1017/S003329171900120X] [PMID: 31179960]

Luomala, H.T., Laaksonen, M. (2000). Contributions from mood research. *Psychol. Mark.,* *17*(3), 195-233.
[http://dx.doi.org/10.1002/(SICI)1520-6793(200003)17:3<195::AID-MAR2>3.0.CO;2-#]

Martin, E.I., Ressler, K.J., Binder, E., Nemeroff, C.B. (2009). The neurobiology of anxiety disorders: brain imaging, genetics, and psychoneuroendocrinology. *Psychiatr. Clin. North Am.,* *32*(3), 549-575.
[http://dx.doi.org/10.1016/j.psc.2009.05.004] [PMID: 19716990]

McIntyre, R.S., Berk, M., Brietzke, E., Goldstein, B.I., López-Jaramillo, C., Kessing, L.V., Malhi, G.S., Nierenberg, A.A., Rosenblat, J.D., Majeed, A., Vieta, E., Vinberg, M., Young, A.H., Mansur, R.B. (2020). Bipolar disorders. *Lancet,* *396*(10265), 1841-1856.
[http://dx.doi.org/10.1016/S0140-6736(20)31544-0] [PMID: 33278937]

Meuret, A.E., Rosenfield, D., Wilhelm, F.H., Zhou, E., Conrad, A., Ritz, T., Roth, W.T. (2011). Do unexpected panic attacks occur spontaneously? *Biol. Psychiatry,* *70*(10), 985-991.
[http://dx.doi.org/10.1016/j.biopsych.2011.05.027] [PMID: 21783179]

Mills, K., Marel, C., Baker, A., Teesson, M., Dore, G., Kay-Lambkin, F., Trimingham, T. (2011). *Mood and Substance Misuse.*. National Drug and Alcohol Research Centre.

Mitchell, P.B. (2012). Bipolar disorder: the shift to overdiagnosis. *Can. J. Psychiatry, 57*(11), 659-665.
[http://dx.doi.org/10.1177/070674371205701103] [PMID: 23149281]

Najafi-Vosough, R., Ghaleiha, A., Faradmal, J., Mahjub, H. (2016). Recurrence in patients with bipolar disorder and its risk factors. *Iran. J. Psychiatry, 11*(3), 173-177.
[PMID: 27928249]

Nehme, E., Obeid, S., Hallit, S., Haddad, C., Salame, W., Tahan, F. (2018). Impact of psychosis in bipolar disorder during manic episodes. *Int. J. Neurosci., 128*(12), 1128-1134.
[http://dx.doi.org/10.1080/00207454.2018.1486833] [PMID: 29888994]

Niles, A.N., Dour, H.J., Stanton, A.L., Roy-Byrne, P.P., Stein, M.B., Sullivan, G., Sherbourne, C.D., Rose, R.D., Craske, M.G. (2015). Anxiety and depressive symptoms and medical illness among adults with anxiety disorders. *J. Psychosom. Res., 78*(2), 109-115.
[http://dx.doi.org/10.1016/j.jpsychores.2014.11.018] [PMID: 25510186]

Olaya, B., Moneta, M.V., Miret, M., Ayuso-Mateos, J.L., Haro, J.M. (2018). Epidemiology of panic attacks, panic disorder and the moderating role of age: Results from a population-based study. *J. Affect. Disord., 241*, 627-633.
[http://dx.doi.org/10.1016/j.jad.2018.08.069] [PMID: 30172214]

Orsolini, L., Pompili, S., Volpe, U. (2020). The 'collateral side' of mood stabilizers: safety and evidence-based strategies for managing side effects. *Expert Opin. Drug Saf., 19*(11), 1461-1495.
[http://dx.doi.org/10.1080/14740338.2020.1820984] [PMID: 32893696]

Pacchiarotti, I., Anmella, G., Colomer, L., Vieta, E. (2020). How to treat mania. *Acta Psychiatr. Scand., 142*(3), 173-192.
[http://dx.doi.org/10.1111/acps.13209] [PMID: 33460070]

Perusini, J.N., Fanselow, M.S. (2015). Neurobehavioral perspectives on the distinction between fear and anxiety. *Learn. Mem., 22*(9), 417-425.
[http://dx.doi.org/10.1101/lm.039180.115] [PMID: 26286652]

Preston, J.D., O'Neal, J.H., Talaga, M.C., Moore, B.A. (2021). *Handbook of clinical psychopharmacology for therapists.* (Newly revised and updated, Ninth edition. ed.). Oakland, CA: New Harbinger Publications..

Rector, N.A., Bourdeau, D., Kitchen, K., Joseph-Massiah, L., Laposa, J.M. (2016). *Anxiety disorders: An information guide..* Centre for Addiction and Mental Health Canada.

Remes, O., Mendes, J.F., Templeton, P. (2021). Biological, psychological, and social determinants of depression: a review of recent literature. *Brain Sci., 11*(12), 1633.
[http://dx.doi.org/10.3390/brainsci11121633] [PMID: 34942936]

Rottenberg, J., Gross, J.J., Wilhelm, F.H., Najmi, S., Gotlib, I.H. (2002). Crying threshold and intensity in major depressive disorder. *J. Abnorm. Psychol., 111*(2), 302-312.
[http://dx.doi.org/10.1037/0021-843X.111.2.302] [PMID: 12003451]

Ruscio, A.M., Hallion, L.S., Lim, C.C.W., Aguilar-Gaxiola, S., Al-Hamzawi, A., Alonso, J., Andrade, L.H., Borges, G., Bromet, E.J., Bunting, B., Caldas de Almeida, J.M., Demyttenaere, K., Florescu, S., de Girolamo, G., Gureje, O., Haro, J.M., He, Y., Hinkov, H., Hu, C., de Jonge, P., Karam, e.g., Lee, S., Lepine, J.P., Levinson, D., Mneimneh, Z., Navarro-Mateu, F., Posada-Villa, J., Slade, T., Stein, D.J., Torres, Y., Uda, H., Wojtyniak, B., Kessler, R.C., Chatterji, S., Scott, K.M. (2017). Cross-sectional comparison of the epidemiology of DSM-5 generalized anxiety disorder across the globe. *JAMA Psychiatry, 74*(5), 465-475.
[http://dx.doi.org/10.1001/jamapsychiatry.2017.0056] [PMID: 28297020]

 Samra, C. K., Torrico, T. J., & Abdijadid, S. (2024). Specific phobia. In StatPearls [Internet]. StatPearls Publishing.

Schoeyen, H.K., Kessler, U., Andreassen, O.A., Auestad, B.H., Bergsholm, P., Malt, U.F., Morken, G., Oedegaard, K.J., Vaaler, A. (2015). Treatment-resistant bipolar depression: a randomized controlled trial of electroconvulsive therapy versus algorithm-based pharmacological treatment. *Am. J. Psychiatry, 172*(1), 41-51.

[http://dx.doi.org/10.1176/appi.ajp.2014.13111517] [PMID: 25219389]

Steer, R. (2011). Self-reported inability to cry as a symptom of anhedonic depression in outpatients with a major depressive disorder. *Psychol. Rep., 108*(3), 874-882.
[http://dx.doi.org/10.2466/02.09.13.15.PR0.108.3.874-882] [PMID: 21879634]

Stein, M.B., Sareen, J. (2015). Generalized anxiety disorder. *N. Engl. J. Med., 373*(21), 2059-2068.
[http://dx.doi.org/10.1056/NEJMcp1502514] [PMID: 26580998]

Tolliver, B.K., Anton, R.F. (2015). Assessment and treatment of mood disorders in the context of substance abuse. *Dialogues Clin. Neurosci., 17*(2), 181-190.
[http://dx.doi.org/10.31887/DCNS.2015.17.2/btolliver] [PMID: 26246792]

Tondo, L., Vázquez, G., Baldessarini, R. (2017). Depression and mania in bipolar disorder. *Curr. Neuropharmacol., 15*(3), 353-358.
[http://dx.doi.org/10.2174/1570159X14666160606210811] [PMID: 28503106]

Trivedi, M.H., Greer, T.L., Mayes, T.L. (2019). 1C1Primer on Depression: Introduction and Overview. In: Trivedi, M.H., Strakowski, S.M., (Eds.), *Depression (pp. 0)..* Oxford University Press.
[http://dx.doi.org/10.1093/med/9780190929565.003.0001]

Van Sprang, E.D., Maciejewski, D.F., Milaneschi, Y., Elzinga, B.M., Beekman, A.T.F., Hartman, C.A., van Hemert, A.M., Penninx, B.W.J.H. (2022). Familial risk for depressive and anxiety disorders: associations with genetic, clinical, and psychosocial vulnerabilities. *Psychol. Med., 52*(4), 696-706.
[http://dx.doi.org/10.1017/S0033291720002299] [PMID: 32624018]

Vieta, E., Berk, M., Schulze, T.G., Carvalho, A.F., Suppes, T., Calabrese, J.R., Gao, K., Miskowiak, K.W., Grande, I. (2018). Bipolar disorders. *Nat. Rev. Dis. Primers, 4*(1), 18008.
[http://dx.doi.org/10.1038/nrdp.2018.8] [PMID: 29516993]

Vorspan, F., Mehtelli, W., Dupuy, G., Bloch, V., Lépine, J.P. (2015). Anxiety and substance use disorders: co-occurrence and clinical issues. *Curr. Psychiatry Rep., 17*(2), 4.
[http://dx.doi.org/10.1007/s11920-014-0544-y] [PMID: 25617040]

Wichniak, A., Wierzbicka, A., Jernajczyk, W. (2012). Sleep and antidepressant treatment. *Curr. Pharm. Des., 18*(36), 5802-5817.
[http://dx.doi.org/10.2174/138161212803523608] [PMID: 22681161]

CHAPTER 7

Eating Disorders Diagnosis, Assessment, and Psychosocial Interventions

Samara Thew[1] and **Tawanda Machingura**[2,*]

[1] *Department of Occupational Therapy, Child Development Centre, Prince George, British Columbia, Canada*

[2] *Head of Discipline Occupational Therapy Program, University of Notre Dame Australia, Sydney, Australia*

Abstract: Currently, one in five Australian children suffer from an eating disorder (ED). Eating Disorder (ED) is a severe mental health condition characterised by severe disturbances in eating behaviours, related thoughts, and emotions (American Psychiatric Association [APA], (2013)). Occupational therapists have a unique skill set to assist with the recovery of an ED. As occupational therapists, we analyse the person, occupation, and environment to provide a variety of interventions to reduce/minimize occupational performance issues (OPI). This chapter will review the diagnostic criteria for the different EDs, the occupational therapy process using the Canadian Model of Occupational Performance and Engagement (CMOP-E) and the Canadian Practice Process Framework (CPPF), and apply the learnings to a case study.

Keywords: Anorexia nervosa, Avoidant-restrictive food intake disorder, Binge eating disorder, Bulimia nervosa, Canadian model of occupational performance and engagement, Case study, Eating disorders – unspecified, Eating disorders, Mental health, Other specified feeding or eating disorder.

INTRODUCTION

Eating disorders are serious and complex mental health conditions that affect individuals of all ages, cultures, races, and economic status across the globe. Many people with eating disorders are desperately attempting to cope with life problems, emotional pain, personal challenges, or societal pressures through an unhealthy relationship with food. The learning objectives for this chapter are:

---

* **Corresponding author Tawanda Machingura:** Head of Discipline Occupational Therapy Program, University of Notre Dame Australia, Sydney, Australia; E-mail: tawanda.machingura@nd.edu.au

1. Understand the different types of eating disorders and the diagnostic criteria.
2. Understand the Occupational Therapy scope of practice within the sector of eating disorders.
3. Understand the Occupational Therapy interventions within the sector of eating disorders.
4. Understand how to use and apply the CPPF and CMOP-E within a case study.

Diagnostic Criteria

According to the International Classification Disease 11th Edition (ICD-11), there are eight different types of feeding and EDs, including anorexia nervosa (AN), bulimia nervosa (BN), binge eating disorder (BED), avoidant-restrictive food intake disorder (ARFID), other specified feeding or eating disorder (OSFED), and feeding or EDs – unspecified (UFED) (World Health Organisation [WHO], 2019). It is important to note that previously, OSFED and UFED were previously known as EDNOS (ED not otherwise specified) as a catch-all category for individuals who did not meet the criteria for AN or BN. Therefore, some individuals may still be diagnosed with EDNOS, now known as OSFED.

ICD-11 describes AN as an ED that presents with a significantly low body weight for an individual's height, age, and developmental stage (WHO, 2019). AN is commonly classified as a body mass index (BMI) under the 5th percentile for children (approximately 18.5 kg/m^2) (WHO, 2019). Low body weight is due to self-induced behaviours, including restricted eating, purging behaviours, and/or increased energy expenditure (*e.g.*, exercise or medication abuse) (WHO, 2019). Individuals present with an intense fear of gaining weight or becoming fat even though they are presenting already at dangerously low weight (APA, 2013). Individuals may also present with body dysmorphia, where they may think their body appears larger than it is (APA, 2013). ICD-11 describes BN as an ED, which presents with frequent and recurrent episodes of binge eating followed by behaviour to prevent weight gain (WHO, 2019). This may include self-induced vomiting, excessive exercise, laxatives, and/or enemas. Individuals with BN are often obsessed with their body shape, weight, and size (WHO, 2019). ARFID is a feeding disorder where an individual avoids and/or restricts the intake of food. This results in energy and/or nutritional deficits, which can impact the physical health of the individual (WHO, 2019). However, ARFID is not related to body weight or shape (WHO, 2019). ARFID usually stems from fear of consequences (*i.e.*, vomiting or choking), sensory sensitivity, and/or lack of interest in food (Thomas & Eddy, 2019). Individuals with OSFED have an ED that does not meet the exact requirements of AN, BN, or BED (APA, 2013). OSFED includes atypical AN, BN, BED, purging disorder, and night eating syndrome (APA,

2013). Presentations now categorised under OSFED and UFED in DSM-V were summarised under the term EDNOS in ICD-11. Individuals with BED experience incidents of binge eating with a lack of control; however, no compensatory behaviours are used to offset the binging episode (APA, 2013).

In the Australian context, one in five children in Australia suffers from an ED (Mitchison *et al.*, 2019). Burt and colleagues (2020) completed a study to investigate the prevalence of ED in children who were Aboriginals compared to non-Aboriginals. A study by Burt *et al.* (2020) identified that the prevalence was similar; however, night-eating syndrome occurred at a higher rate within the Aboriginal population. Hay and Carriage (2012) found Aboriginals were at a higher risk of binge eating episodes compared to non-Aboriginals. Hay and Carriage (2012) discovered Aboriginals are more at risk of disordered eating in relation to body weight concerns associated with obesity. Interestingly, Burt and colleagues (2020) found that individuals who were not presenting as underweight were often overlooked, leading to a delayed diagnosis and treatment. Therefore, it is crucial to assess the whole individual rather than just their weight (Burt *et al.*, 2020).

MODES OF THERAPY

Cognitive Behavioural Therapy

Cognitive behavioural therapy (CBT) has the foundation that one's behaviour, thoughts, and feelings are interconnected, influencing one's reaction and response to a situation (Wilding & Milne, 2010). Enhanced Cognitive Behavioural Therapy (CBT-E) is an evidence-based practice to assist with treating EDs (Grave *et al.*, 2019). CBT-E focuses on the individual and their ED rather than external factors (*i.e.*, family dynamics) (Grave *et al.*, 2019). CBT-E is designed for the individual to take control over their recovery rather than being dependent on others to do the work (Grave *et al.*, 2019). CBT-E is an individual-based practice where there is honesty and agreement about the treatment the individual is participating in. CBT-E addresses the individual's beliefs about shape and weight regarding their body. CBT-E also addresses one's eating behaviours and their relation to their ED. CBT-E utilises cognitive and behavioural strategies to provide the individual with education to address the ED thoughts and behaviours (Grave *et al.*, 2019).

Cognitive Behavioural Therapy for Avoidant/Restrictive Food Intake Disorder (CBT-AR) is a specific form of CBT designed for individuals diagnosed and struggling with ARFID. There are four stages to CBT-AR:

- **Stage one:** It includes psychoeducation regarding ARFID and the treatment of ARFID (Thomas & Eddy, 2019). The parent/carer(s) will be asked to monitor the child's food intake (Thomas & Eddy, 2019). The child and the therapist will work on establishing a pattern of regular meals and normalising hunger cues (Thomas & Eddy, 2019). The child will be encouraged to increase the volume and variety of food (Thomas & Eddy, 2019). The therapist will also address the driving force of the ARFID (sensory sensitivity, fear of consequences, and/or lack of interest in food (Thomas & Eddy, 2019).

- **Stage two**: The child will continue to work on increasing the volume and variety of foods (Thomas & Eddy, 2019).
- **Stage three**: It addresses sensory sensitivity, fear of consequences, and lack of interest in food/eating (Thomas & Eddy, 2019). This can include desensitisation of foods, psychoeducation, and exposure therapy (Thomas & Eddy, 2019).
- **Stage four**: The child and therapist work on relapse prevention and continue treatment as required (Thomas & Eddy, 2019).

Maudsley Family-based Treatment

Maudsley Family-based treatment (MFBT) uses the fundamental philosophy that parents are a vital requirement to the success of the child's success in recovery (Lock *et al.*, 2012). MFBT has been more effective up to a year post-treatment than individual therapy (Couturier *et al.*, 2013). It is predicted that this may be due to parents stepping into the therapist role at home (Couturier *et al.*, 2013). MFBT has also been shown to focus on ED behaviours; therefore, it is recommended to be the first line of treatment (Couturier *et al.*, 2013). MFBT has been integrated into meal support, which has been shown to be effective (Herscovici *et al.*, 2017).

Nyman-Carlsson and colleagues (2020) completed a study that analysed the effectiveness of CBT compared to MFBT. The CBT group had a 64.9% weight restoration rate, and the MFBT group had a rate of 83.8%. Post-treatment showed a recovery rate of 76% in both groups, with 89% of CBT participants recovering at follow-up versus 81% of MFBT participants recovered.

Meal Support Intervention

Meal Support Intervention (MSI) exposes individuals to food in a supportive environment to gain coping strategies for regulation (Biddiscombe *et al.*, 2018). Biddiscombe and colleagues (2018) used a behaviour experiment framework to analyse individuals attending a practical food group. Within the therapy sessions, participants were exposed to food (including fear foods), eating in facilitated environments, educated on portion sizing and nutritional requirements, and taught coping strategies. Participants identified that this group was a valuable and necessary component to their treatment and recovery. MSI can also be integrated into MFBT. MSI and MFBT include the individual, their parent/carers, and a therapist (Godfrey *et al.*, 2014). The therapist attempts to implement strategies to encourage the parent/carers to assist with mealtime (Godfrey *et al.*, 2014). These strategies included room rearrangement, behavioural statements, and supportive strategies (empathising, encouragement, and externalisation) (Godfrey *et al.*, 2014). Godfrey and colleagues (2014) completed a study utilising a therapist to redefine and strengthen the parenting foundation.

Dialectical Behaviour Therapy

Dialectical Behaviour Therapy (DBT) stems from CBT to help individuals with emotional regulation (Dimeff & Linehan, 2001). DBT utilises mindfulness with validation and acceptance-based strategies to illicit change in the individual (Dimeff & Linehan, 2001). DBT includes behavioural analysis, problem-solving techniques, skill training, cognitive modification, and exposure-based interventions (Dimeff & Linehan, 2001). DBT interventions may consist of mindful eating and food diary cards (Ritschel *et al.*, 2015). DBT has also been shown to be effective in other diagnoses that may be present when diagnosed with an ED, such as self-harm, depression, substance abuse, post-traumatic stress disorder, and borderline personality disorder (Ritschel *et al.*, 2015). Currently, there is limited research on the effectiveness of DBT in children (Reilly *et al.*, 2020). However, in adults diagnosed with AN and BN, there have been promising results of DBT improving one's emotional regulation skills, showing significant improvements when assessed using the Difficulties in Emotion Regulation Scale (Brown *et al.*, 2020).

Measures

Some common measures occupational therapists may want to utilize when working with children with EDs are: Strengths and Difficulties Questionnaire (SDQ), Children Global Assessment Scale (CGAS), Health of The Nation Outcome Scales for Children and Adolescents (HoNOSCA), Participation and Environment Measure for Children and Youth (PEM-CY), Depression Anxiety Stress Scale – 21 (DASS-21)/ Mood and Feeling Questionnaire (MFQ)/ Spence Children Anxiety Scale (SCAS), ED Examination Questionnaire (EDE-Q)/ Pica, ARFID, and Rumination Disorder Interview – Avoidant/Restrictive Food Intake Disorder Questionnaire (PARDI-AR-Q), Systemic Clinical Outcome and Routine Evaluation (SCORE-15), Child Outcome Rating Scale (CORS), Children's Yale-Brown Obsessive-Compulsive Scale (CY-BOCS), and Compulsive Exercise Test (CET). These assessment tools are summarised in Table **1**.

The SDQ is a self-reported behavioural screening questionnaire (Goodman *et al.*, 1998). The measure includes 25 items divided into five categories (Goodman *et al.*, 1998). The categories include conduct problems, hyperactivity, emotional symptoms, peer problems, and prosocial behaviours (Goodman *et al.*, 1998). There are two different types of the questionnaire. One is directed for parents or teachers to complete regarding children (aged 4 to 16) (Goodman *et al.*, 1998). The other is for the child (aged 11-16) to complete. Both forms are the same; however, the parent/teacher is worded in the third person, whereas the child questionnaire is worded in the first person (Goodman *et al.*, 1998). The questions are answered with a scale of "Not True", "Somewhat True", and "Certainly True" (Goodman *et al.*, 1998). The internal reliability is assessed across the five categories and overall using a Cronbach's alpha coefficient, which includes total (0.82), emotional symptoms (0.75), conduct problems (0.72), hyperactivity (0.69), prosocial behaviours (0.65), and peer problems (0.61) (Goodman *et al.*, 1998). Therefore, the reliability ranges from good (0.82) to questionable (0.61). The validity of the SDQ is satisfactory as it can distinguish between high and low-risk populations (Goodman *et al.*, 1998). Table **1** below details common assessment tools used when working with people with eating disorders.

Table 1. Summary of common assessment tools used with people with eating disorders

Assessment – Categories	Outcome Measure – Health	Outcome Measure –Behaviours	Outcome Measure – Emotional	Outcome Measure – Social	Outcome Measure – Occupational
HoNOSCA					
Behaviour		X			
Impairments	X				
Symptoms	X				
Social				X	
Informational					X
CGAS					
Overall Function				X	X
SDQ					
Hyperactivity		X			
Conduct Problems		X			
Emotional Symptoms			X		
Peer Problems				X	
Prosocial Behaviours				X	
PEM-CY					

(Table 1) cont.....

Assessment – Categories	Outcome Measure – Health	Outcome Measure –Behaviours	Outcome Measure – Emotional	Outcome Measure – Social	Outcome Measure – Occupational
School Environment					X
Community Environment					X
Home Environment					X
DASS-21					
Depression Symptoms			X		
Anxiety Symptoms			X		
Stress Symptoms			X		
MFQ					
Total			X		
SCAS					
Separation Anxiety			X		
Social Phobia			X		
Obsessive Compulsive Problems			X		
Panic/Agoraphobia			X		
Generalised Anxiety/Overanxious Symptoms			X		
Fear of Physical Injury			X		
EDE-Q					
Restraint		X			
Eating Concern		X			
Shape Concern		X			
Weight Concern		X			
PARDI-AR-Q					
Severity of Impact		X			
Sensory Based Avoidance		X			
Lack of Interest		X			
Concern about Aversive Consequences		X			
SCORE-15					
Overall Family Function			X	X	
CORS					
Individual	X	X	X		
Interpersonal				X	

(Table 1) cont.....

Assessment – Categories	Outcome Measure – Health	Outcome Measure –Behaviours	Outcome Measure – Emotional	Outcome Measure – Social	Outcome Measure – Occupational
Social				X	X
Overall	X	X	X	X	X
Y-BOCS					
Total		X			
CET					
Avoidance and Rule-Driven Behaviour		X			
Weight-control Exercise		X			
Mood Improvement			X		
Lack of Exercise Enjoyment			X		
Exercise Rigidity		X			
Bloodwork					
Chem 20	X				
Biochemistry	X				
FBC	X				
Vitamin A	X				
Vitamin B	X				
Vitamin D	X				
Vitamin E	X				
Scans					
DEXA	X				
BIA	X				

The HoNOSCA is a measure completed by a health professional to assess the function of children within the mental health sector (Gowers *et al.*, 1999a). The HoNOSCA measures 15 items divided into five categories: behaviour, impairments, symptoms, social, and information (Gowers *et al.*, 1999a). The questions are answered on a scale from zero to four (0 = no problems; 1 = minor impairment; 2 = mild impairment; 3 = moderately severe; 4 = severe impairment; 9 = not known or not applicable) (Gowers *et al.*, 1999b). The HoNOSCA has an overall interrater reliability of 0.8, demonstrating good reliability (Gowers *et al.*, 1999a). The HoNOSCA demonstrated satisfactory face validity (Gowers *et al.*, 1999a). Clinicians are trained in the HONOSCA rating.

The CGAS is a measure completed by a health professional to assess the child's overall functioning at home and school and with peers (Shaffer *et al.*, 1983). The CGAS is intended for children aged 4 to 16 (Shaffer *et al.*, 1983). The measure uses a scale from 1 to 100, all representing different levels of care or support required (Shaffer *et al.*, 1983). A total number above 70 represents a slight impairment to superior functioning; therefore, little to no intervention is needed (Shaffer *et al.*, 1983). The test-retest reliability of the CGAS measured a coefficient of 0.87 to 0.95, therefore representing excellent reliability (Shaffer *et al.*, 1983). The CGAS also has satisfactory discriminant and concurrent validity (Shaffer *et al.*, 1983).

The PEM-CY is a parent/carer-reported measure to examine a child's participation within the home, school, and community environment (Coster *et al.*, 2011). The PEM-CY is intended for children aged 5 to 17 years old. The measure can be utilised for children/you with and without a disability (Coster *et al.*, 2011). The measure reviews how often the child participates in set activities, their level of involvement, and the level of change the parent/carer would like (Coster *et al.*, 2011). This process applies to all three environments, including home, school, and community. The PEM-CY has satisfactory reliability and validity (Coster *et al.*, 2011).

The SCORE-15 measure is a self-reported questionnaire to assess an individual's family dynamics (Hamilton *et al.*, 2015). The SCORE-15 is intended for individuals 12 years old or older. There is a child version of the SCORE 15 for children aged 7 to 11 (Hamilton *et al.*, 2015). The SCORE-15 analyses family strengths, difficulties, and communication (Hamilton *et al.*, 2015). The SCORE-15 has satisfactory internal consistency reliability, test-retest reliability, and criterion validity (Hamilton *et al.*, 2015). The child SCORE-15 also has satisfactory internal consistency and test-retest reliability.

The CORS is a self-reported scale used for children aged 6 to 15 to measure psychosocial functioning (Casey *et al.*, 2020). The CORS utilises a visual analogue scale for the child to mark how they feel in each category (individual, interpersonal, social, and overall) (Casey *et al.*, 2020). The score ranges from 0 (poor psychosocial functioning) to 40 (excellent psychosocial functioning). The recommended cut-off score is 28 (Casey *et al.*, 2020). The CORS has satisfactory sensitivity, internal consistency, and validity (Casey *et al.*, 2020).

Depending on the child's age, there will be administration of an anxiety/mood questionnaire. The DASS-21 will be utilised for individuals over the age of 15. For individuals under the age of 15, the MFQ and SCAS will be utilised. The DASS-21 is a self-reported measure thatmeasures the subcategories of depression, anxiety, and stress (Lovibond & Lovibond, 1995). The DASS-21 consists of 21 questions where the individual reports how often the statement applies to them in the past week. The DASS-21 has score cut-offs from normal to extremely severe in all subcategories. The DASS-21 is valid for individuals 14 years or older. The DASS-21 has satisfactory validity and reliability (Henry & Crawford, 2005).

For individuals under 15 years of age, the MFQ and SAS will be utilised. The MFQ is a self-reported questionnaire completed by the child and/or the parent/carer(s) (Costello & Angold, 1988). MFQ analyses the child's depressive symptoms over 2 weeks utilising a three-point scale (0 = not true; 1 = sometimes; 2 = true) (Costello & Angold, 1988). The MFQ has a mean cut-off of less than or equal to 28 (Thabrew *et al.*, 2018). If the individual scores 28 or less, there is a high likelihood of depression (Thabrew *et al.*, 2018). The MFQ has satisfactory internal reliability, content validity, convergent validity, and criterion validity (Thabrew *et al.*, 2018). The SCAS is a self-reported questionnaire completed by the child and/or the parent/carer(s) (Spence, 1997). The SCAS has 45 items to analyse six subscales, including separation anxiety, social phobia, obsessive-compulsive problems, panic/agoraphobia, generalised anxiety/overanxious symptoms, and fear of physical injury (Spence, 1997). The SCAS is scored from 0 to 114 (Spence, 1997). The higher the score, the greater the severity of anxiety symptoms. The scores are converted into percentiles. If a subscale or total score has a percentile score greater than 84, this indicates clinically significant anxiety symptoms are present (Spence, 1997). The SCAS has satisfactory internal consistency, test-retest reliability, convergent validity, and discriminant validity (Spence, 1998).

Depending on the participant's diagnosis, the EDE-Q or PARDI-AR-Q will be administered to analyse ED behaviour. The EDE-Q is a self-reported questionnaire regarding restricting, eating concerns, shape concerns, and weight concerns. The EDE-Q was originally valid for individuals 14 years and older. However, there have been studies conducted supporting the use of EDE-Q in the child population (Binford *et al.*, 2005). The EDE-Q explores the child's thoughts and behaviours that contribute to their ED in the last 28 days (Fairburn & Beglin, 1994). The EDE-Q has satisfactory reliability and validity (Berg *et al.*, 2012).

The PARDI-AR-Q is a self-reported questionnaire completed by the child (14 years or older) and/or the parent/carer(s) (Bryant-Waugh *et al.*, 2019). The PARDI-AR-Q is based on the semi-structured interview. It is a 32-item questionnaire analysing the severity of impact, sensory-based avoidance, lack of interest, and concern about aversive consequences (Bryant-Waugh *et al.*, 2019). The PARDI has satisfactory validity and reliability. Currently, data is limited regarding the validity and reliability of the PARDI-AR-Q.

The CY-BOCS is a self-report/semi-structured interview for children between the ages of 6-17 (Scahill *et al.*, 1997). The CY-BOCS is completed with the child and may require parent/carer assistance. The CY-BOCS contains three sections, including a symptom checklist, target symptom list, and severity rating. The symptom checklist looks at current and past obsession and compulsive behaviour (Scahill *et al.*, 1997). Obsessive behaviour includes the sub-categories of contamination, aggressive, sexual, hoarding/saving, magical thought/superstitious, somatic, religious, and miscellaneous (Scahill *et al.*, 1997). Compulsive behaviour includes the sub-categories of washing/cleaning, checking, repeating rituals, counting, ordering/arranging, hoarding/saving, excessive games/superstitions, rituals involving other people, and miscellaneous (Scahill *et al.*, 1997). The target symptom list is completed for both obsession and compulsive behaviour (Scahill *et al.*, 1997). The individual is required to rate the top 4 most severe behaviour (Scahill *et al.*, 1997). The severity rating is where the interviewer asks the individual questions regarding their obsessive and compulsive behaviour. This includes 10 questions rating from 0 (none) to 4 (extreme). The CY-BOCS total is scored from 0 (subclinical) to 40 (extreme) (Scahill *et al.*, 1997). The CY-BOCS has satisfactory validity and reliability (Scahill *et al.*, 1997).

The CET is a self-reported questionnaire to analyse an individual's exercise compulsivity in relation to their ED. Although the CET was not intended for children, there has been a study confirming it is valid and reliable for children between the ages of 12 to 14 (Goodwin *et al.*, 2011). The questionnaire consists of five subcategories, including avoidance and rule-drive behaviour, weight control exercise, mood improvement, lack of exercise enjoyment, and exercise rigidity (Taranis *et al.*, 2011). Each question is answered on a scale from 0 (never true) to 5 (always true). The CET is scored from a subcategory and total score perspective. The total score can range from 0 to 120; the higher the score, the more likely an ED's impact on exercise behaviour (Taranis *et al.*, 2011).

It is important that the physician orders and monitors the client's bloodwork. This will include biochemistry, chem20, and full blood count (FBC). For participants diagnosed with AN or BN, vitamins B, D, and E will be analysed. For participants diagnosed with ARFID, vitamin A will be analysed. In some settings, the physician may order a DEXA and/or BIA scan will be conducted to analyse the bone density, muscle, fat, and water mass.

Canadian Practice Process Framework

The Canadian Practice Process Framework (CPPF), Fig. (**1**) assists with guiding the Occupational Therapy process (Polatajko *et al.*, 2007a).

Enter/Initiate

Enter/Initiate is the client and occupational therapist's first interaction. The therapist receives the referral, and it will be determined if it is appropriate for occupational therapy services. If deemed appropriate, this will be the client and therapist's first point of contact. When contacting the client, the therapist will explain the occupational therapist's role, scope of practice, and duty to report to the client. The goal is to have the client identify the occupational performance issues and occupational performance goals using a client-centred approach. The hope with this stage is to start to build a therapeutic relationship with the client.

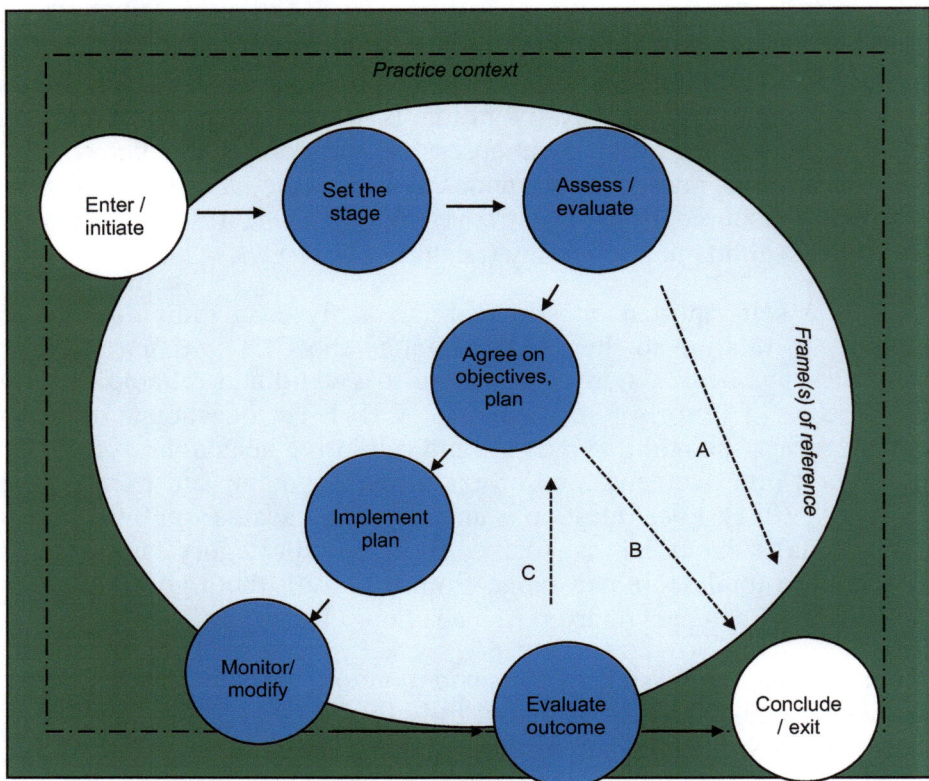

Fig. (1). The Canadian Practice Process Framework (Polatajko *et al.*, 2007a)

Set the Stage

The goal of setting the stage is to build rapport and continue to build on the therapeutic relationship with the client. The occupational therapist may start to engage in conversations with the client's family, loved ones, and other healthcare professionals. It must be ensuredthat you receive consent to obtain and release information before speaking to others. During this stage, you will start to complete the CMOP-E to process and organize the information (Polatajko *et al.*, 2007b). Using the CMOP-E, you will gather the details required to identify occupational performance issues and goals.

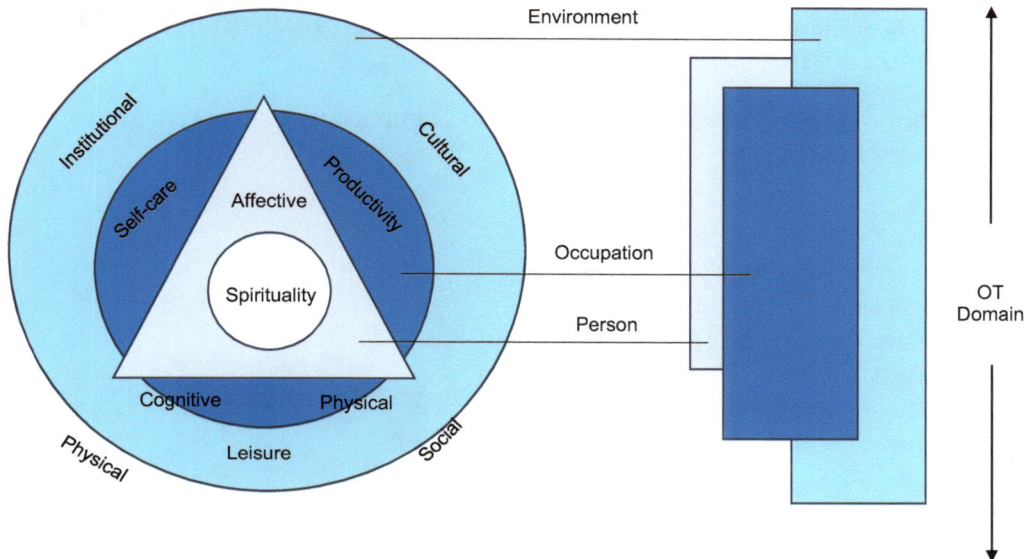

Fig. (2). Canadian Model of Occupational Performance and Engagement (Polatajko *et al.*, 2007b).

Spirituality: focus on inner motivation and identify values and things that give meaning and purpose to the person's life. Spirituality is at the centre of the person as shown in Fig. (**2**) above.

- What does the person value?
- What is important to them?

Person: focus on personal factors that impact their ability to engage in daily occupations.

- Affective
    - How is the client's mood?
    - Does the client have co-morbidity of anxiety, depression, OCD, *etc*?
- Physical
    - Is the client stable? Are they on bed rest? Do they have any physical limitations?
    - What is the diagnosis?

- ○ Any other diagnoses we should be aware of?
- ○ Current ED behaviours?
- Cognitive
  - ○ How is their cognition?
  - ○ How are their memory, attention/concentration, orientation, and level of consciousness?

Occupation: the focus is on assessing valued occupations that they want to, need to, or are expected to do.

- Self-care
  - ○ How is their hygiene?
  - ○ How is their ED impacting them?
  - ○ How are they feeding?
- Productivity
  - ○ Do they have a job or go to school?
  - ○ Do they do sports or extra curriculum activity?
- Leisure
  - ○ What do they do for fun?

Environment: the focus is on assessing environmental factors that impact the person's ability to engage in their daily occupations.

- Physical
  - ○ Where do they live?
  - ○ What type of dwelling do they live in?
  - ○ Who lives in the dwelling with the individual?
  - ○ How do they access their home?
- Cultural
  - ○ Any cultural/religious beliefs we should know about
- Social
  - ○ Do they have friends?
  - ○ Do they value social connection?
  - ○ Do they live with anyone?
  - ○ Has their social connection decreased with ED behaviours?

Assess/Evaluate

The goal of assessment/evaluation is to assess the occupational performance issues identified from setting the stage. The occupational therapist is required to draw on their clinical expertise, knowledge, and experience to decide how to assess and evaluate the client's occupational performance issues. The occupational therapist may decide to use clinical observation, questionnaires, or functional assessments. For example, if there are concerns regarding depression and anxiety, you may decide to do the DASS-21. If the client is having difficulties completing meal preparation, you may complete an observation of a meal preparation session to assess what the difficulties are. After the assessment/evaluation, the occupational therapist will create a working hypothesis on why the occupational performance issue exists. The occupational therapist will discuss the findings with the client, relevant stakeholders, and support personnel.

Agree on Objectives and Plans

The goal of agreeing on objectives and plans is to collaborate with the client, relevant stakeholders, and support personnel to create, adapt, and support the plan to achieve the client's goal. As the occupational therapist, it is your job to ensure the client has the opportunity to work on the goal within a realistic timeframe. It is important the client has opportunities to engage in different settings. For example, if the client is in a day program, he can engage in meal preparation at the hospital versus in the client's home. This helps translate the goal to a setting where the client will be after discharge. The occupational therapist will be able to assess facilitators and barriers in the home and make the appropriate recommendations to ensure the client is successful.

Implement the Plan

The goal of implementing the plan is to start to work on the agreed objectives from the above stage. The occupational therapist may assist with implementing the plan through direct interventions, advocating for the client, coaching, providing adaptations to the environment, and providing education to the client and others.

Monitor and Modify

The goal of monitoring and modifying is to continue to review the objectives and plans along with the client's progress. As the occupational therapist, it is critical you review the plan and the strategies regularly to ensure the client is progressing. If the plan is not working, you will have to modify it by providing more education, making adaptations, coaching, and/or advocating for the client. You will also collaborate with the client on the next steps in the plan to progress the client to their goal.

Evaluate the Outcome

The goal of evaluating the outcome is to review the objectives and plan to see if the client has reached their identified goals. The occupational therapist will have to re-assess using a standardized assessment or re-observing the client's engagement in the occupation. From this stage, as the occupational therapist, you will either determine:

1. The client has met his goals and no longer requires services
2. The client has met his goals but has other occupation performance issues; you will repeat the process to address the new goals.
3. The client has not met the goals, and the client and therapist work together to develop the next steps.

Conclude/Exit

From evaluating the outcome, the occupational therapist will collaborate with the client on the next steps. With the consideration of the three options above, you may discharge the client or create new goals. This also depends on the setting you work in as the occupational therapist, if you work in the hospital and the client is getting discharged, you may refer the client to a community therapist.

The checklist presented in Table 2 may be a useful guide.

Table 2. CMOP-E Checklist

Enter/Initiate
✓ Review Referral ✓ Contact Client ✓ Introduce yourself to the client ✓ Explain the role of occupational therapy and the scope of practice ✓ Identify goals
Set the Stage
✓ Consent to obtain and release information ✓ Complete the intake using an occupational therapy model such as the CMOP-E ✓ Receive informed consent for services ✓ Re-identify goals if needed
Assess/Evaluate
✓ Standardized assessments, if needed ✓ Observations ✓ Questionnaires
Agree on Objectives and Plan
✓ Collaborate with the client, stakeholders, and support personnel
Implement Plan

(Table 2) cont.....

Enter/Initiate
✓ Implement the plan through direct interventions, advocating, coaching, adaptations, and education
Monitor and Modify
✓ Monitor the client's progress ✓ Modify when necessary
Evaluate the Outcome
✓ Re-assess the client ✓ Determine where the client is at with their goals
Conclude/Exit
✓ Discharge the client, set up new objectives, and plan or refer to a community therapist

Occupational Therapy Interventions

Along with CBT-E, CBT-AR, MFBT, MSI, and DBT, there are direct interventions occupational therapists can utilize to assist clients with EDs. The following are some interventions occupational therapists may utilize to assist with occupational performance and engagement during ED recovery.

- Grocery Shopping
- Meal preparation support
- Engagement in occupations
- Learning how to dress
- Setting up a routine/schedule
- Exposure Therapy

Meal Planning / Grocery Shopping / Meal Preparation

Grocery shopping, meal preparation, and meal support can be a scary occupation to engage in during recovery from an ED. Some clients may have a fear of food and may not have engaged in these occupations for a long period of time. Occupational therapists have a unique role where we can support and provide adaptations that may assist with making grocery shopping, meal preparation, and meal support easier for the client. An occupational therapist can provide the following strategies for the client:

Assist with meal planning: This may include creating a meal plan, making a grocery list, and going grocery shopping with the client. As the occupational therapist, you may need to collaborate with a dietitian to ensure the client is meeting their caloric intake during recovery. Creating a meal plan can be challenging for the client as it may include foods they have feared or have not eaten in a long time. We can support the feelings that may come up and coach and educate the client through the importance of eating. We can also provide strategies such as having 3-4 meal plans ready so the client can rotate between the meal plans.

Grocery shopping: Grocery shopping can be challenging for clients. They may have not grocery shopped in a few months to years. Occupational therapists can support clients and provide strategies for how to grocery shop again. Strategies may include making a grocery list together with details of brand and quantity, organizing the list to ensure efficiency in the store, which will decrease the time to spend in store, planning the time of day to go grocery shopping, creating a grocery budget, breaking up the grocery trip into several trips if a large grocery list is too much to handle, and using online grocery shopping and delivery. Some clients may be hyper-focus on the calories, so we can provide education on removing the label or taping over the label when the food enters the house.

Meal Preparation: Making the meal is another additional step. Some clients may not have cooked a meal for a long period of time. Occupational therapists can provide education on how to complete meal preparation and provide adaptations when necessary to make this step easier. For example, they may find completing meal preparation daily difficult, so occupational therapists may suggest setting aside one day to complete all the meal preparation for the week. Creating freezer meals is another adaptation as they are quick and easy to defrost when busy or having a difficult day. Some clients may have challenges regarding the quantity of food they require. We can support clients with portion sizing.

Engagement in Occupations

When recovering from an ED, some clients have disengaged from occupations such as school, sport, work, social gatherings, *etc*. As occupational therapists, we know the importance occupations provide in one's life and how the occupations give clients meaning and purpose. It is critical to re-engage the client in desired occupations as soon as possible. This can be done through adaptations, coaching, advocating, and education. Coelho and colleagues (2020) found through the COPM that individuals in recovery identified the following occupations to re-engage in: school, work, volunteer, leisure activities, socialization, community management, personal care, and treatment/recovery.

Learning How to Dress

During ED recovery, clients may gain or lose weight depending on their diagnosis. This may impact the size of clothes, which can be challenging for a client. occupational therapists, can provide strategies for how to shop and purchase clothes that fit the client's new body shape and size. Some clients may be fixated on the size and may be upset if they go up a size. Occupational therapists can provide strategies for how to shop for clothes again and find the style the client wants to wear. Strategies may include shopping online and trying clothes on at home, going to one or two stores to figure out the client's new size in basic tops and bottoms, and providing education that size does not matter but what matters is what the client's body feels good and comfortable in.

Setting up a Routine/Schedule

Routine and schedule are important for everyone. Sometimes, during ED recovery, clients may not have a routine/schedule anymore. Developing a routine/schedule with a client will assist with providing the client with purpose and meaning in their life. This will also assist with re-engagement in occupations. As an occupational therapist, you can assist with creating a daily or weekly schedule with the client and support engagement in occupations.

Exposure Therapy

Some clients may have difficulties facing a fear of food, going back to school or work, going shopping, entering social events, *etc*. When this comes up, occupational therapists can provide support with exposure therapy. For example, maybe a client wants to eat a fear food. Clinicians can provide support with exposure to the fear of the food and help the client work through the feelings and emotions. Some clients may have difficulties entering school again, but we can provide support with going to the school for the first time. Clinicians can assist clients to work through anxiety that may come up and provide strategies and education. This may include sitting at the back of the class, coming to class just when the class starts and leaving immediately when the class ends, and providing education on why certain thoughts may be coming up and how to reduce those thoughts.

Sensory Processing

Occupational therapists can assess a client's sensory processing system to assist with regulation and functioning. Some clients may present with difficulties with regulation and sensory processing differences. As occupational therapists, we can assess the client's sensory system, including visual, olfactory, auditory, proprioception, tactile, gustatory, vestibular, and interoception. Occupational therapists can help provide strategies to assist with sensory processing functioning and well-being. Some interventions may include awareness, education, and adaptations. For example, for a client who has tactile defensiveness to soft foods, occupational therapists can provide adaptations so they do not need to touch the food with their hands. They can also provide education on how to clean the client's hands after touching the soft food. Occupational therapists can also work with the client towards tolerating touching soft foods through client-led exposure and experience. Sensory processing intervention is especially important for neurodiverse clients.

Sensory interventions can also be utilised before, during, or after challenges to assist the client in learning to regulate their body. Sensory interventions can also be utilised to re-establish regulation prior to and during interventions. For example, a weighted blanket can provide proprioceptive feedback to help reduce anxiety.

Case Study

Emily is a 20-year-old female who has anorexia nervosa, generalized anxiety disorder, and depression. She has been participating in an outpatient day program for the last 12 weeks. Her weight is stable, and she is getting ready to be discharged in the next four weeks. She is currently on medication to assist with the anxiety and depression symptoms. Prior to the day program, she was attending university to complete her bachelor's degree. Due to her ED and treatment, she has had to take a leave of absence. However, she is excited to return to school and complete her degree. On her multidisciplinary team are a psychologist, psychiatrist, paediatrician, dietitian, and case manager. The team has referred Emily to Occupational Therapy services to assist with discharge planning.

You have received the referral and have consent for services from Emily. Emily has never worked with an OT before and is unsure what Occupational Therapy can do for her.

Enter / Initiate: As the occupational therapist, you have introduced yourself to Emily and have explained what Occupational Therapy is and how you can assist her with discharge. Through discussions, Emily has identified her goals are to stay in recovery, return to school, and establish a routine.

Set the Stage: As the occupational therapist, you are now working on completing Emily's occupational profile using the CMOP-E Model. Through discussion, you have established the following occupational profile:

Spirituality

• Emily is a University Student. She wants to finish her degree. It is important for her to stay in recovery in order to finish her degree.

Person

- Affective: Emily identified that her mood has improved since being on medication. She describes her mood as mostly happy and excited to be discharged. She is able to identify warning signs of anxiety and depression symptoms, such as decreased engagement in activities of daily living, skipping class, and not responding to texts or phone calls.
- Physical: Emily is preparing for discharge. She has no physical limitations. She is worried about re-entering school. She has to be cautious and aware of meal times as she sometimes skips meals.
- Cognitive: During the session, the occupational therapist completed a mental status exam, which resulted in no cognitive impairment.

Occupation

- Self-care: Emily is now engaging in self-care tasks more regularly. She reported she is worried about continuing to prioritize self-care tasks when she is discharged. She is also worried about meal planning and grocery shopping to ensure she continues to progress with her recovery. Emily and her dietitian have worked together to create different meal options but Emily reports she is unsure of how to execute them when she is discharged. Emily also reports she is worried about her wardrobe. She reports most of her clothes do not fit her anymore, and she is scared to go clothes shopping alone.
- Productivity: Emily had to take a leave of absence from school this past semester. She is excited to go back to school. Emily does not work as she wants to focus on school and keeping her grades.
- Leisure: Emily used to go out with her friends often; however, she stopped due to her ED. She has identified that this is something she wants to return to. She also enjoys being around her pet dog.

Environment

- Physical: Emily currently lives in a rental apartment near the university. She lives on her own. Her parents live approximately 3 hours away. There are no concerns with her accessing her home.
- Cultural: Emily does not identify as religious. She has not shared any cultural beliefs at this time.
- Social: Emily used to love to hang out with her friends. She reports when her ED worsened, she lost the connection with her friends. It was hard for her to go out to restaurants, so she stopped all social interactions. This is something Emily would like to change, and she would like to re-establish her previous

friendships.

Assess/Evaluate

By setting the stage, Emily has identified the following priorities:

• Prioritizing self-care tasks
• Meal planning
• Clothes shopping
• Returning to University
• Re-establishing previous friendships
• Eating out in restaurants

Through the Occupational Therapy assessment, we will complete a meal planning, grocery shopping, and meal preparation assessment. We will discuss how she is currently completing her self-care tasks and how she plans for her routine post-discharge.

Through the assessment, it was identified Emily has significant anxiety in the grocery store. She also has difficulties with portion sizing. The completion of the self-care tasks is primarily done through reminders from others. Emily does not have a routine outside of the day program she is currently in.

Agree on Objectives and Plan

Through discussion with Emily, we have collaborated and made the following plan:

• OT's focus will be on meal planning, grocery shopping, and meal preparation.
　○ Developing independence with the task
　○ Reducing anxiety in grocery shopping
　○ Developing skills in portion sizing
• We will also focus on developing a routine post-discharge that fosters self-care tasks, returning to university, and socialization with friends.
• We will also work on how to purchase new clothes and reduce the anxiety around clothes shopping.

Monitor and Modify

Over the next four weeks prior to discharge, the occupational therapist and Emily will have regular sessions to work on the objectives above. Emily and the occupational therapist will work together in developing a realistic routine to support self-care tasks and university demands, developing skills in meal planning, grocery shopping, and meal preparation, and developing strategies for shopping for new clothes. The occupational therapist will continue to monitor and modify depending on Emily's progress.

Interventions Provided

- Meal planning, grocery shopping, and meal preparation:
    - Develop a variety of meals, including a list of ingredients. This way, Emily can rotate through the meals as needed.
    - Create strategies for the grocery store, including online shopping; creat the grocery list in order by the aisles; tape over the calorie label once purchased; grocery shopping weekly.
    - Meal preparation: Emily decided meal preparation once a week would work best for her. Emily decided Sundays would work best for her. We have created strategies for portion sizing through measurements with Emily's bowls and plates, as well as through reassurance and practice.
    - Meal support in restaurants: We discussed looking at the menu ahead of time and deciding what to eat before going to the restaurant to reduce anxiety and pressure.
- Clothes Shopping:
    - Emily and OT went clothes shopping together. We figured out the sizing of tops and bottoms for Emily in a few different stores. We wrote down the sizes so Emily could order online with more confidence. We also discussed bringing a comfortable top and matching the size with other shirts to reduce the need to try on the clothes in the store, as that causes Emily anxiety.
- Routine:
    - Emily and the occupational therapist developed a routine to foster self-care and university demands. Emily started engaging in the routine prior to discharge to ensure success. Adjustments were made as needed.
- Socialization
    - During Emily's discharge planning, she reached out to her friends and went out for dinner. Using the strategies provided during the meal support in a restaurant, Emily was successful with her friends.

Evaluate the Outcome

The occupational therapist re-evaluated Emily. She reported she feels more confident with meal planning, grocery shopping, and meal preparation. However, she fears that she will go back to her old ways of skipping meals. We discussed strategies, including following the established routine and setting alarms on her phone to remind her to eat. It has been determined that she has met her goal; however, she would benefit from further Occupational Therapy services through the outpatient program to continue to monitor.

Conclude/Exit

Emily has been discharged from the day program; however, outpatient follow-up will occur. We will develop a new objective and plan at the next session.

SUMMARY

This chapter described the types of feeding and EDs, including anorexia nervosa (AN), bulimia nervosa (BN), binge eating disorder (BED), avoidant-restrictive food intake disorder (ARFID), other specified feeding or eating disorder (OSFED), and feeding or EDs – unspecified. This chapter also highlighted the evidence-based therapy frameworks, including Cognitive behavioural therapy (CBT), Maudsley Family-based treatment (MFBT), Meal Support Intervention (MSI), and Dialectical Behaviour Therapy (DBT). The chapter has also highlighted common measures occupational therapists may utilise when working with children with EDs, such as the Strengths and Difficulties Questionnaire (SDQ), Children Global Assessment Scale (CGAS), and many others. The chapter ended by presenting a comprehensive case study using the Canadian Practice Process Framework (CPPF) to guide the occupational therapy process.

Key Points

- There are several different types of eating disorders that clients may present with.
- There are evidence-based therapy frameworks that are useful when working with people with eating disorders, including Cognitive behavioural therapy, Maudsley Family-based treatment, Meal Support Intervention, and Dialectical Behaviour Therapy.
- Using the Canadian Practice Process Framework (CPPF) to guide the occupational therapy process is beneficial.

REFERENCES

American Psychiatric Association *Diagnostic and statistical manual of mental disorders.* [http://dx.doi.org/10.1176/appi.books.9780890425596]

Berg, K.C., Peterson, C.B., Frazier, P., Crow, S.J. (2012). Psychometric evaluation of the eating disorder examination and eating disorder examination-questionnaire: A systematic review of the literature. *Int. J. Eat.*

Disord., *45*(3), 428-438.
[http://dx.doi.org/10.1002/eat.20931] [PMID: 21744375]

Biddiscombe, R.J., Scanlan, J.N., Ross, J., Horsfield, S., Aradas, J., Hart, S. (2018). Exploring the perceived usefulness of practical food groups in day treatment for individuals with eating disorders. *Aust. Occup. Ther. J.,* *65*(2), 98-106.
[http://dx.doi.org/10.1111/1440-1630.12442] [PMID: 29270987]

Binford, R.B., Le Grange, D., Jellar, C.C. (2005). Eating Disorders Examination versus Eating Disorders Examination-Questionnaire in adolescents with full and partial-syndrome bulimia nervosa and anorexia nervosa. *Int. J. Eat. Disord.,* *37*(1), 44-49.
[http://dx.doi.org/10.1002/eat.20062] [PMID: 15690465]

Brown, T.A., Cusack, A., Berner, L.A., Anderson, L.K., Nakamura, T., Gomez, L., Trim, J., Chen, J.Y., Kaye, W.H. (2020). Emotion regualtion difficulties during and after partial hospitalisation treatment across eating disorders. *Behav. Ther.,* *51*(3), 401-412.
[http://dx.doi.org/10.1016/j.beth.2019.07.002] [PMID: 32402256]

Bryant-Waugh, R., Micali, N., Cooke, L., Lawson, E.A., Eddy, K.T., Thomas, J.J. (2019). Development of the Pica, ARFID, and Rumination Disorder Interview, a multi-informant, semi-structured interview of feeding disorders across the lifespan: A pilot study for ages 10–22. *Int. J. Eat. Disord.,* *52*(4), 378-387.
[http://dx.doi.org/10.1002/eat.22958] [PMID: 30312485]

Burt, A., Mitchison, D., Dale, E., Bussey, K., Trompeter, N., Lonergan, A., Hay, P. (2020). Prevalence, features and health impacts of eating disorders amongst First-Australian Yiramarang (adolescents) and in comparison with other Australian adolescents. *J. Eat. Disord.,* *8*(1), 10.
[http://dx.doi.org/10.1186/s40337-020-0286-7] [PMID: 32190326]

Casey, P., Patalay, P., Deighton, J., Miller, S.D., Wolpert, M. (2020). The Child Outcome Rating Scale: validating a four-item measure of psychosocial functioning in community and clinic samples of children aged 10–15. *Eur. Child Adolesc. Psychiatry,* *29*(8), 1089-1102.
[http://dx.doi.org/10.1007/s00787-019-01423-4] [PMID: 31659441]

Coelho, J.S., Fernandes, A., Suen, J., Keidar, A., Cairns, J. (2020). Perceived occupaitonal performance in youth with eating disorders: Treatment-related changes. *Can. J. Occup. Ther.,* *87*(5), 423-430.
[http://dx.doi.org/10.1177/0008417420953229] [PMID: 32911969]

Costello, E.J., Angold, A. (1988). Scales to assess child and adolescent depression: checklists, screens, and nets. *J. Am. Acad. Child Adolesc. Psychiatry,* *27*(6), 726-737.
[http://dx.doi.org/10.1097/00004583-198811000-00011] [PMID: 3058677]

Coster, W., Bedell, G., Law, M., Khetani, M.A., Teplicky, R., Liljenquist, K., Gleason, K., Kao, Y.C. (2011). Psychometric evaluation of the participation and environment measure for children and youth. *Dev. Med. Child Neurol.,* *53*(11), 1030-1037.
[http://dx.doi.org/10.1111/j.1469-8749.2011.04094.x] [PMID: 22014322]

Couturier, J., Kimber, M., Szatmari, P. (2013). Efficacy of family-based treatment for adolescents with eating disorders: A systematic review and meta-analysis. *Int. J. Eat. Disord.,* *46*(1), 3-11.
[http://dx.doi.org/10.1002/eat.22042] [PMID: 22821753]

Dimeff, L., Linehan, M.M. (2001). Dialectical behavioural therapy in a nutshell. *The California Psychologist,* *34*(1), 10-13. Available from: https://www.dbtselfhelp.com/dbtinanutshell.pdf

Fairburn, C.G., Beglin, S.J. (1994). Assessment of eating disorders: Interview or self-report questionnaire? *Int. J. Eat. Disord.,* *16*(4), 363-370.
[http://dx.doi.org/10.1002/1098-108X(199412)16:4<363::AID-EAT2260160405>3.0.CO;2-#]   [PMID: 7866415]

Godfrey, K., Rhodes, P., Miskovic-Wheatley, J., Wallis, A., Clarke, S., Kohn, M., Touyz, S., Madden, S. (2015). Just one more bite: a qualitative analysis of the family meal in family-based treatment for anorexia nervosa. *Eur. Eat. Disord. Rev.,* *23*(1), 77-85.

[http://dx.doi.org/10.1002/erv.2335] [PMID: 25469661]

Goodman, R., Meltzer, H., Bailey, V. (1998). The strengths and difficulties questionnaire: A pilot study on the validity of the self-report version. *Eur. Child Adolesc. Psychiatry, 7*(3), 125-130.
[http://dx.doi.org/10.1007/s007870050057] [PMID: 9826298]

Goodwin, H., Haycraft, E., Taranis, L., Meyer, C. (2011). Psychometric evaluation of the compulsive exercise test (CET) in an adolescent population: Links with eating psychopathology. *Eur. Eat. Disord. Rev., 19*(3), 269-279.
[http://dx.doi.org/10.1002/erv.1109] [PMID: 21584919]

Gowers, S.G., Harrington, R.C., Whitton, A., Lelliott, P., Beevor, A., Wing, J., Jezzard, R. (1999). Brief scale for measuring the outcomes of emotional and behavioural disorders in children. *Br. J. Psychiatry, 174*(5), 413-416. a
[http://dx.doi.org/10.1192/bjp.174.5.413] [PMID: 10616607]

Dalle Grave, R., Eckhardt, S., Calugi, S., Le Grange, D. (2019). A conceptual comparison of family-based treatment and enhanced cognitive behavior therapy in the treatment of adolescents with eating disorders. *J. Eat. Disord., 7*(1), 42.
[http://dx.doi.org/10.1186/s40337-019-0275-x]

Hamilton, E., Carr, A., Cahill, P., Cassells, C., Hartnett, D. (2015). Psychometric properties and responsiveness to change of 15- and 28-item versions of the SCORE: A family assessment questionnaire. *Fam. Process, 54*(3), 454-463.
[http://dx.doi.org/10.1111/famp.12117] [PMID: 25585671]

Hay, P.J., Carriage, C. (2012). Eating disorder features in indigenous Aboriginal and Torres Strait Islander Australian peoples. *BMC Public Health, 12*(1), 233.
[http://dx.doi.org/10.1186/1471-2458-12-233] [PMID: 22439684]

Henry, J.D., Crawford, J.R. (2005). The short-form version of the Depression Anxiety Stress Scales (DASS-21): Construct validity and normative data in a large non-clinical sample. *Br. J. Clin. Psychol., 44*(2), 227-239.
[http://dx.doi.org/10.1348/014466505X29657] [PMID: 16004657]

Herscovici, C.R., Kovalskys, I., Orellana, L. (2017). An exploratory evaluation of the family meal intervention for adolescent anorexia nervosa. *Fam. Process, 56*(2), 364-375.
[http://dx.doi.org/10.1111/famp.12199] [PMID: 26596997]

Lock, J., Le Grange, D., Russel, G. (2013). *Treatment manual for anorexia nervosa: A family-based approach.* The Guilford Press.

Lovibond, P.F., Lovibond, S.H. (1995). The structure of negative emotional states: comparison of the depression anxiety stress scales (DASS) with the beck depression and anxiety inventories. *Behav. Res. Ther., 33*(3), 335-343.
[http://dx.doi.org/10.1016/0005-7967(94)00075-U] [PMID: 7726811]

Mitchison, D., Mond, J., Bussey, K., Griffiths, S., Trompeter, N., Lonergan, A., Pike, K.M., Murray, S.B., Hay, P. (2020). DSM-5 full syndrome, other specified, and unspecified eating disorders in Australian adolescents: prevalence and clinical significance. *Psychol. Med., 50*(6), 981-990.
[http://dx.doi.org/10.1017/S0033291719000898] [PMID: 31043181]

Nyman-Carlsson, E., Norring, C., Engström, I., Gustafsson, S.A., Lindberg, K., Paulson-Karlsson, G., Nevonen, L. (2020). Individual cognitive behavioral therapy and combined family/individual therapy for young adults with Anorexia nervosa: A randomized controlled trial. *Psychother. Res., 30*(8), 1011-1025.
[http://dx.doi.org/10.1080/10503307.2019.1686190] [PMID: 31709920]

Polatajko, H.J., Craik, J., Davis, J., Townsend, E.A. (2007). Canadian practice process framework: Amplifying the process. In: Townsend, E.A., Polatajko, H.J., (Eds.), *Enabling Occupation II: Advancing an Occupational Therapy Vision for Health, Well-Being, & Justice through Occupation.* Canadian Association of Occupational Therapists. a

Polatajko, H.J., Townsend, E.A., Craik, J. (2007). Canadian model of occupational performance and engagement (CMOP-E). In: Townsend, E.A., Polatajko, H.J., (Eds.), *Enabling Occupation II: Advancing an Occupational Therapy Vision for Health, Well-Being, & Justice through Occupation.* Canadian Association of Occupational Therapists. b

Reilly, E.E., Orloff, N.C., Luo, T., Berner, L.A., Brown, T.A., Claudat, K., Kaye, W.H., Anderson, L.K. (2020). Dialectical behavioral therapy for the treatment of adolescent eating disorders: a review of existing work and proposed future directions. *Eat. Disord., 28*(2), 122-141.
[http://dx.doi.org/10.1080/10640266.2020.1743098] [PMID: 32301680]

Ritschel, L.A., Lim, N.E., Stewart, L.M. (2015). Transdiagnositc applications of DBT for adolescents and adults. *Am. J. Psychother., 69*(2), 111-128.
[http://dx.doi.org/10.1176/appi.psychotherapy.2015.69.2.111] [PMID: 26160618]

Scahill, L., Riddle, M.A., McSWIGGIN-HARDIN, M.A.U.R.E.E.N., Ort, S., King, R.A., Goodman, W.K., Cicchetti, D., Leckman, J.F. (1997). Children's yale-brown obsessive compulsive scale: Reliability and validity. *J. Am. Acad. Child Adolesc. Psychiatry, 36*(6), 844-852.
[http://dx.doi.org/10.1097/00004583-199706000-00023] [PMID: 9183141]

Shaffer, D., Gould, M.S., Brasic, J., Ambrosini, P., Fisher, P., Bird, H., Aluwahlia, S. (1983). A children's global assessment scale (CGAS). *Arch. Gen. Psychiatry, 40*(11), 1228-1231.
[http://dx.doi.org/10.1001/archpsyc.1983.01790100074010] [PMID: 6639293]

Spence, S.H. (1997). Structure of anxiety symptoms among children: A confirmatory factor-analytic study. *J. Abnorm. Psychol., 106*(2), 280-297.
[http://dx.doi.org/10.1037/0021-843X.106.2.280] [PMID: 9131848]

Spence, S.H. (1998). A measure of anxiety symptoms among children. *Behav. Res. Ther., 36*(5), 545-566.
[http://dx.doi.org/10.1016/S0005-7967(98)00034-5] [PMID: 9648330]

Taranis, L., Touyz, S., Meyer, C. (2011). Disordered eating and exercise: Development and preliminary validation of the compulsive exercise test (CET). *Eur. Eat. Disord. Rev., 19*(3), 256-268.
[http://dx.doi.org/10.1002/erv.1108] [PMID: 21584918]

Thabrew, H., Stasiak, K., Bavin, L.M., Frampton, C., Merry, S. (2018). Validation of the mood and feelings questionnaire (MFQ) and short mood and feelings questionnaire (SMFQ) in New Zealand help-seeking adolescents. *Int. J. Methods Psychiatr. Res., 27*(3), e1610.
[http://dx.doi.org/10.1002/mpr.1610] [PMID: 29465165]

Thomas, J.J., Eddy, K.T. (2019). *Cognitive behavioural therapy for avoidant/restrictive food intake disorders for children, adolescents, and adults..* Cambridge University Press.

Wilding, C., Milne, A. (2010). *Cognitive Behavioural Therapy.* Hodder Education Group.

World Health Organisation *International Classification of Diseases for Mortality and Morbidity Statistics.* Available from: https://icd.who.int/

CHAPTER 8

Assessment and Treatment of Personality Disorders in Occupational Therapy Practice

Zonia Weideman[1,*]

[1] *Department of Allied Health and Therapies, Metro North Hospital and Health Service, Brisbane, Queensland, Australia*

Abstract: This chapter focuses on the unique role of occupational therapy in the assessment and treatment of personality disorders. Integrating occupational therapy assessments and interventions within existing assessment and treatment approaches can improve functional outcomes for people with personality disorders. Occupational therapy plays a pivotal role in multidisciplinary areas and across generic therapeutic approaches, for example, Dialectical Behaviour Therapy (DBT). Occupational therapists are experts in assessing the performance of daily activities and functioning across the lifespan. Therefore, occupational therapist makes a valuable contribution to the recovery journey of people with personality disorders. This review introduces the role of occupational therapy in the management of personality disorders as defined by the Alternative Model of Personality Disorders (AMPD) in the Diagnostic and Statistical Manual of Mental Disorders version 5 (DSM-5). Assessment and treatment options unique to the profession are also described.

Keywords: AMPD, Multidisciplinary treatment approach, Mental health services, Pccupational therapist, Personality disorders.

INTRODUCTION

People with a Personality Disorder (PD) often remain undiagnosed, or a diagnosis is delayed due to stigma in the community and within health services (Stiles, 2023). Personality disorders have their onset in adolescence, which provides an opportunity to start treatment as soon as possible, according to Sharp (2018). However, diagnosing adolescents with personality disorders does not tend to be the norm. More often, diagnoses of personality disorders are made once a person has developed ineffective coping strategies to manage their distress, such as frequent presentations to emergency departments, self-harming, and suicide attempts (Lewis, 2019: Meuldijk, 2017). Delays in diagnoses and treatment

_____

[*] **Corresponding author Zonia Weideman:** Department of Allied Health and Therapies, Metro North Hospital and Health Service, Brisbane, Queensland, Australia; E-mail: Zonia.Weideman@health.qld.gov.au

Tawanda Machingura (Ed.)

increase the risk of impaired psychosocial functioning, with reduced participation in meaningful activities such as work and relationships. The person with personality disorder then feels increasingly disconnected from their social environment, which can contribute to the worsening of their symptoms.

Definition

The fifth edition of the American Psychiatric Association's *Diagnostic and Statistical Manual of Mental Disorders* (DSM-5) (American Psychiatric Association, 2013) defines a personality disorder as a person's way of thinking and feeling about themselves and others that significantly and adversely affects how they function in many aspects of daily life. The DSM-5 retained the same categorical approach that was included in the DSM-IV and differentiated 10 distinct types of personality disorders: paranoid, schizoid, schizotypal antisocial, borderline, histrionic, narcissistic, avoidant, dependent, and obsessive-compulsive.

The ICD-11 Classification of Personality Disorder also includes impairments to self, interpersonal functioning (with different levels of dysfunction), and domain qualifiers: negative affectivity, detachment, disinhibition, and anankastia. The Personality Trait domains are similar in the ICD-11 and the DSM-5 despite being developed independently. The main difference is the inclusion of anankastia in the ICD-11 and the psychotic domain in the DSM-5. Both the ICD-11 and the DSM AMPD are veering away from categories towards a dimensional model with greater emphasis on psychosocial functioning.

The DSM-5 Personality and Personality Disorder working group recommended an Alternative Model of Personality Disorders (AMPD). The AMPD was published in Section III of the DSM-5's 'Emerging Measures and Models' (Skodol, 2015). The inclusion of the AMPD in the DSM-5 has assisted clinicians in utilising descriptions of a person's personality, thus facilitating enhanced treatment planning (Widiger, 2013; Widiger, 2007.). Thus, the AMPD model of personality disorders will be described.

The AMPD is designed to be flexible and aligns with occupational therapy's core philosophy that daily functioning within your environment is a priority. The AMPD defines personality disorder as a combination of clinically significant problems in daily functioning and psychopathology. The AMPD considers the person more holistically, which also aligns with occupational therapy's philosophy and includes the consideration of comorbidities such as substance use, the person's developmental stage, and their sociocultural environment (Krueger, 2020).

The AMPD includes criteria A to G. Criterion A defines the level of personality functioning, where functioning is described as impairments in their sense of self and interpersonal functioning. Criterion B includes pathological personality traits. Criterion C and D refer to the pervasiveness and stability of impairments of functioning and psychopathology - personality traits are severe yet remain relatively stable. Criteria E, F, and G discuss alternative explanations of personality pathology, which includes differential diagnoses and other medical conditions. Other explanations considered are their developmental stage, for example, adolescence.

Aetiology

The aetiology or cause of personality disorder is complex. Childhood trauma is often a major theme for people living with personality disorders. However, not all children who have lived through traumatic experiences develop a personality disorder (Beatson, 2010). Dialectical behaviour therapy uses the biosocial model to explain the aetiology of borderline personality disorder (BPD) (Linehan, 1993). The biosocial model provides people with a great sense of relief when they hear the explanation. This model is a no-blame model, transactional, and provides threads of hope that can benefit a person in their recovery journey. The 'bio' in biosocial refers to the biological attributes of someone with BPD and sensitivity to emotional cues, experiencing stronger emotions longer and more often, as well as impulsivity. The "social" refers to the person's social and living environment. Within this environment, the person experiences invalidation and lack of role-modeling of effective expression of emotion. These interactions become 'transactional' and reinforce emotional expression and intensity. The primary function of emotions is to communicate. When the emotional message is not received or the message is invalidated, the communicator escalates the intensity of their communication style (Linehan, 2015). The biosocial model is one method of explaining the aetiology of BPD. Other models include the development of maladaptive schemas from adverse childhood experiences and impaired mentalising (seeing multiple perspectives) due to attachment trauma (Sharp, 2022).

Prevalence

People with a diagnosis of personality disorder account for a high economic cost to society through frequent presentations to emergency departments and accessing a significant proportion of specialist psychiatric services (Bender, 2001; Meuldijk, 2017; Soeteman, 2008). An Australian study by Lewis *et al.* (2018) confirmed that over 20% of people presenting to the emergency department and 25% of mental health inpatient admissions had a diagnosis of personality disorder. Lewis found that people with a diagnosis of personality disorder were 2.3 times more likely to re-present within 28 days of their first presentation than people with other mental health diagnoses, second only to people experiencing psychosis. People with personality disorders are also more likely to be brought to the emergency department by police after-hours and have a higher length of stay than other mental health patient groups (Penfold, 2016).

People with personality disorder, specifically BPD, account for 9.3% of all suicides, as found in a Coroner's investigation in Victoria from 2009 to 2013. This places PD on par with diagnoses like schizophrenia, bipolar disorder, and depressive disorder (Broadbear, 2020). 99% of people who died by suicide had been in contact with emergency and mental health services within 12 months of their death, with 88% seeking help from services in the six weeks leading up to their death, highlighting the importance of service contacts with people with personality disorders (Broadbear, 2020).

Broadbear (2020) also described other important characteristics of people with a diagnosis of BPD who died by suicide; some of these characteristics include:

- Male suicides peaked between ages 25-34, and females between ages 35-44
- Higher unemployment rate
- Decreased ability to work
- Not in an intimate relationship
- Higher rates of separation
- Increased domestic violence
- Higher levels of interpersonal conflict within families
- Elevated concerns around sexual identity and sexuality
- Increased substance misuse and dependence
- Higher prevalence of a friend or loved one who died by suicide.

Treatment Guidelines

Several international and national guidelines specify the treatment of people with PD across both community and inpatient services. However, the role of OTs is not specified. Examples of treatment guidelines include Project Air's treatment guidelines and the National Health & Medical Research Council's (NH&MRC) clinical practice guidelines on the management and care of people with BPD. OTs were not included in the Organising Committee in the development of the NH&MRC guidelines. Yet the guidelines note that mental health OTs should utilise the guide, and no occupational therapy-specific recommendations were made. OTs were included in the service evaluation and development of the Project Air guideline. However, no specific references were made to occupational therapy assessment and intervention. In 2019, the National Institute of Health and Clinical Excellence (NICE) convened a committee to review the guidelines for self-harm. Once again, occupational therapists were not included. However, this time, occupational therapists all over the world rallied and demanded a place at the table (Harding, 2020). The role of occupational therapy in gold-standard treatments like Dialectical Behaviour Therapy is very limited or is grouped under mental health clinicians and not specified (Linehan, 2014).

Why are OTs not regularly included in the care of people with a personality disorder? This is a multifaceted answer and requires more investigation. However, some contributing factors include limited literature, the relatively small voice of OTs in the Mental Health (MH) workforce, the focus on manualised psychotherapies, which have been proven to be highly effective without the role of occupational therapy specified in that treatment, and the lack of public knowledge around the role of an OT. We, therefore, have a patient population who are high users of the mental health system and a workforce that can make a difference. How do we cross this chasm? Can this chasm be bridged, and what can we as OTs do to carve out a rung in the ladder with the ultimate focus in mind of assisting people with PD along their recovery journey? One possible solution is to make the role of an OT in the treatment and assessment of a person with PD clear to link it to both diagnostic manuals and international guidelines and to demonstrate OT's effectiveness. Within this chapter, the role of an OT in the treatment of PD will be discussed.

Occupational Therapy-Specific Theory Related to the AMPD Criteria

Occupational therapy is defined as 'the therapeutic use of everyday life activities (occupations) with individuals or groups to enhance or enable participation in roles, habits, and routines in home, school, workplace, community, and other settings" (American Occupational Therapy Association, 2014; Wasmuth, 2020). OTs are trained to deeply examine the relationships between a person, their occupations, environmental contexts, and internal experiences. OTs are well-placed to assess and treat the key elements of pathological personality functioning.

A key component of occupational therapy is adaptability or flexibility (AMPD – criteria C and D). As summarised by Hagedorn (2012), 'Changes occur as part of normal growth, maturation and aging and as a response to the demands of the physical or social environment and the challenges of living. Without change, normal life is impossible. Basic survival depends on it." People who cannot learn (attend to, perceive, store, and recall information and relate situations) cannot adapt. OTs hold the primary assumption that adaptability is essential for survival and well-being (Schkade & Schultz, 1992). Adaptation relies on an accurate perception of stimuli and learning new responses when required. Adaptability can be enhanced by improving a person's perception, interpretation, problem-solving ability, planning skills, and successful engagement in the environment (Schkade & Schultz, 1992). The person with PD is relatively inflexible, and this leads to reduced functioning in social, occupational, and daily living skills. The AMPD (DMS5, p 882) notes that individuals with PD "are unable to modify their thinking or behaviour, even in the face of evidence that their approach is not working." Occupational therapists can support a person with a personality disorder by completing cognitive screens, facilitating cognitive rehabilitation, and engaging them in meaningful activities that provide opportunities for feedback.

Criteria E, F, and G include eliminating alternative explanations, including a developmental stage that may explain functioning. Occupational therapists are experts in understanding the impact of developmental stages on daily functioning (Hocking, 2004). A definition of developmental stages is a "Process of growth and maturation of humans that occurs over the lifespan that can be divided into physical, cognitive, emotional, and social. A largely biomedical and psychological construct, it is used extensively in occupational therapy, although the concept occupational development has emerged.' (Molineux, 2017). It is, therefore, important that occupational therapists assess a person's developmental history, identify delays, and plan a strategy with the person to address any areas for further development. Areas for improvement can include establishing a meaningful daily routine and better engagement in self-care activities.

Also included in Criteria E, F, and G is eliminating sociocultural environments as a possible explanation for behaviour. OTs add a holistic perspective to patient care that translates to and addresses the diversity among various cultures and localities (Wasmuth, 2020). Including a cultural assessment and formulation in treatment planning will assist in identifying the problem/concerns of the person with PD, avoid misdiagnoses, obtain information pertaining to risks, protective factors, and possible response to treatment in terms of improved engagement in daily living skills, enhance therapeutic relationships, improve patient outcomes, and inform further research (DSM5, 2013).

PSYCHOSOCIAL INTERVENTIONS

Therapeutic Modalities

Publications regarding psychosocial interventions for BPD dominate current research. A recent systematic review and meta-analysis was conducted on the effectiveness of outpatient and community treatments for people with a diagnosis of PD (Katakis, 2023). 54 trials were analysed, 37 described interventions for

BPD and 16 studies included non-BPD studies. Katakis *et al.* found that all the intervention types described were equally effective in treating the symptoms of PD and were more effective than treatment as usual. The duration and intensity of different treatments did not provide clinically significant variations. The treatments discussed were Cognitive Behaviour Therapy (CBT), Psychodynamic therapies, DBT, Mentalisation-Based Therapy (MBT), Schema Therapy, and Transference-Focussed Psychotherapy (TFP). It is generally accepted that OTs form part of the Multidisciplinary Team (MDT) that delivers these interventions; however, their specific roles are mostly not stipulated.

Medication

To date, there is insufficient evidence for the efficacy of prescribing psychotropic medications for people with PD. Clinical guidelines from around the world, including the United Kingdom and Australia, state that medication should not be prescribed to treat the symptoms of personality disorder long-term and that medication for comorbidities should be prescribed cautiously (NICE, 2009. NHMRC, 2012). However, in practice, there are high rates of polypharmacy, defined as five or more medications prescribed, seen within this cohort (Tennant, 2023. Dudley, 2021). The most prescribed medications for people with personality disorders were designed to treat the symptoms of mental illnesses such as schizophrenia, acute manic episodes, anxiety, insomnia, and major depressive disorder.

Dean Mercer and Paul Links (2019, p. 188) argued that the message that psychotherapy is the intervention of choice does not assist individuals with BPD who are in crisis and suffering (Choi-Kain, 2019). They may even have commenced psychotherapy; however, they have not seen the results yet. The therapeutic alliance when working with people with personality disorders is of utmost importance (Mercer & Links, YEAR). Medications should be an adjunct to psychotherapy.

Therapeutic Alliance and the Therapist-Patient Relationship

The strength of a therapist-patient alliance is often what keeps people with PD in therapy and sometimes alive (Linehan, 1993). The presence of a positive therapeutic alliance may prevent the person with PD from responding with opposition, frustration, or other therapy-interfering behaviours during treatment. Linehan (1993, p 514) described the importance of the therapeutic relationship with an analogy: "The relationship is the vehicle through which the therapist can affect the therapy; it *is* also the therapy." The practical guide of Good Psychiatric Management for BPD lists the cornerstones of alliance building as providing psychoeducation, showing concerned attention, emphasising the need for collaboration, and being active and not reactive (Choi-Kain, 2019, p 189). Linehan (1993) describes the ideal therapist as compassionate, sensitive, flexible, non-judgemental, accepting, and patient. Grenyer outlined key principles for working with people with PD: demonstrate empathy, listen to their current experiences, validate their current emotional state, take the person seriously (noting verbal and non-verbal communication), be non-judgemental, stay calm, remain respectful and caring, engage in open communication, be human (acknowledge both the serious and funny side of life), foster trust, be clear, consistent, and reliable, remember that aspects of behaviour have survival value, and convey encouragement and hope (Grenyer, 2014).

The above characteristics seem obvious; however, treating people with PD comes with certain challenges. This group exhibits some of the most stressful patient behaviours to manage: suicide attempts, suicidal threats, self-harm, interpersonal hostility, and splitting behaviours. And, due to their emotional sensitivity, the person will pick up when a therapist is not authentic or certain. Linehan (1993, p 425) describes the importance of consultation: "Patients often inadvertently reinforce therapists for engaging in ineffective therapy and punish them for engaging in effective therapy." And "In individual therapy, a patient usually does not want to discuss targeted behaviours, such as parasuicide, therapy-interfering behaviours, or behavioural patterns seriously interfering with the quality of life. If she does so, she wants to have a heart-to-heart discussion about her feelings or the therapist's behaviour, rather than analysing her behaviour or engaging in more adaptive problem-solving. The power struggle that ensues is usually very aversive to the therapist. It is much easier to let the patient control the agenda." It is extremely important that OTs, therefore, seek support/supervision/consultation to be an effective therapist to the person with PD.

Another important skill to acquire when caring for a person with PD is a balanced communication style. It is balancing acceptance with change, nurturing with benevolent demanding and unwavering centeredness with compassionate flexibility (Linehan, 1993). Balancing acceptance and change is often a skill that new OTs need to develop, which is best done within structured supervision sessions. Appropriate self-disclosure by OTs assists the person with PD to normalise and validate their feelings and to understand that challenges arise, even therapists can make mistakes, and reflection and adaption are a lifelong process, and to assist with possible problem-solving strategies. It assists in creating therapist authenticity, role modelling effective emotional experiences, and fostering hope (Linehan, 1993; Gunderson, 2014; Project Air Strategy, 2015).

RECOVERY AND REHABILITATION

The Importance of Hope

Facilitating hope is as important as the therapeutic relationship. Challenging health professional's pessimism and therapeutic nihilism is vital, especially considering there are intervention options available. The person with PD will benefit from all healthcare providers relaying a message of hope. The stigma around people with PD, often perpetuated by a workforce that does not have the essential skills to care for these people, can lead to people disengaging or losing faith in health services and then not attending effective treatment. Therefore, having a consistent and organised approach, especially at points of entry into services, is important. However, caring for a person with PD in an ED environment can be challenging. People with BPD can elicit feelings of anger, frustration, anxiety, and fear and sometimes rescue fantasies in clinicians (Gunderson, 2014). It is, therefore, important that all OTs are trained in basic principles of care for people with a personality disorder, as making clinical decisions based on feelings can lead to iatrogenic harm.

Diagnostic Disclosure (Improving Insight)

OTs are integral to the MDT and making a diagnosis of PD, as discussed above. Providing psychoeducation about a diagnosis can help people with personality disorders come to terms with their suffering. Disclosing the diagnoses effectively can facilitate hope and bring relief to the person with PD and their carers and loved ones (Lester, 2020; Gunderson, 2014). Diagnosis can facilitate the person with PD to access effective treatment. The stigma around the diagnoses and delay in diagnosing causes the person with PD to access treatment with poor outcomes and delays in the recovery journey as trust in the health service needs to be restored.

Goal Setting / Treatment Planning

This section discusses approaches to treatment planning. People with PD have often been through different forms of psychotherapy. Generally, the first step is goal setting. Goal setting is difficult for people who struggle with their identity and often cannot see out of the haze of their current distress. Goal setting can be viewed by people with a personality disorder negatively because of prior failures in accomplishing desired occupations or meeting goals (Wasmuth, 2020). DBT starts with setting treatment targets and focusing on the therapeutic relationship and commitment and orientation of the person with PD to the treatment (Linehan, 1993). Treatment targets are outlined: suicidal, parasuicidal, and life-threatening behaviours are the top priority. Therapy-interfering behaviours are second, followed by behaviours that impact a person's quality of life.

Collaborative care planning is completed with the person with PD and their carers. Care plans include safety planning through the identification of triggers, helpful strategies, skills to use in a crisis, and who to phone in the event of an emergency. Devising the care plan provides an opportunity for the person with PD to take responsibility for their own treatment, be actively involved, enhance their problem-solving options and decision-making strategies, reflect on what strategies have worked in the past and what did not, and be aware of their progress (Project Air Strategy, 2015). Care planning also provides the OT the opportunity to enhance the therapeutic relationship, identify the person's level of risk, identify all other service providers, clarify everyone's roles, and start exploring what a quality life will look like for the person with PD. Involving carers can enable support for the person with PD by providing carers with strategies to manage a crisis, knowing that the person with PD agreed to these strategies ahead of time. Carer contributions are then valued as part of treatment andinstill a sense of hope.

Contracting as a suicide intervention practice is no longer the best practice. However, to achieve therapist-patient transparency, agreements are still used with people with BPD. It is very important that therapy does not commence without the therapist and patient agreeing on how therapy will proceed and, if necessary, terminate. People with PD will communicate their desperation for therapy, and the therapist may feel compelled to assist. However, therapy is more effective when both parties are clear on what can be expected. Agreements, especially with people with BPD, work well, as limits are clearly stated. The treatment agreement also provides the therapist an opportunity to make every reasonable effort to assist the person with BPD to stay within these limits. Agreements typically include timeframes of therapy, circumstances for termination, contact agreement, confidentiality, and contact with other healthcare providers involved in care, crisis guidelines, and participation agreement.

Risk Management

People with PD can exhibit challenging behaviours when they are in crisis. Behaviours may include suicide attempts, self-harming, and other risk-taking behaviours (DSM5, 2013). It is important to appropriately respond to these behaviours. Yet, a balance is required by the OT. "Paying too much attention to these behaviours may inadvertently reinforce self-destructive behaviours" (Project Air Strategy, 2015). Always assess risk and manage risk as much as possible according to the care plan. Working with people with PD does include some therapeutic risk-taking, but this should only be used within an effective therapeutic relationship and only after a psychosocial assessment has been completed. The NICE guidelines on Self-harm developed in 2022 include a section on therapeutic risk-taking, and the Project Air Treatment Guidelines for Personality Disorder include a section on tolerating risk (NICE, 2022. Project Air Strategy, 2015). In DBT, all suicidal behaviours are seen by the therapist as "maladaptive problem-solving behaviours" and by the person with BPD as one possible solution (Linehan, 1993, p. 128). Therapeutic risk-taking provides the person with PD the opportunity to take control of their lives, understand the function of risky behaviours, replace ineffective behaviours with skilled behaviours, and receive validation or reinforcement for skills used.

Sensory Modulation and Emotion Regulation

Emotional dysregulation is one of the core symptoms of BPD and often leads to restrictive practices in inpatient units. Sensory modulation is, therefore, used in inpatient units, generally through "activity-based sensory interventions and sensory equipment" and mostly to reduce people's anxiety and agitation and to "assist with emotional regulation" (Wright, 2022).

Emotional dysregulation leads to crisis, and personalised sensory modulation strategies should be included in care planning (O'Sullivan, 2018). Sensory strategies are embedded in DBT as the dive reflex or intense exercise, as well as self-soothing and distraction (Linehan, 2015). Other potential strategies that can be used to regulate emotions include blankets, wraps, ice packs, ear plugs, music, and rocking or massage chairs (Champagne, 2011). It is important that people with PD are provided with sensory options and test those options prior to a crisis.

It is recommended that the OT completes the following steps when using the Sensory Modulation approach (O'Sullivan, 2018):

- Sensory assessment
- Sensory profile
- The design of a sensory space for an organisation
- Purchasing of sensory modulation items
- Identifying sensory triggers to trauma
- Assist in developing sensory strategies when sensory sensitivities influence occupations
- When the person is engaging in behaviours that may be explained through using a sensory lens.

Establishing routines and Activities of Daily Living (ADL)

People with PD often experience challenges with maintaining a meaningful routine, engagement in self-car tasks and ADLs, and participation in purposeful and meaningful activities (Larivière, 2016). Lack of participation may be due to reduced intrinsic motivation, or people with personality disorders may find these activities "meaningless" or "tedious", or a feeling of inadequacy may arise (Potvin, 2019). Potvin (2019) also notes that "just like the general public, people living with a PD engage in self-care activities largely to seek social approval rather than finding intrinsic motivation or meaning". Disruptions to this routine also occur when in crisis or throughout a hospital admission (Birken, 2017). Even though a person with PD life may seem balanced objectively, they may not perceive their activity levels as balanced (Kennon, 2010). It is therefore important for the OT to understand the person with PD's values, interests, and meaning derived from activities and then collaboratively identify the barriers and strategies to overcome these (Larivière, 2016). Another strategy may be to compare routines on weekends to weekdays and to analyse a 24-hour day to identify the amount of time spent working, sleeping, and participating in recreational activities (Kennon, 2010). Comparing this to peers within a group or even to the therapist's day may assist with normalisation and problem-solving.

Vocational Rehabilitation

Occupation is the core concept on which occupational therapy is built. Yet, the definition has changed over the years. Occupation is complex, multifaceted and means different things to different people. The book "Illuminating the Dark Side of Occupation" (Mercer, 2021, p xvii) identified the importance of including "marginalised, deviant, unhealthy or ignored occupations, their characteristics and relationships to occupational justice, and their connections to individual and cultural narratives as these reveal needs, situations and lifestyles" Mercer (2021, p 74). Self-defeating behaviour can be viewed from an occupational perspective. Self-defeating behaviours and their value to the person need to be closely examined and incorporated into occupational therapy assessment and treatment planning. 'Dark occupations' may include violence, addiction, eating disordered behaviour, self-harm, and suicide attempts (Wasmuth, 2020). Less obvious behaviours to participation in meaningful activities could be accessing health services frequently and behaviour that conflicts with their life goals, such as not attending work (Mercer, 2021).

Getting a job sometimes seems like an impossible task for people with PD. However, getting a job is a highlight for people, and they, in turn, feel productive and better able to cope with their symptoms (Wasmuth, 2020). Preliminary research suggests a relationship between occupational balance and emotional regulation (Romero-Ayuso, 2023). Engagement in productive pursuits can help people with PD get a break from their invading thoughts, focus on a tangible and meaningful activity, and maintain connections and relationships (Potvin, 2019). Occupational participation can provide opportunities for people with PD to develop identity, meaning, and a sense of purpose while exercising competencies and contributing to the community. "This concept can also be defined as full participation in occupations for purposes of doing what one needs and wants to do, being, becoming who one desires to be, and belonging, through shared occupations in communities" (Potvin, 2019). Wasmuth *et al.* (2020) stated that OTs can promote occupational engagement through social participation, which can create and sustain support environments. OTs are also well-placed to assist people with PD to apply the skills they learn through therapy into everyday life (Wasmuth, 2020)

Groups

Occupational therapists have been facilitating groups since the origin of the profession. Occupational therapists are well-placed to facilitate group therapy for people with PD. There are several therapeutic modalities that incorporate group therapy or can be delivered within a group format for people with PD: DBT, Acceptance Commitment Therapy (Wise Choices), Schema Therapy, and Good Psychiatric Management.

Groups are, however, only sporadically available to people with PD due to complications around implementation and sustainability (Weideman, 2024). People with BPD often resist group therapy as they fear what others may think of them, or they want their therapist's undivided attention (Gunderson, 2014). Gunderson noted that this resistance usually diminishes if the main therapist endorses group therapy or makes attending the group contingent on individual therapy.

Family-Based Interventions

Families, partners, and carers of people with PD are now routinely involved in the care of people with PD (Project Air Strategy, 2019). Incorporating families and carers into care planning can assist them within their roles and improve relationship skills. Sensory modulation yields the best results when a process of co-creation is followed by the person with PD and their families (Williamson, 2020).

Environmental Restructuring

One of the core skills of our profession as OTs is adapting individuals to their environments. In the treatment of people with PD, the OT is well-equipped to identify how a social environment influences functioning and to be explicit in our goal of promoting functioning. Within DBT, this is called "Environmental Intervention Strategies" (Linehan, 1993). Environmental restructuring should only be done if the person with PD is unable to solve their own problems if the person with PD does not have the power or capability to do so and always in collaboration.

OTs can also be equally confident in challenging restrictive environments that promote life-threatening ways of coping, for example, inpatient units, community centres, homes, and schools. "For physical health problems, we have no problems in identifying hazards and adapting environments to ensure that people are able to do what they want and need to do" and "… we can be the profession that calls for the environment to change rather than calling for more restriction or medication for individuals" (Harding, 2016).

CASE STUDY

Rosie was referred to a team specalising in the treatment of BPD by the Acute Care Team after she presented to the Emergency Department for the third time in two weeks. When the OT met with Rosie for the first time, she was angry and did not trust the health service as she felt that she did not receive the care she required within the ED department. Rosie also informed the OT that she was not aware that she was given a diagnosis of BPD. This was contradictory to her medical notes, in which it was stipulated that her diagnosis of BPD was disclosed to her. An approach of gentle curiosity was used with Rosie. Questions like, 'What do you understand is a diagnosis of BPD?' were used rather than engaging with her around her perspectives of ED or ACT. The OT did not promote splitting behaviours between health professionals. Rosie's current emotional state and her ability to seek help were validated . However, self-harm and suicidal behaviour were recognised as behaviour that had survival value and were not validated. The Biosocial theory from DBT was used to explain the BPD diagnosis to Rosie. She related the diagnoses with phrases like "Yep, that sounds like me".

Rosie identified through the Care planning process that anger was affecting her relationships with friends and family. A reflection (chain analysis) of her last 'anger outburst' was completed, and she could identify that she was more vulnerable to her emotions towards the end of the day when she was tired. Rosie identified strategies that she had tried before that were less-than-helpful, such as getting together with her friends, watching television, and eating snacks. Rosie wanted to try other sensory strategies that were suggested by the OT: a cool pack on her eyes, showering using her favourite lavender shower gel, and listening to her favourite music on her way to see her friends. Rosie reported back that showering rejuvenated her and made her feel calm prior to social events with her friends. This was added to Rosie's care plan.

Rosie was also referred to a comprehensive DBT program. However, the skills that were taught to her in the group to her home environment were not generalised. The OT conducted a cognitive screen, and it was established that Rosie did not have the cognitive capability to apply new information in different contexts without assistance. Through the adaption of the DBT program, shorter individual sessions, regular phone coaching with a focus on skill utilisation, and wallet-size reminders of DBT skills, she was able to implement some strategies outside of therapy and completed modified DBT. This led to Rosie reducing her visits to the ED and an extended period of no self-harm.

Rosie then identified a goal of returning to work and eventually completing a trade. She and her OT discussed some of the barriers to exploring this new role. Rosie saw the self-harm scars on her forearms as a barrier to employment. We discussed possible solutions, and Rosie noted that she wanted to get her forearms tattooed to hide the scars. She would show the OT already selected tattoo designs, which enhanced her motivation to continue to improve her functioning in daily life. We discussed how tattoos can only be done on skin that has not been injured in 12 months. This then became Rosie's next goal towards a more meaningful and productive life.

FUTURE DIRECTIONS

Advancements in Treatment

OTs inclusion in the MDT for the care of people with PD are occurring more frequently as they have a unique role to play. This facilitates future research opportunities on the role and effectiveness of teams with an OT and comparably without an OT. The inclusion of occupational therapy within the development of the NICE guidelines on self-harm is an important step forward. OTs are essential as they are experts in development, understanding activity, functioning, and environmental adaptations. However, work is still required within the profession to promote the value of the profession.

Research on Personality Disorders

Further research on the specific role within PD of OT needs to be conducted and translated into minimum requirements of knowledge for OT students. This will assist in placing occupational therapy at the forefront of the management of personality disorders.

CONCLUSION

OTs are well placed to assist in both the assessment and treatment of people with PD,; however, this is not well documented. OTs are an integral part of the MDT and can offer varied assessment data to firstly determine if a person meets the criteria of a PD according to the AMPD and, secondly to treat people with a PD. Treating this population group does come with certain challenges; however, mitigating strategies are already incorporated into how OTs practice with supervision and continued professional development embedded in the profession.

OTs are now incorporated in the design and evaluation of both international and national guidelines for people with PD. OTs are also well placed to utilise different treatment approaches like DBT, GPM, *etc.* This capitalises on a workforce that has the expertise, especially as people with PD are high-service users, and each presentation has the potential to save a life.

REFERENCES

American Psychiatric Association. (2013). *Diagnostic And Statistical Manual of Mental Disorders: DSM-5 (5th Ed.)*.

Beatson, J., Rao, S., Watson, C., Victoria, S.P.D.S.F. (2010). *Borderline Personality Disorder: Towards Effective Treatment.*. Australian Postgraduate Medicine.

Bender, D.S., Dolan, R.T., Skodol, A.E., Sanislow, C.A., Dyck, I.R., McGlashan, T.H., Shea, M.T., Zanarini, M.C., Oldham, J.M., Gunderson, J.G. (2001). Treatment utilization by patients with personality disorders. *Am. J. Psychiatry, 158*(2), 295-302.
[http://dx.doi.org/10.1176/appi.ajp.158.2.295] [PMID: 11156814]

Birken, M., Harper, S. (2017). Experiences of people with a personality disorder or mood disorder regarding carrying out daily activities following discharge from hospital. *Br. J. Occup. Ther., 80*(7), 409-416.
[http://dx.doi.org/10.1177/0308022617697995]

Birken, M., Morley, M. (2016). Testing an Evidence-Based Intervention for Adults with a Personality or Mood Disorder. *Br. J. Occup. Ther., 79*, 104-104.Https://Search.Ebscohost.Com/Login.Aspx?Direct=True&Authtype=Ip,Athens&Db=Ccm&AN=117819538&Site=Eds-Live

Broadbear, J.H., Dwyer, J., Bugeja, L., Rao, S. (2020). Coroners' investigations of suicide in Australia: The hidden toll of borderline personality disorder. *J. Psychiatr. Res., 129*, 241-249.
[http://dx.doi.org/10.1016/j.jpsychires.2020.07.007] [PMID: 32823217]

Champagne, T. (2011). *Sensory Modulation & Environment: Essential Elements of Occupation: Handbook & Reference (Third Edition Revis Ed.)*.. Pearson Australia Group..

Choi-Kain, L.W., Gunderson, J.G. (2019). *Applications Of Good Psychiatric Management for Borderline Personality Disorder: A Practical Guide.*. American Psychiatric Pub..
[http://dx.doi.org/10.1176/appi.books.9781615379309]

Dudley, B., Bellam, S., Lawrie, A. (2021). Audit of pharmacological management of borderline personality disorder as per NICE clinical guidelines CG78. *BJPsych Open, 7*(S1), S319-S319.
[http://dx.doi.org/10.1192/bjo.2021.841]

Gunderson, J.G. (2014). *Handbook of Good Psychiatric Management for Borderline Personality Disorder..* American Psychiatric Pub..
[http://dx.doi.org/10.1176/appi.books.9781615378432]

Hagedorn, R. (1997). *Foundations For Practice in Occupational Therapy.* Churchill Livingstone.

Harding, K. (2020). Enhancing the occupational therapy role around 'personality disorder' and self-harm. *Br. J. Occup. Ther., 83*(9), 547-548.
[http://dx.doi.org/10.1177/0308022620947642]

Hocking, C., Erik Ness, N. (2004). WFOT Minimum Standards for the Education of Occupational Therapists: Shaping the Profession. *World Federation of Occupational Therapists Bulletin, 50*(1), 9-17.
[http://dx.doi.org/10.1179/otb.2004.50.1.003]

Katakis, P., Schlief, M., Barnett, P., Rains, L.S., Rowe, S., Pilling, S., Johnson, S. (2023). Effectiveness of outpatient and community treatments for people with a diagnosis of 'personality disorder': systematic review and meta-analysis. *BMC Psychiatry, 23*(1), 57-57.
[http://dx.doi.org/10.1186/s12888-022-04483-0] [PMID: 36681805]

Krueger, R.F., Hobbs, K.A. (2020). An Overview of the DSM-5 Alternative Model of Personality Disorders. *Psychopathology, 53*(3-4), 126-132.
[http://dx.doi.org/10.1159/000508538] [PMID: 32645701]

Larivière, N., Denis, C., Payeur, A., Ferron, A., Levesque, S., Rivard, G. (2016). Comparison of Objective and Subjective Life Balance Between Women With and Without a Personality Disorder. *Psychiatr. Q., 87*(4), 663-673.
[http://dx.doi.org/10.1007/s11126-016-9417-3] [PMID: 26875106]

Lester, R., Prescott, L., McCormack, M., Sampson, M. (2020). Service users' experiences of receiving a diagnosis of borderline personality disorder: A systematic review. *Pers. Ment. Health, 14*(3), 263-283.
[http://dx.doi.org/10.1002/pmh.1478] [PMID: 32073223]

Lewis, K.L., Fanaian, M., Kotze, B., Grenyer, B.F.S. (2019). Mental health presentations to acute psychiatric services: 3-year study of prevalence and readmission risk for personality disorders compared with psychotic, affective, substance or other disorders. *BJPsych Open, 5*(1), e1.
[http://dx.doi.org/10.1192/bjo.2018.72] [PMID: 30575497]

Linehan, M. (2014). *DBT? Skills Training Manual..* Guilford Publications.

Linehan, M.M. (1993). *Skills Training Manual for Treating Borderline Personality Disorder..* Guilford Press.

Mercer, S. (2020). Self-defeating behaviour in an individual with borderline personality disorder from an occupational perspective. *Illuminating The Dark Side of Occupation.* Routledge.
[http://dx.doi.org/10.4324/9780429266256-10]

Meuldijk, D., McCarthy, A., Bourke, M.E., Grenyer, B.F.S. (2017). The value of psychological treatment for borderline personality disorder: Systematic review and cost offset analysis of economic evaluations. *PLoS One, 12*(3), e0171592.
[http://dx.doi.org/10.1371/journal.pone.0171592] [PMID: 28249032]

Molineux, M. (2017). *A Dictionary of Occupational Science and Occupational Therapy..* Oxford University Press.
[http://dx.doi.org/10.1093/acref/9780191773624.001.0001]

National Health and Medical Research Council (NHMRC). (2012). *Clinical Practice Guideline for The Management of Borderline Personality Disorder.*

NICE: National Institute for Health and Care Excellence (2009). *Borderline Personality Disorder: Recognition and Management - Clinical Guideline (CG78).*Https://Www.Nice.Org

NICE: National Institute for Health and Care Excellence. (2022). *Self-Harm: Assessment, Management and Preventing Recurrence (NG225).*Https://Www.Nice.Org

Nott, A. (2014). Understanding Persons with Personality Disorders: Intervention in Occupational Therapy. In: Crouch, R., Alers, V., (Eds.), *Occupational Therapy in Psychiatry and Mental Health.* Wiley Blackwell. [http://dx.doi.org/10.1002/9781118913536.ch26]

O'Sullivan, J.F. (2018). *Carolyn..* Sensory Modulation.

Project Air. (2015). *A Personality Disorder Strategy..* Treatment Guidelines for Personality Disorders.

Project Air. (2019). *A Personality Disorder Strategy..* Family, Partner and Carer Intervention Manual For Personality Disorders.

Penfold, S., Groll, D., Mauer-Vakil, D., Pikard, J., Yang, M., Mazhar, M.N. (2016). A retrospective analysis of personality disorder presentations in a Canadian university-affiliated hospital's emergency department. *BJPsych Open, 2*(6), 394-399. [http://dx.doi.org/10.1192/bjpo.bp.116.003871] [PMID: 27990295]

Potvin, O., Vallée, C., Larivière, N. (2019). Experience of Occupations among People Living with a Personality Disorder. *Occup. Ther. Int., 2019*, 1-11. [http://dx.doi.org/10.1155/2019/9030897] [PMID: 31049046]

Romero-Ayuso, D.M., Toledano-González, A., Pinilla-Cerezo, M., Sánchez-Rodríguez, Ó., García-Arenas, J.J., Triviño-Juárez, J.M., Ortíz-Rubio, A. (2023). Occupational balance and emotional regulation in people with and without serious mental illness. *Canadian Journal of Occupational Therapy.*Https://Doi.Org/10.1177/00084174231178440

Sheldon, K.M., Cummins, R., Kamble, S. (2010). Life balance and well-being: testing a novel conceptual and measurement approach. *J. Pers., 78*(4), 1093-1134. [http://dx.doi.org/10.1111/j.1467-6494.2010.00644.x] [PMID: 20545821]

Schkade, J.K., Schultz, S. (1992). Occupational adaptation: toward a holistic approach for contemporary practice, Part 1. *Am. J. Occup. Ther., 46*(9), 829-837. [http://dx.doi.org/10.5014/ajot.46.9.829] [PMID: 1514569]

Schultz, S., Schkade, J.K. (1992). Occupational adaptation: toward a holistic approach for contemporary practice, Part 2. *Am. J. Occup. Ther., 46*(10), 917-925. [http://dx.doi.org/10.5014/ajot.46.10.917] [PMID: 1463064]

Sharp, C. (2017). Bridging the gap: the assessment and treatment of adolescent personality disorder in routine clinical care. *Arch. Dis. Child., 102*(1), 103-108. [http://dx.doi.org/10.1136/archdischild-2015-310072] [PMID: 27507846]

Skodol, A.E., Morey, L.C., Bender, D.S., Oldham, J.M. (2015). The Alternative DSM-5 Model for Personality Disorders: A Clinical Application. *Am. J. Psychiatry, 172*(7), 606-613. [http://dx.doi.org/10.1176/appi.ajp.2015.14101220] [PMID: 26130200]

Soeteman, D.I., Hakkaart-van Roijen, L., Verheul, R., Busschbach, J.J.V. (2008). The economic burden of personality disorders in mental health care. *J. Clin. Psychiatry, 69*(2), 259-265. [http://dx.doi.org/10.4088/JCP.v69n0212] [PMID: 18363454]

Stiles, C., Batchelor, R., Gumley, A., Gajwani, R. (2023). Experiences of Stigma and Discrimination in Borderline Personality Disorder: A Systematic Review and Qualitative Meta-Synthesis. *J. Pers. Disord., 37*(2), 177-194. [http://dx.doi.org/10.1521/pedi.2023.37.2.177] [PMID: 37002935]

Tennant, M., Frampton, C., Mulder, R., Beaglehole, B. (2023). Polypharmacy in the treatment of people diagnosed with borderline personality disorder: repeated cross-sectional study using New Zealand's national databases. *BJPsych Open, 9*(6), e200. [http://dx.doi.org/10.1192/bjo.2023.592] [PMID: 37881020]

Wasmuth, S., Mokol, E., Szymaszek, K., Gaerke, K.J., Manspeaker, T., Lysaker, P. (2020). Intersections of occupational participation and borderline personality disorder: A grounded theory approach. *Cogent Psychol., 7*(1), 1803580.

[http://dx.doi.org/10.1080/23311908.2020.1803580]

Widiger, T.A., Costa, P.T., Gore, W.L., Crego, C. (2013). *Five-Factor Model Personality Disorder Research.* American Psychological Association.
[http://dx.doi.org/10.1037/13939-006]

Widiger, T.A., Trull, T.J. (2007). Plate tectonics in the classification of personality disorder: Shifting to a dimensional model. *Am. Psychol., 62*(2), 71-83.
[http://dx.doi.org/10.1037/0003-066X.62.2.71] [PMID: 17324033]

Williamson, P., Ennals, P. (2020). Making sense of it together: Youth & families co☐create sensory modulation assessment and intervention in community mental health settings to optimise daily life. *Aust. Occup. Ther. J., 67*(5), 458-469.
[http://dx.doi.org/10.1111/1440-1630.12681] [PMID: 32648269]

Wright, L., Meredith, P., Bennett, S. (2022). Sensory approaches in psychiatric units: Patterns and influences of use in one Australian health region. *Aust. Occup. Ther. J., 69*(5), 559-573.
[http://dx.doi.org/10.1111/1440-1630.12813] [PMID: 35706333]

Part 3
Occupational Therapy Interventions in Mental Health Practice

• Summary of the various occupational therapy interventions used in mental health practice

• Discussion of how occupational therapists can select and use the most appropriate intervention for each client and situation

• Explanation of the importance of evidence-based practice in occupational therapy interventions in mental health practice.

I worked with a psychiatrist once who asked me, "What do occupational therapists do in mental health anyway?" On the spot, it was difficult for me to come up with a 3-minute elevator pitch for him, and I am afraid I fumbled more than I would have liked.

In mental health settings, occupational therapists are a fundamental part of the interdisciplinary team in delivering a range of interventions, like psychoeducation, cognitive behavioural therapy, dialectical behavioural therapy, solution-focused therapy, family therapy, group therapy, stress management, social skills training, health and fitness interventions, and even medication. While many of these interventions are considered in this text, we particularly focussed on interventions commonly led by occupational therapists. These include occupation analysis and related therapeutic media, supported employment, leisure and recreational therapy, and sensory modulation.

CHAPTER 9

Foundations of Occupational Therapy Practice in Mental Health

Tawanda Machingura[1,*], Charleen Machingura[2] and Robert Pereira[3]

[1] *Head of Discipline Occupational Therapy Program, University of Notre Dame Australia, Sydney, Australia*

[2] *Department of Mental Health Services, Gold Coast Hospital and Health Service, Gold Coast, Queensland, Australia*

[3] *Department of Occupational Therapy, University of Canberra, Canberra, ACT, Australia*

Abstract: This chapter provides an overview of occupational therapy practice in mental health. Occupational therapists often find themselves working in a multidisciplinary team. The occupational therapist (OT) enables and promotes consumers to obtain the skills needed to enhance their ability to participate in or modify the environment to support their participation in everyday occupations. This chapter introduces the occupational therapy process and discusses some common interventions used in mental health, such as supported employment. The chapter concludes by discussing emerging and future mental health occupational therapy practice opportunities.

Keywords: Biopsychosocial approach, Health promotion, Occupation, Occupational therapy, Supported employment.

INTRODUCTION

In 1914, George Barton introduced the term 'occupational therapy', with the discipline being officially founded in 1917 at Clifton Springs, New York, in the USA. Considering that it has been just over 100 years since the profession was founded, it is still considered in the infancy stage of development (Paterson, 2008). Despite this, the occupational therapy profession has flourished internationally, with over 110 member organisations across the Global North and South representing 633,000 occupational therapists (World Federation of Occupational Therapists, 2024). The underpinnings of the therapeutic use of occupation, the profession's therapeutic medium, have their origins in mental health (Paterson, 2008).

* **Corresponding author Tawanda Machingura:** Head of Discipline Occupational Therapy Program, University of Notre Dame Australia, Sydney, Australia; E-mail: tawanda.machingura@nd.edu.au

Historically, mental health care has, to a large extent, been dependent on social, medical, political, and economic factors. The founders of the profession of occupational therapy were influenced by many key public personalities in the 1700s, including the French psychiatrist Phillipe Pinel and the British philanthropist William Tuke, who in the late 1700s advocated for the 'unshackling of patients' and instead providing them with activities to occupy their minds, which included arts and crafts. Pinel and Tuke are widely recognised for spearheading the moral treatment movement (Paterson, 2008). In the early 1900s, Dr. Adolf Meyer, a Swiss-born American Psychiatrist, viewed mental illness as a person's maladaptive interaction with the environment, and this became the basis of what we now know as the biopsychosocial model adopted by many in the field of psychiatry in the 20th century (Paterson, 2008). The other founders of the occupational therapy profession independent of Meyer were Americans William Rush Dunton (psychiatrist), Susan Tracy (nurse), Eleanor Clarke Slagle (social worker), Thomas Kidner (Architect), and George Barton (Architect and lived Experience Expert). The pioneers of the profession of occupational therapy had a background in a variety of disciplines, and today, occupational therapy remains a unique blend of the various health and technical professions, with occupational therapy being described as embracing the art and science of practice (Dirette, 2016). It appears as if the pioneers realised a gap in what they were all collectively providing to their patients at the time.

Currently, occupational therapy is a profession that aims to promote health and well-being through the therapeutic use of occupation. Occupations are the activities that people do in life across various contexts and environments that are meaningful, purposeful, personal, or collective in nature and that shape an identity over time (Pereira & Whiteford, 2022). The primary objective of occupational therapy is to support people to perform and engage in activities of everyday life, and occupational therapists assist people to enhance their ability to participate or modify the environment to better support their participation in these occupations (WFOT, 2007).

To work effectively in mental health, the occupational therapist requires some core skills, knowledge, and attitudes, including:

- An understanding of the biopsychosocial approach.
- Knowledge and understanding of common mental health conditions, including signs, symptoms, and interventions.
- Knowledge and understanding of the Mental Health Act, relevant laws, and other legislative instruments that commonly apply to mental health clients.
- An understanding of occupational therapy theories, frameworks, and processes.

These are discussed in detail in other chapters of this book.

- An ability to conduct a comprehensive initial assessment (this includes mental state and risk assessment, personal and family history, history of presenting illness, and an intervention/crisis management plan).
- Skills and abilities to work in partnership with the consumer (mental health client) and this includes therapeutic use of self and other interpersonal skills.
- Skills in evidence-based occupational therapy and other psychosocial interventions.
- Skills and knowledge of promoting occupational justice.
- Skills and knowledge of recovery-oriented and community development approaches.
- Knowledge of community services and resources.

The focus of OT services is to improve one's ability to engage in meaningful activities (including, but not limited to, play, leisure, work, education, social interaction, activities of daily living [ADLs], instrumental ADLs, sleep, and rest) in a range of settings, including homes, workplaces, communities, schools, residential facilities, and healthcare facilities.

The first pertinent question to ask is, "What do OTs do in mental health?". Here are a few considerations to start to answer this question, which are explored further in this chapter:

- Evaluate the client's condition and needs by reviewing their medical, personal, social, and family history, asking questions, and observing them doing tasks, activities, and/or occupations.
- Assess the client's physical environment, for *e.g.*, home or workplace, based on their health needs, *e.g.*, labelling kitchen cabinets for a person with poor memory.
- Develop a treatment plan with the client, identifying specific goals and the relevant occupations that will be used to support them in working towards or reaching those goals.
- Teach alternative ways to perform tasks or new skills, for *e.g.*, teaching a person with poor social skills how to communicate with others.
- Modify routines and habits, and sometimes, introducing and promoting new ones.
- Recommend special equipment, such as sensory equipment or electronic reminders, and instruct clients on how to use such equipment.
- Advocate for clients or supporting self-advocacy.

Occupational therapists assist individuals in resuming past roles or learning new ones.The actual "doing" of occupations enables continuous personal development and growth. It is understood to be transformative, encourages adaptation and the formation of social and personal identities, and links people into communities.The use of 'occupations'

Occupations have special significance and value to a client's (individual, group, or population) identity, competence, and general well-being. According to WFOT (2012a), para. 2, occupations refer to the everyday activities that people engage in as individuals, families, and communities to pass the time and give their lives meaning and purpose. They include things people need to, want to, and are expected to do. According to Wilcock (2014), p. 542, "occupation is everything people want, need, or have to do, whether of a physical, mental, social, sexual, political, or spiritual nature, and includes sleep and rest". It refers to all aspects of human doing, being, becoming, belonging, and connecting (Pereira & Whiteford, In press).

Occupation can be used in two distinct fashions: as a 'means' and as an 'end' in and of itself (Gray, 1998). Ultimately, occupation can be employed in therapy as a tool to help clients reach their goals. "Occupation as ends" refers to the client's goals of participation in specific occupations. For example, a child who is 6 or 7 years old may have difficulty with the occupation of handwriting, which is necessary for their occupational role as a student. Another example is where the occupational therapist may observe that the child has difficulty with their posture and sitting still, or the child may have some difficulty with the grip on their pencil. In both examples, the occupational therapist could then use the occupation of play, doing lots of fun activities to work on the child's ability to sit up straight and control the pencil. Play can also be used in working on grip and control of the fingers. Working in mental health, clients may have difficulty in looking after themselves and preparing healthy food or difficulty with social skills. The occupational therapist may then run groups such as a cooking group so that clients can learn new skills and practice cooking healthy food, or a photography group, where clients can learn a skill for leisure and learn and develop skills in socialising with others in affirming ways.

Occupation as an end is more straightforward. For instance, the occupational therapist may be working with someone unable to get a job themselves. This could be because of low motivation or poor communication and interaction skills due to a major psychiatric disorder. The goal of occupational therapy is to work with the individual on pre-vocational skills to support job readiness and support different work trials and exposure to different workplace environments so that they can obtain a permanent and sustainable job. Here, the occupation of choosing and getting a job is being used as the ends and the means of therapy.

Approaches and Frameworks

Occupational therapists who work in mental health use the biopsychosocial approach. Fig. (1) is a diagrammatic representation of the model.

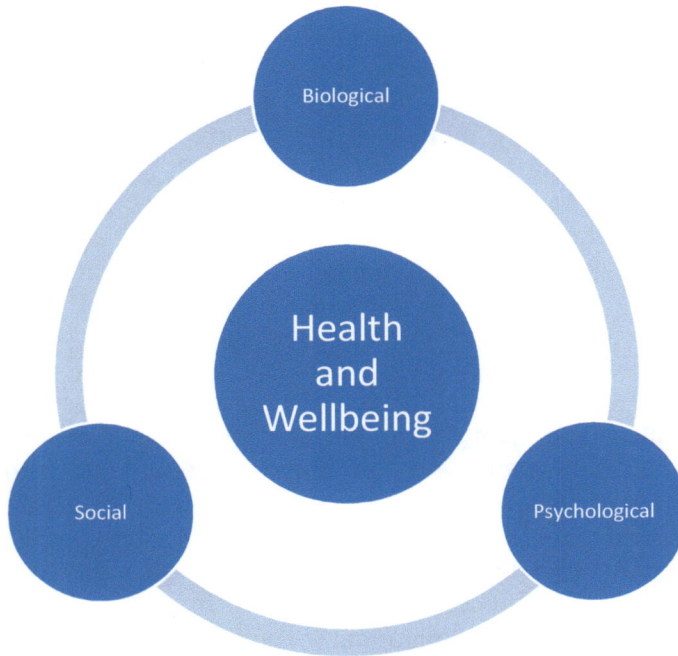

Fig. (1). Biopsychosocial approach

In mental health practice, OTs may use a behavioural theory approach to apply behavioural approaches to assist clients to:

- Adopt changes to their occupations or lifestyle.
- Develop planning and organisational skills.
- Develop or compensate for memory and attention difficulties.
- Develop skills to help with sequencing activities.
- Support with modifying behaviours through supportive and neuroaffirming ways (Dallman *et al.*, 2022).

The Occupational Therapy Process Based on OTPF-4ᵗʰ Edition

Occupational therapists use the OTPF as a framework that provides a foundation or structure upon which to develop practice. (**"Framework"; AOTA, 2020).** The OTPF creates a shared understanding of the fundamental ideas and concepts that underpin occupational therapy practice. In conjunction with the available and relevant evidence and information pertinent to occupation and occupational therapy, the OTPF–4 acts as a guide for practice within the identified practice areas with the appropriate clients. The two main sections of the OTPF-4 are the (1) domain, which defines the scope of the profession and the fields in which its members have a body of established knowledge and expertise, and the (2) process, which outlines the steps practitioners take to provide client-centred, occupation-focused services.

All components of the domain are dynamically connected. Each aspect has equal significance and interacts with one another to affect one's engagement in life, health, and sense of occupational identity. Context is a broad concept defined as the personal and environmental factors unique to each client, which impact participation and engagement in occupations. The quality of and satisfaction with performance, as well as their access to occupations, are influenced by the context (Christiansen, 2024). Practitioners understand that individuals must not only function but also engage securely within their unique combination of contexts to achieve full participation, meaning, and purpose.

Environmental Factors encompass the natural environment and human-made modifications to the environment. Products and technology, relationships and social support, attitudes, services, systems, and policies are also included.

Personal Factors include chronological age, sexual orientation, gender identity, ethnicity, race, attitudes and cultural identification, socioeconomic standing, childhood and life events, habits, historical and contemporary behavioural trends, distinctive personal qualities, and coping mechanisms.

Performance Patterns are those behaviours, rituals, or habits that people tend to follow in their lives. They can help or inhibit performance and satisfaction when doing daily activities. Performance patterns are also described as 'doing in time' (Eklund *et al.*, 2017). People do daily activities at certain times depending on their personal circumstances and culture, and these patterns contribute to fulfilling lifestyles and occupational balance (Eklund *et al.*, 2017).

Performance skills include motor, process, and social interaction abilities that are observable, goal-directed activities (Fisher & Griswold, 2019). Occupational therapists assess and analyse performance skills during the real performance of activities (smaller components of occupations) to determine a client's capacity to carry out activities (Fisher & Marterella, 2019).

Client factors are skills, traits, or beliefs that exist within an individual, community, or population and impact work performance (Table **9**). The existence or lack of illness, disease, deprivation, and handicap, in addition to life stages and experiences, all have an impact on client factors. These elements can influence performance skills in various ways. For instance, a person might experience limited mobility in their left leg (a client factor), making it challenging to climb stairs (a motor and process skill). Similarly, a student with hearing impairment (a client factor) may struggle to follow verbal instructions in class (a motor and process skill). Continuous interaction between evaluation, intervention, and outcomes is a fundamental part of the occupational therapy process.

Evaluation The unique perspective of occupational therapy practitioners enhances the therapy process through professional reasoning, analysing occupations and activities, and collaborating with clients. This process begins with evaluation. The *first step* in the evaluation of the client's needs is establishing an occupational profile. The OT must establish why the client is seeking services, the client's occupational history, the occupations the client feels successful in, the enablers and barriers to occupational performance and engagement, personal and environmental or contextual, the client's goals and priorities, and their occupational performance patterns. The recommended way to obtain this information is by interviewing the client and their significant others.

The *second step* in evaluation is analysing occupational performance. In this phase, the occupational therapist analyses findings from the client's occupational profile to determine their priorities and goals. To determine the demands of the intended occupations and activities on the client, the OT must also do an occupational analysis or activity analysis on the desired occupations. The OT must complete specific assessments, keeping in mind the client's intended occupations, to evaluate the client's context, performance patterns, or performance skills, identify any shortcomings, and ascertain the efficacy of the performance.

The third step is synthesizing the information. This involves interpreting the assessment data to identify barriers and enablers to occupational performance while considering the client's values and preferences. It includes formulating a hypothesis about the client's occupational performance and deficits (case formulation), determining desired outcomes with the client, setting collaborative goals to achieve these outcomes, and selecting appropriate outcome measures.

Intervention

Intervention Plan

The occupational therapist (OT) uses their evaluation to inform the intervention plan, which is a dynamic process that can evolve. The intervention plan should include objective, measurable, and specific occupation-based goals (Fisher & Marterella, 2019). The OT also determines intervention strategies, which may aim to maintain, establish, restore, prevent, create, promote, or modify various aspects of the client's occupational performance (Townsend & Polatajko, 2007). Additionally, the OT must consider service plans and potential discharge plans to ensure a comprehensive approach to the client's care and progression.

Intervention Implementation

Selecting and implementing interventions is crucial in mental health care. These interventions encompass a range of strategies, such as therapeutic use of occupations, psychoeducation, skills training, and advocacy. For instance, OTs must continually assess and adapt interventions based on the client's response through collaborative and relationship-focused ways (Egan & Restall, 2022). This adaptive approach ensures that the treatment remains effective and tailored to the client's needs throughout the therapy process.

Intervention Review

After implementing an intervention, the OT proceeds to review the intervention plan. This review is pivotal as it helps the OT assess the effectiveness of the intervention and ascertain whether ongoing interventions are necessary. During this stage, the OT also evaluates if any services should be continued or discontinued based on the client's progress and evolving needs.

Outcomes

Ultimately, the OT utilises the outcome measures chosen at the outset to gauge progress. The crucial aspect here lies in the specificity, measurability, and reliability of these outcome measures. By employing such metrics, the OT can effectively track the client's advancements and setbacks. Subsequently, these results serve as the foundation for informed decision-making regarding the future course of action (Pereira *et al.*, 2020).

Summary

Understanding the intrinsic connection between the domain and process of occupational therapy is essential (AOTA, 2020). This comprehension guides the intricate decision-making process inherent in everyday mental health practice within occupational therapy. It also enriches practitioners' utilisation of professional reasoning. By recognising and appreciating this interrelation, occupational therapists can navigate the complexities of their field with greater efficacy, ensuring the provision of high-quality care tailored to individual needs.

Fig. (**2**) below summarises the OT Process.

Operationalizing the Occupational Therapy Process

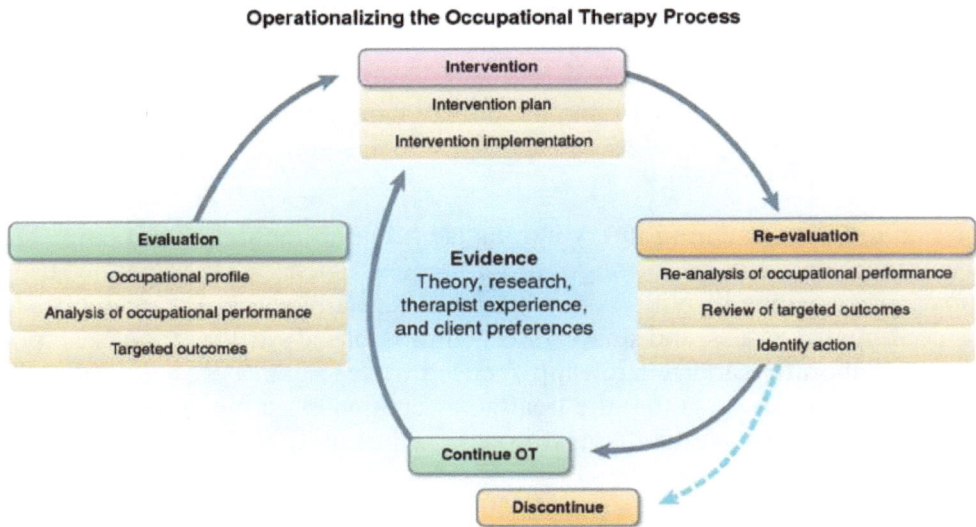

Fig. (2). Occupational therapy process (*used with permission*)

Working in Multidisciplinary Teams

Typically a generic role, OTs working in mental health often work in multidisciplinary team (MDT) settings, which may include the following professions:

- Consultant psychiatrist
- Consumer advocates/ consultants
- Psychiatric registrars and interns
- Nurses (RN/CN/CNC/NUM)
- Psychologists
- Social Workers
- Occupational Therapists
- Speech Pathologists
- Administration Officers and
- Peer-support workers.

Psychiatric Rehabilitation (PsR)

In many contexts, occupational therapists often work in the community, with their key role being to coordinate mental health rehabilitation for allocated consumers. In some countries like Australia, this role is often embedded in a case management role. In other countries, particularly countries in the majority world, such as those in the Global South, this role is often embedded in community-based rehabilitation (CBR) initiatives. The term "psychiatric rehabilitation' is often not used because it is seen by many as being rooted in the medical reductionist model. However, the concepts within this model are very much recovery-oriented. We present the Boston Psychiatric Rehabilitation Approach (BPsR)) approach to the reader so they can assess and reflect on their current approach and how that might be similar or different to this approach (Farkas & Anthony, 2010; Rogers *et al.*, 2006). The aim of rehabilitation is to enable people to live meaningful and satisfying lives in environments of their choosing (Farkas & Anthony, 2010).

Psychiatric rehabilitation comprises two key intervention strategies. The first approach is client-centred and focused on improving the client's ability to interact in an emotionally intensive setting. The second, an ecological approach, focuses on creating environmental resources that reduce possible stressors (Farkas & Anthony, 2010). Most will require a combination of the two methods. Overall, psychiatric rehabilitation aims to help people acquire the intellectual, social, and emotional abilities necessary to live, learn, and work in the community with the least professional care (Farkas *et al.*, 2007; Farkas & Antony, 2010). Recognising that rehabilitation is centred around the individual within the context of their unique surroundings is the first step towards developing a sufficient grasp of the subject. Supporting the individual in determining their objectives is the second phase. In this process, people do not simply list their needs. It is preferable to conduct motivational interviews highlighting a client's unique costs and benefits related to the demands mentioned. As a result of this, determining each person's level of change preparedness is also essential. The client's strengths are the focus of the rehabilitation planning procedure. Regardless of the level of psychopathology exhibited by a particular client, the clinician must engage with the healthy aspect of the ego since there is always a portion of the ego that is intact and can be targeted for rehabilitation and treatment (Cohen *et al.*, 2002). To this end, consumer and practitioner processes are summarised in Table **1** below.

Successful rehabilitation requires collaboration and partnership between the practitioner and the consumer (Egan & Restall, 2022). This means the consumer is a valued partner, and the practitioner must support their autonomy throughout the recovery process (Bevitt *et al.*, 2022). The concept of recovery embodies these rehabilitation ideals.

PsR Interventions

It is now well understood that mental health consumers share the same aspirations as anyone else in their society or culture. They seek respect as autonomous individuals and aim to live as normal a life as possible. Typically, they desire:

a. Their own housing,
b. Adequate education and a meaningful career,
c. Fulfilling social and intimate relationships, and
d. Full participation in community life with all associated rights.

Table 1. Psychiatric rehabilitation process

Person responsible	Choosing what role/goal to focus on	Achieving the role/ goal	Maintaining the role
Consumer Role: The actions, steps, and processes the consumer takes.	**Choose:** The consumer chooses a valued role such as being a worker, being a student, being a homemaker, or being a friend.	**Get:** The consumer finds out more information about their valued role; they develop specific skills such as job searching skills, study skills, or budgeting skills; they need and take action towards the achievement of their chosen goal within their chosen role.	**Keep:** The consumer takes actions to develop skills such as dealing with stress at work, developing communication skills, and engaging with support to maintain their chosen role.
Practitioner Role: The actions, steps, and processes the practitioner takes.	**Engage:** The practitioner engages with the consumer and develops a rapport and trust with the consumer.	**Link:** The practitioner links the consumer to existing services, resources, and opportunities they need that are specific to the consumer's desired role/ goal.	**Skills Assessment:** The practitioner assesses and determines the critical skills, deficits, strengths the consumer has, and resources the client needs to maintain success and satisfaction in their role.
	Assess: The practitioner works collaboratively with the consumer to determine their readiness to set an achievable goal in their chosen role..	**Create** Where services, resources, and opportunities do not exist, the practitioner creates new opportunities and/or resources for the consumer.	**Skills Training:** The practitioner provides skills training to enable the client to develop the necessary skills and resources.
	Set rehabilitation Goal: The practitioner then works with the consumer to develop specific, measurable, achievable, realistic, and time-framed (SMART) goals in line with their chosen role.	**Advocate:** The practitioner advocates for the client to assist the client in achieving their goal.	**Developing Supports:** The practitioner surrounds the consumer with the natural and formal support they need to maintain their chosen role. This often includes *peer support,* among others.

*Arrows indicate suggested direction of actions and focus

PsyR interventions currently blend evidence-based practices, promising practices, and emerging methods. These can be effectively integrated using the PsyR process framework, which assists individuals with serious mental illnesses in choosing, obtaining, and maintaining valued roles. Combined with complementary treatment-oriented psychosocial interventions, this approach provides a comprehensive strategy for facilitating recovery.

Supported Housing

The ideal solution would be to offer a residential continuum (RC) with a variety of housing options. Supported housing (or supported accommodation), which is independent housing combined with the provision of support services, is now the most promising housing model. It first appeared as an alternative to an independent community (RC) in the 1980s. Depending on the needs of the individual, supported housing provides personalised and flexible services. Most people who move into supported housing remain there and are less likely to become hospitalised, and research shows that results from other outcomes are inconsistent.

Supported Employment

Supported employment (SE) is the most promising approach to vocational rehabilitation. The conceptualisation of SE was greatly influenced by the work of Deborah Becker and Robert Drake. As soon as possible, individuals are put in competitive employment by their preferences under their Individual Placement Model, and they get all the assistance required to keep their position. The assistance is given for an unlimited amount of time. Benefits of SE include non-vocational outcomes like enhanced relationships, self-worth, social integration, and control over substance misuse, as well as improved standard of living, cognition, and symptom control. Findings on SE are positive, but there are still a few significant issues that must be addressed. Many people in SE work part-time occupations that require little competence. Since most of the research only assessed brief follow-up times (12–18 months), the long-term effects are still unknown.

Supported Education

Like how supported housing and employment are provided to people with psychiatric impairments who pursue post-secondary education or training, supported education also adopts a rehabilitative approach by offering advocacy and support to clients (Farkas *et al.*, 2007).

Social Skills Training

Social skills training is most effective when the client's environment recognises and supports their transformed behaviour and when the learned skills are applied to their everyday life. This approach enhances community and social occupational performance and engagement (Lloyd & 2010). Unlike the immediate effects of medication, the benefits of skill training develop gradually. For favourable outcomes, long-term training is also necessary. It has been demonstrated that social skills training is generally beneficial for the development, maintenance, and application of skills in everyday life.

Child and Youth Interventions

Families and carers are examples of support networks that offer context-dependent learning in natural settings, which is crucial for recovering occupational competence. Programmes for family and carer intervention are successful in lowering relapse rates, enhancing psychosocial functioning, and reducing the burden on families. When carers have less social support and fewer coping tools, they frequently feel more burdened.

An OT works in a multi-disciplinary team to help young people maximize their independence in meaningful and purposeful activities identified by themselves, their families, or their carers. The OT provides support and advice to children and young people who have difficulty with daily activities and life roles. The primary goal is to assess both the individual and their environment to facilitate engagement in activities that hold significance for the young person. For example, an OT might work with a child with autism who finds it challenging to participate in classroom activities. By evaluating the classroom environment and the child's specific needs, the OT can suggest modifications such as sensory tools or seating arrangements. These changes help the child engage more effectively in their educational activities, improving their learning experience and overall well-being.

Interventions in Inpatient Services

Acute inpatient services aim to stabilise the mental state or reduce risks (Lloyd *et al.*, 2014). The OT collaborates with the client to devise and implement an intervention plan focusing on occupational goals. The OT typically supports the consumer with occupational and social goals as well as helps address presenting symptoms by working with other members of the multidisciplinary team, carers, and families.

Interventions in Community Mental Health Services

Consumers of mental health services typically have severe and complex mental health issues that significantly impact their daily function or quality of life. Interventions in community mental health services include medication management, occupational, social, and vocational support, psychosocial support, psychotherapies, and community interventions.

Individuals receiving mental health occupational therapy services often face severe and multifaceted mental health challenges that substantially affect their daily functioning and quality of life. Interventions in this field encompass a variety of approaches, including activity-based therapies, cognitive-behavioural techniques, social skills training, life skills development, environmental modifications, and psychoeducation. These interventions aim to support the individual's overall well-being and enhance their ability to participate meaningfully in daily activities.

Emerging and Future Mental Health Occupational Therapy Practice

The definition of health has changed over time. The current contemporary view is that health is no longer just the absence of disease but 'a complete state of physical, mental and social wellbeing and not merely the absence of disease or infirmity' (WHO, 1946). Current and future health professionals must recognise and develop a holistic understanding of how health and well-being are created, how people cope with illness, and how different health professions work together to shape the health and well-being of consumers (Keleher & Murphy, 2016).

Suggested Future Approaches

Approach	Possible OT Approach
Primary Health Care Approach	Occupational therapists must consider aiming to advance equity, access, empowerment, community self-determination, and intersectoral collaboration .
Determinants Approach	Occupational therapists must consider situating health and social problems in the broader social, structural, and cultural conditions of our society.
Health Promotion Approach	Occupational therapists to consider enabling people to increase control over and improve their health. Health promotion work is strongly influenced by the knowledge derived from the determinants of health approach.
Ecological Approach	Occupational therapists must consider the relationships between the health of the planet and the health of populations.
Population Health Approach	Occupational therapists must consider the dual purpose of improving the health of the entire population while targeting the reduction of health inequities among population groups .

(Table) cont....

Approach	Possible OT Approach
Indigenous Approaches	Occupational therapists must understand that one cannot separate health from life, social and spiritual relations, and the environment, particularly when working with Indigenous people and people from non-Western backgrounds.
Participatory Occupational Justice Framework	Occupational therapists must adopt an occupational justice lens when addressing social and occupational injustices related to participation in occupations.

Mental health practitioners need to focus on all these areas. Some specific examples of future and emerging areas of practice or interventions include:

- *Physical*: Increased focus on the development and promotion of physical health, including evidenced-based ways of promoting physical activity and other occupations to better physical health for consumers.
- *Mental*: increased focus on the development of new occupational therapy interventions, including those aimed at promoting cognitive functioning/cognitive rehabilitation *e.g.*, cognitive remediation.
- *Social*: A renewed focus on social determinants of health. Health is influenced by genetic, environmental, social, and political circumstances.
- *Wellbeing*: An increased focus on health promotion and public health. OTs will need to consider how they can consider and influence the broader social, economic, and political factors and the distribution of resources.

Occupational Justice

Research evidence suggests that occupational justice can be used to inform practice when that practice is about addressing occupational injustices (Malfitano *et al.*, 2019). Occupational justice is a concept used to describe situations where engagement in occupations is prevented, limited, or restricted to an individual or group (Wilcock & Townsend, 2000). Various other associated terms, such as occupational alienation, occupational imbalance, occupational marginalisation, and occupational apartheid, are described in occupational therapy literature (Malfitano *et al.*, 2019; Wilcock & Townsend, 2000). Addressing these injustices for at-risk individuals and populations such as refugees, migrants, prisoners, people in aged care facilities, and patients admitted to hospitals is needed. There are emerging frameworks that have been developed for occupational therapists to use when promoting occupational justice, such as the Participatory Occupational Justice Framework (POJF: Townsend & Wilcock, 2004; Whiteford & Townsend, 2011). There is potential for occupational therapy practice to be more informed by the POJF now and into the future.

The Dark Side of OT

Another focus must be on the 'dark occupations'. Occupational therapists need to consider how they will enable occupational performance when working with people who engage in what society regards as unhealthy, illegal, and/or deviant (Kiepek *et al.*, 2019). OTs will need to consider how they work with clients who have goals, some of which they might not personally agree with or support, such as those who engage in:

- Alcohol, tobacco, and other drug use
- Serial offending and criminal behaviour
- Sex work and prostitution
- Self-harm
- Graffiti, and
- War and war crimes.

Some of these clients may wish to continue to participate in these occupations. Occupational therapists need to understand that how occupations are defined is influenced by cultural identity and cultural context including social and cultural norms, expectations, law, and environment.

CONCLUSION

- There is an intrinsic connection between the domain and method of occupational therapy, which guides the decision-making process inherent in everyday mental health practice.
- Social and community functioning improves when the environment recognises and supports that changed behaviour, and the trained skills apply to the client's everyday life.
- The most effective vocational rehabilitation model is supported employment.
- The occupational therapist working with children and young people will offer support and advice to young people who are having difficulty in their daily activities and life roles.
- Mental health consumers have the same life aspirations as any other person in their society or culture.
- Occupational therapists must recognise and develop a holistic understanding of how health and well-being are created, how people cope with illness, and how different health professions work together to shape health and well-being.

REFERENCES

American Occupational Therapy Association. (2020). Occupational therapy practice framework: Domain and process (4th ed.). *American Journal of Occupational Therapy*

[http://dx.doi.org/10.5014/ajot.2020.74S2001]

Anthony, W.A., Cohen, M., Farkas, M., Gagne, C. (2002). *Psychiatric rehabilitation.* Boston University, Center for Psychiatric Rehabilitation.

Australian Institute of Health Welfare. (2022). *Mental health services in Australia.* Available from: https://www.aihw.gov.au/reports/mental-health-services/mental-health-services-in-australia.

Barbato, A., D'Avanzo, B. (2000). Family interventions in schizophrenia and related disorders: a critical review of clinical trials. *Acta Psychiatr. Scand., 102*(2), 81-97.
[http://dx.doi.org/10.1034/j.1600-0447.2000.102002081.x] [PMID: 10937780]

Bevitt, T., Isbel, S., Pereira, R.B., Bacon, R. (2022). Australian occupational therapists' perspectives of consumers authentically contributing to student learning during practice placements: 'It just makes sense!' but 'we need a process'. *Aust. Occup. Ther. J., 69*(6), 753-765.
[http://dx.doi.org/10.1111/1440-1630.12853] [PMID: 36372902]

Bond, G.R. (2004). Supported employment: evidence for an evidence-based practice. *Psychiatr. Rehabil. J., 27*(4), 345-359.
[http://dx.doi.org/10.2975/27.2004.345.359] [PMID: 15222147]

Christiansen, C.H., Bass, J., Baum, C.M. (2024). *Occupational therapy: Performance, participation, and well-being..* Taylor & Francis.
[http://dx.doi.org/10.4324/9781003522997]

Dallman, A.R., Williams, K.L., Villa, L. (2022). Neurodiversity-affirming practices are a moral imperative for occupational therapy. *Open J. Occup. Ther., 10*(2), 1-9.
[http://dx.doi.org/10.15453/2168-6408.1937]

Dirette, D.P. (2016). Personalized medicine and evidence-based practice: Merging the art and science of OT. *Open J. Occup. Ther., 4*(2), 1.
[http://dx.doi.org/10.15453/2168-6408.1269]

Egan, M., Restall, G. (2022). *Promoting occupational participation: Collaborative relationship-focused occupational therapy..* CAOT Publications.

Eklund, M., Orban, K., Argentzell, E., Bejerholm, U., Tjörnstrand, C., Erlandsson, L.K., Håkansson, C. (2017). The linkage between patterns of daily occupations and occupational balance: Applications within occupational science and occupational therapy practice. *Scand. J. Occup. Ther., 24*(1), 41-56.
[http://dx.doi.org/10.1080/11038128.2016.1224271] [PMID: 27575654]

Farkas, M., Anthony, W.A. (2010). Psychiatric rehabilitation interventions: A review. *Int. Rev. Psychiatry, 22*(2), 114-129.
[http://dx.doi.org/10.3109/09540261003730372] [PMID: 20504052]

Farkas, M., Jansen, M.A., Penk, W.E. (2007). Psychosocial rehabilitation: Approach of choice for those with serious mental illnesses. *J. Rehabil. Res. Dev., 44*(6), vii-xxi.
[http://dx.doi.org/10.1682/JRRD.2007.09.0143] [PMID: 18075935]

Fisher, A.G., Marterella, A. (2019). *Powerful practice: A model for authentic occupational therapy..* Center for Innovative OT Solutions, Inc..

Gray, J.M. (1998). Putting occupation into practice: occupation as ends, occupation as means. *Am. J. Occup. Ther., 52*(5), 354-364.
[http://dx.doi.org/10.5014/ajot.52.5.354] [PMID: 9588260]

Grove, B. (1994). Reform of mental health care in Europe. Progress and change in the last decade. *Br. J. Psychiatry, 165*(4), 431-433.
[http://dx.doi.org/10.1192/bjp.165.4.431] [PMID: 7804654]

Keleher, H., MacDougall, C. (2016). Concepts of health. In: Keleher, H., MacDougall, C., (Eds.), *Understanding health.* Oxford University Press.

Kiepek, N.C., Beagan, B., Rudman, D.L., Phelan, S. (2019). Silences around occupations framed as

unhealthy, illegal, and deviant. *J. Occup. Sci., 26*(3), 341-353.
[http://dx.doi.org/10.1080/14427591.2018.1499123]

Kopelowicz, A., Wallace, C.J., Liberman, R.P. (2007). Psychiatric rehabilitation. In: Gabbard, G.O., (Ed.), *Treatments of psychiatric disorders.* American Psychiatric Publishing.

Leufstadius, C., Eklund, M., Erlandsson, L.K. (2009). Meaningfulness in work – Experiences among employed individuals with persistent mental illness. *Work, 34*(1), 21-32.
[http://dx.doi.org/10.3233/WOR-2009-0899] [PMID: 19923673]

Leufstadius, C., Erlandsson, L.K., Eklund, M. (2006). Time use and daily activities in people with persistent mental illness. *Occup. Ther. Int., 13*(3), 123-141.
[http://dx.doi.org/10.1002/oti.207] [PMID: 16986774]

Liberman, R.P., Glynn, S., Blair, K.E., Ross, D., Marder, S.R. (2002). *in vitro* amplified skills training: promoting generalization of independent living skills for clients with schizophrenia. *Psychiatry, 65*(2), 137-155.
[http://dx.doi.org/10.1521/psyc.65.2.137.19931] [PMID: 12108138]

Liberman, R.P., Hilty, D.M., Drake, R.E., Tsang, H.W.H. (2001). Requirements for multidisciplinary teamwork in psychiatric rehabilitation. *Psychiatr. Serv., 52*(10), 1331-1342.
[http://dx.doi.org/10.1176/appi.ps.52.10.1331] [PMID: 11585949]

Lloyd, C., King, R., Machingura, T. (2014). An investigation into the effectiveness of sensory modulation in reducing seclusion within an acute mental health unit. *Adv. Ment. Health, 12*(2), 93-100.
[http://dx.doi.org/10.1080/18374905.2014.11081887]

Lloyd, C., Lee Williams, P. (2010). Occupational therapy in the modern adult acute mental health setting: a review of current practice. *Int. J. Ther. Rehabil., 17*(9), 483-493.
[http://dx.doi.org/10.12968/ijtr.2010.17.9.78038]

Malfitano, A. P. S., de Souza, R. G. da M., Townsend, E. A., Lopes, R. E. (2019). Do occupational justice concepts inform occupational therapists' practice? A scoping review. *Canadian Journal of Occupational Therapy (1939), 86*(4), 299-312.
[http://dx.doi.org/10.1177/0008417419833409]

Mitchell, R., Unsworth, C.A. (2005). Clinical reasoning during community health home visits: Expert and novice differences. *Br. J. Occup. Ther., 68*(5), 215-223.
[http://dx.doi.org/10.1177/030802260506800505]

Mueser, K.T., Bond, G.R., Drake, R.E., Resnick, S.G. (1998). Models of community care for severe mental illness: a review of research on case management. *Schizophr. Bull., 24*(1), 37-74.
[http://dx.doi.org/10.1093/oxfordjournals.schbul.a033314] [PMID: 9502546]

Onken, S.J., Dumont, J.M., Ridgway, P. Mental health recovery: what helps and what hinders? A national research project for the development of recovery facilitating system performance indicators. Available from: https://www.researchgate.net/publication/242469660.

Paterson, C.F. (2008). A short history of occupational therapy in psychiatry. In: Creek, J., Lougher, L., (Eds.), *Occupational therapy and mental health.* Churchill Livingstone.

Pereira, R.B., Whiteford, G., Hyett, N., Weekes, G., Di Tommaso, A., Naismith, J. (2020). Capabilities, Opportunities, Resources and Environments (CORE): Using the CORE approach for inclusive, occupation-centred practice. *Aust. Occup. Ther. J., 67*(2), 162-171.
[http://dx.doi.org/10.1111/1440-1630.12642] [PMID: 31957045]

Pereira, R.B., Whiteford, G.E. (2022). Enabling inclusive occupational therapy through the Capabilities, Opportunities, Resources and Environments (CORE) approach. In: Liamputtong, P., (Ed.), *Handbook of social inclusion: Research and practices in health and social sciences..* Cham: Springer.
[http://dx.doi.org/10.1007/978-3-030-89594-5_97]

Pereira, R.B., Whiteford, G.E. The Capabilities, Opportunities, Resources and Environments (CORE) approach for inclusive and occupation-centred practice. In: Ikiugu, M., Kantartzis, S., Taff, S., Pollard, N.,

(Eds.), *Theories, models, and concepts in occupational therapy: Foundations for sustaining the profession..* SLACK Inc.. In press
[http://dx.doi.org/10.4324/9781003526766-14]

Rebeiro, K.L. (1998). Occupation-as-means to mental health: A review of the literature, and a call for research. *Can. J. Occup. Ther., 65*(1), 12-19.
[http://dx.doi.org/10.1177/000841749806500102]

Roder, V., Zorn, P., Müller, D., Brenner, H.D. (2001). Improving recreational, residential, and vocational outcomes for patients with schizophrenia. *Psychiatr. Serv., 52*(11), 1439-1441.
[http://dx.doi.org/10.1176/appi.ps.52.11.1439] [PMID: 11684737]

Rog, D.J. (2004). The evidence on supported housing. *Psychiatr. Rehabil. J., 27*(4), 334-344.
[http://dx.doi.org/10.2975/27.2004.334.344] [PMID: 15222146]

Rüesch, P., Graf, J., Meyer, P.C., Rössler, W., Hell, D. (2004). Occupation, social support and quality of life in persons with schizophrenic or affective disorders. *Soc. Psychiatry Psychiatr. Epidemiol., 39*(9), 686-694.
[http://dx.doi.org/10.1007/s00127-004-0812-y] [PMID: 15672288]

Rüsch, N., Angermeyer, M.C., Corrigan, P.W. (2005). Mental illness stigma: Concepts, consequences, and initiatives to reduce stigma. *Eur. Psychiatry, 20*(8), 529-539.
[http://dx.doi.org/10.1016/j.eurpsy.2005.04.004] [PMID: 16171984]

Salyers, M.P., Becker, D.R., Drake, R.E., Torrey, W.C., Wyzik, P.F. (2004). A ten-year follow-up of a supported employment program. *Psychiatr. Serv., 55*(3), 302-308.
[http://dx.doi.org/10.1176/appi.ps.55.3.302] [PMID: 15001732]

Schell, B.A.B., Gillen, G. (2019). *Willard & Spackman's occupational therapy.* Wolters Kluwer.

Townsend, E., Polatajko, H. (2007). *Enabling occupation II: Advancing an occupational therapy vision for health, well-being & justice through occupation..* CAOT Publications.

Townsend, E., Wilcock, A.A. (2004). Occupational justice and client-centred practice: a dialogue in progress. *Can. J. Occup. Ther., 71*(2), 75-87.
[http://dx.doi.org/10.1177/000841740407100203] [PMID: 15152723]

Unsworth, C., Baker, A. (2016). A systematic review of professional reasoning literature in occupational therapy. *Br. J. Occup. Ther., 79*(1), 5-16.
[http://dx.doi.org/10.1177/0308022615599994]

Whiteford, G. (2000). Occupational deprivation: Global challenge in the new millennium. *Br. J. Occup. Ther., 63*(5), 200-204.
[http://dx.doi.org/10.1177/030802260006300503]

Whiteford, G., Townsend, E. (2011). Participatory occupational justice framework (POJF 2010): Enabling occupational participation and inclusion. *Towards an Ecology of Occupation-Based Practices* In F. Kronenberg, N. Pollard & D. Sakellariou (Eds.), Occupational therapies without borders. London, UK: Elsevier..

Whiteford, G., Jones, K., Weekes, G., Ndlovu, N., Long, C., Perkes, D., Brindle, S. (2020). Combatting occupational deprivation and advancing occupational justice in institutional settings: Using a practice-based enquiry approach for service transformation. *Br. J. Occup. Ther., 83*(1), 52-61.
[http://dx.doi.org/10.1177/0308022619865223]

Wilcock, A.A. (1999). Reflections on doing, being and becoming. *Aust. Occup. Ther. J., 46*(1), 1-11.
[http://dx.doi.org/10.1046/j.1440-1630.1999.00174.x]

Williams, P.L., Lloyd, C. (2012). Social skills and employment. In: King, R., Lloyd, C., Meehan, T., Deane, F.P., Kavanagh, D.J., (Eds.), *Manual of psychosocial rehabilitation.* John Wiley & Sons, Ltd..
[http://dx.doi.org/10.1002/9781118702703.ch11]

World Federation of Occupational Therapists. (2024). List of member organisations. Available from: https://wfot.org/membership/organisational-membership/list-of-wfot-member-organisations.

World Health Organization *International Classification of Functioning, Disability and Health (ICF)..* Geneva: World Health Organization.

World Health Organization. (2021). *Comprehensive Mental Health Action Plan 2013–2030..* Geneva: World Health Organization.

World Health Organization. (1946). *Preamble to the Constitution of the World Health Organization as adopted by the International Health Conference.*New York, NY: World Health Organisation..

CHAPTER 10

Psychosocial Interventions

Tawanda Machingura[1,*] and **Last Machingura**[2]

¹ Head of Discipline Occupational Therapy Program, University of Notre Dame Australia, Sydney, Australia

² Occupational Therapist, Unworthy Therapeutic Services, Cape Town, South Africa

Abstract: This chapter offers a thorough examination of psychosocial therapies used in occupational therapy, with an emphasis on cognitive behavioural therapy (CBT), acceptance and commitment therapy (ACT), and family therapy. Giving readers a thorough grasp of these strategies and how to use them in occupational therapy practice is the main goal. This chapter explores the theoretical underpinnings, guiding principles, and practical applications of each intervention through the lens of evidence-based practice, emphasising the intervention's applicability in resolving a range of psychosocial issues that people encounter in their lives. The chapter emphasizes the holistic approach to client care by clarifying the integration of psychosocial therapies with the scope of occupational therapy, drawing on recent research and clinical experiences.

Drawing on current research and clinical insights, the chapter elucidates the integration of psychosocial interventions within the scope of occupational therapy, emphasizing the holistic approach to client care. Special attention is given to the role of occupational therapists in facilitating meaningful engagement and participation in daily activities through the implementation of tailored interventions.

Practical case examples and vignettes are employed throughout the chapter to illustrate the application of psychosocial interventions in real-world occupational therapy contexts. By the conclusion of this chapter, readers will not only gain a nuanced understanding of key psychosocial interventions but also develop the necessary skills to critically evaluate and select evidence-based approaches in their clinical practice.

Keywords: Acceptance and commitment therapy (ACT), Cognitive behaviour therapy (CBT), Family therapy, Occupational therapy, Psychosocial interventions.

INTRODUCTION TO COGNITIVE BEHAVIOUR THERAPY

CBT is a form of "talk therapy" that helps patients manage problems by changing their relationships with their thoughts and opening the way for behavioural alter-

---
* **Corresponding author Tawanda Machingura:** Head of Discipline Occupational Therapy Program, University of Notre Dame Australia, Sydney, Australia; E-mail: tawanda.machingura@nd.edu.au

natives. A variety of issues, such as depression, anxiety disorders, issues with alcohol and drugs, marital issues, eating disorders, and other serious mental illnesses, have been shown to respond well to cognitive behavioral therapy (CBT), a type of psychological treatment (Gajecki *et al.*, 2014).

CBT is aligned with occupational therapy practice in many ways. Firstly, it is a short-term, goal-oriented treatment that takes a hands-on, practical approach to problem-solving as the tenet of most occupation-based interventions. Secondly, CBT is present-focused and acknowledges the role of learned patterns of thought and behaviour. This is similar to occupational therapy practice, where the OT would explore the past, present, and future occupations and occupational patterns to assist the client with present and future occupational engagement.

Origins

CBT emerged in the 1950s and 1960s. CBT was developed by Aaron T Beck and Albert Allis. It has its roots in psycho-analytic psychotherapy and behaviour therapy. It is a highly effective strategy for dealing with many psychological problems. CBT offers a theoretical framework to comprehend how people's perceptions of their experiences might contribute to the emergence and perpetuation of psychological disorders like depression and anxiety.

Key Features

The main tenet of CBT is that thoughts, feelings (physical sensations and emotions), and behaviours are interrelated. What we THINK affects how we act and feel (THOUGHTS). What we DO affects how we think and feel (BEHAVIOUR). How we FEEL affects what we think and do (EMOTIONS). This is often referred to as the Cognitive Triad, which is shown in Fig. (**1**) below.

Thoughts include:

- Thoughts about self
- About others
- About our partners/family/friends
- About our colleagues
- About our work
- About our clients

Thoughts are important contributors to our lens on the world. CBT provides techniques to interrupt the automatic patterns that keep patients in destructive and often self-defeating cycles.

The therapist uses this approach by identifying and modifying cognitive distortions as important goals of treatment. The therapist helps a patient to critically examine whether their response to a situation is justified. CBT is not about replacing negative thinking with positive thinking. Rather, CBT is a problem-solving process. The focus of treatment is on how problems are being maintained in the present and how different symptoms interact with each other. CBT allows clients to break patterns and substitute them with helpful alternatives. This cognitive triad is shown in Fig. (**1**) below.

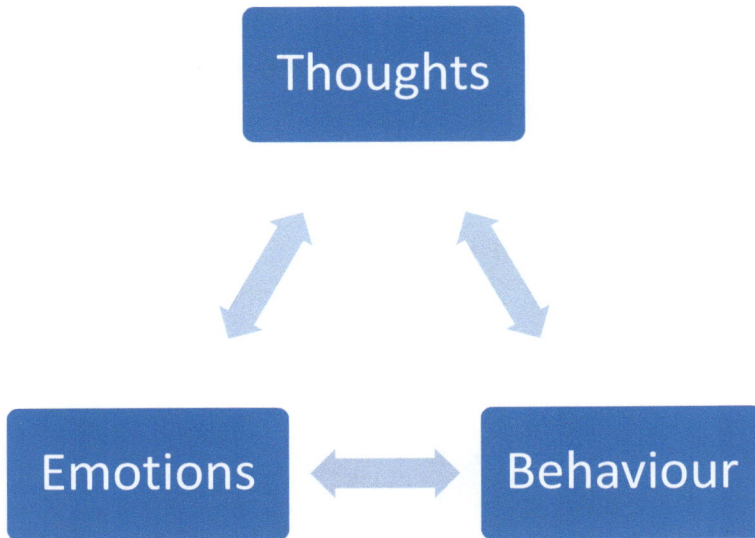

Fig. (1). Cognitive Triad.

CBT is defined precisely and has a structure that is followed by practitioners:

- Time-limited (set number of sessions)
- Operational manual
- Set agenda at the beginning of each session
- Clients are given homework
- Use of standardised measures

CBT requires high levels of collaboration between practitioner and client.

General Process

The CBT process generally involves establishing rapport and then working sequentially with the client to identify, challenge, and substitute unhelpful thoughts, as shown in Fig. (**2**) below.

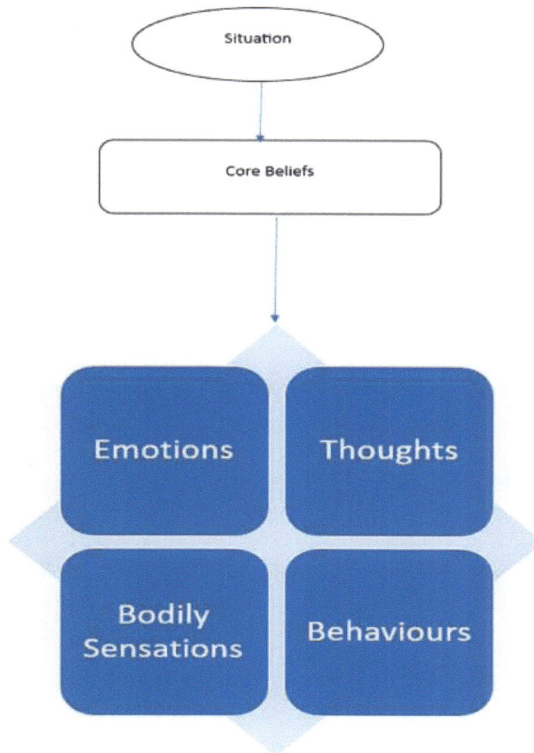

Fig. (2). CBT General Process.

There are certain assumptions in using this approach:

Assumption 1: There are mental belief systems or schemas that represent established ways of seeing ourselves and the world. These are influenced by cognitive distortions or unhelpful thinking styles, which include:

- Filtering
- Polarised thinking
- Overgeneralisation
- Jumping to conclusions
- Catastrophising
- Personalisation
- Control Fallacies
- Fairness fallacy
- Blaming
- Should and musts

- Emotional reasoning
- Fallacy of change
- Global labelling
- Always being right
- Heaven's reward

Assumption: Cognitions (thoughts, beliefs, and images that people's minds contain) have an impact on emotions, behaviour, and physical symptoms. An example of this would be:

Situation: You wave at an acquaintance, and they carry on walking without acknowledging you.

Thought A: What have I done wrong, and why are they not fond of me?

Thought B: They appear distracted; I wonder what's bothering them.

CBT Strategies

Put simply, we first take note of the thought and associated feeling and identify the distortion by questioning our own thoughts *e.g.*, where is the evidence? Is there an alternate point of view? What happens when I believe this thought? And what happens when I open to alternatives?

Fig. (**3**) below shows these beliefs in a Belief Driven Formulation flow chart.

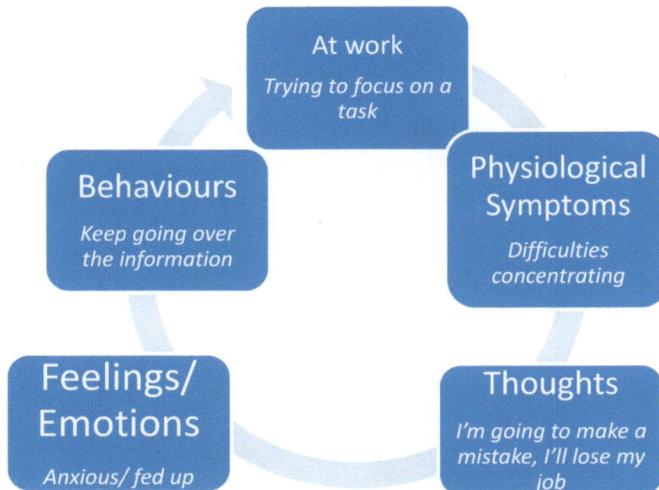

At work
Trying to focus on a task

Physiological Symptoms
Difficulties concentrating

Thoughts
I'm going to make a mistake, I'll lose my job

Feelings/ Emotions
Anxious/ fed up

Behaviours
Keep going over the information

Fig. (3). Belief Driven Formulation.

CBT with Depression and Anxiety

Fig. (4) below shows an example of a maintenance cycle for someone who is struggling to keep a job:

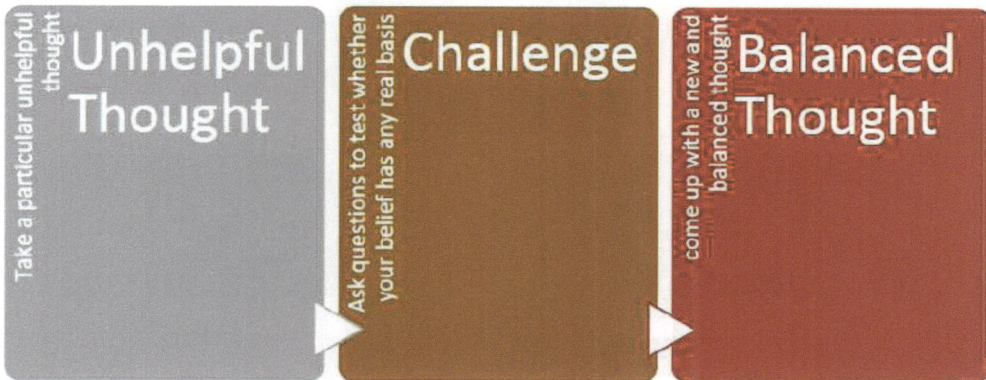

Fig. (4). Maintenance cycle.

Thought Diary

Thought diaries are used to help the client break a problematic maintenance cycle. These are very visual and useful tools when using CBT in practice. An example of this would be:

Situation: At work, you made a mix-up with one of your appointments.

Thought: I'm rubbish at my job.

Another example of this would be:

Thought B: You were supposed to go shopping with your partner but couldn't make it, so they went alone.

These two examples are mentioned in Table **1** below:

Table 1. Thought Diary

Date	situation	emotion	Negative thought
Mon 2 june	*At work, I made a mix-up with one of my appointments*	*Anxious 6/10 Down 7/10*	*I'm rubbish at my job*
Tues 9 june	*Supposed to go shopping with my partner but couldn't make it so they went alone*	*Miserable 8/10 Anxious 5/10*	*I'm a bad partner/spouse*

Challenging Unhelpful Thoughts

The process for challenging unhelpful thoughts is shown in Fig. (**5**) below.

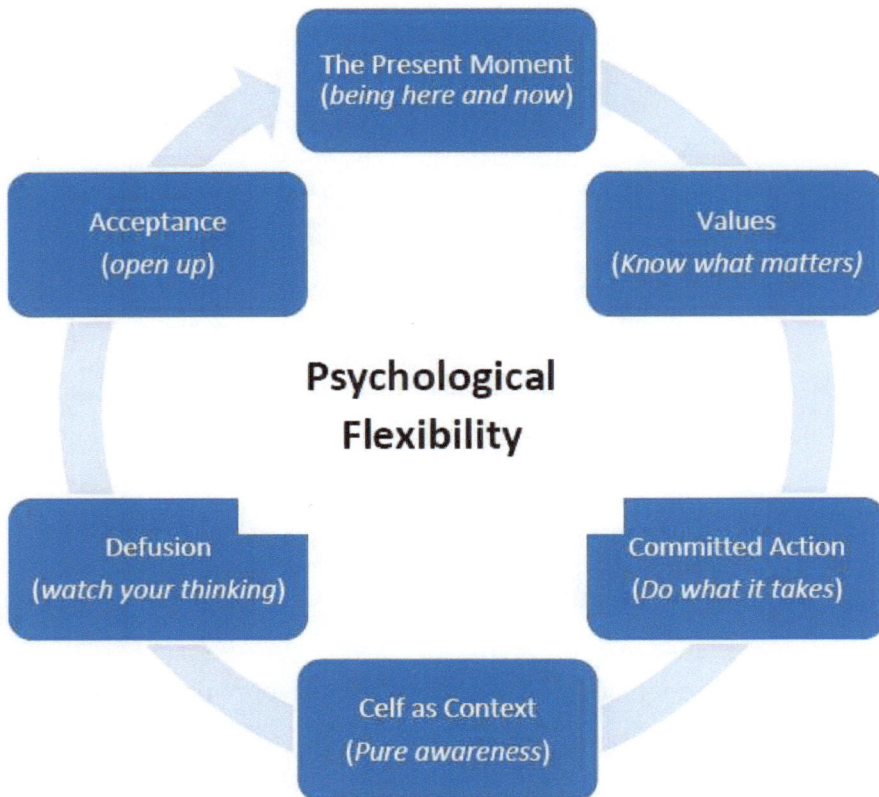

Fig. (5). Challenging unhelpful thoughts.

Case Study

Tara (35), a physical education teacher, injured her back at a school ski camp in July 2017. After ignoring the injury for several weeks, hoping the pain would subside, Tara followed medical advice and had surgery to repair the bulging disc.

Tara is currently on a four-weeks leave and will return to work on restricted duties later in the year. Tara separated from her husband in January this year and shares custody of her son, Panashe (11).

Tara has struggled with a restriction of movement following the surgery and reports symptoms of depression and anxiety in a severe range. She reports feeling very low and is reluctant to leave the house on the days when her son is staying with his father.

Commenced occupational therapy but has not been engaging in recommended activities at home. Motivation is low.

What **thoughts** might Tara be having?

- I'm not coping; I'm old and unattractive; I'm going to lose my job; even my son prefers to be with his dad; my friends are bored with me; I'll never get back to normal.

What **Emotions** might Tara be having?

- Lonely, afraid, sad, angry, irritable, anxious/worried, guilty, resentful

What **feelings** might Tara be having?

- Overwhelming fatigue, stomachaches, headaches, tears, agitation, sleeping difficulties

What **behaviours** might Tara be displaying?

- Stay at home, watch television, eat junk food, write angry letters to ex-husband, drink alcohol with pain medication

Mindfulness CBT

Reflect

- How much of your time is spent thinking about the past?
- What are these thoughts?
- How much of your time is spent thinking about the future?
- What are these thoughts?
- How much of your time is spent in the present moment?

Mindfulness = A mental state achieved by focusing one's awareness on the present moment while calmly acknowledging and accepting one's feelings, thoughts, and bodily sensations

Acceptance Commitment Therapy

According to Levin *et al.* (2020), the main objective of Acceptance and Commitment Therapy (ACT) is to improve psychological flexibility, which is the capacity to act in a way that is consistent with one's values even in the face of negative thoughts and emotions and to be mindful of experiences in the present moment in a way that is accepting and nonjudgmental. The focus is on acceptance of thoughts as opposed to deliberating challenging thoughts, recognising the struggle that occurs as we attempt to "control our thoughts", extensive use of metaphors, diffusion techniques, and value identification and alignment to promote value-guided action. Through six main phases of change, acceptance and commitment therapy (ACT) seeks to reduce suffering and promote well-being (Gloster *et al.*, 2020).

The main stages of ACT are summarised in the figure below.

Knowledge Check

1. What is the goal of CBT?
2. Name and provide two examples of cognitive distortions.
3. What is the major difference between traditional CBT and ACT?
4. How might these approaches be useful to you in your work with clients?

Family Therapy

Origins

It was developed by Murray Bowen (1913-1990). It is based on the theory of human behaviour that views the family as an emotional unit. The therapy uses a systems approach to understanding psychological well-being. This therapy is based on the assumption that any change in a system will be predictably followed by reciprocal changes in others within the system. Any psychotherapeutic endeavour that specifically focuses on changing interactions between or among family members and aims to enhance the functioning of the family as a whole, its subsystems, and/or the individual family members can be referred to as family therapy (Cottrell & Boston, 2002). From the standpoint of systems theory, interdependence fosters the unity and cooperation needed by families to provide food, shelter, and security for their members. However, conflicts, particularly anxiety-provoking ones, can exacerbate the mechanisms that sustain harmony and collaboration while upending the family structure. The overall goal is to help the family become experts to help themselves without the need for professional experts.

Key Features

Anxiety

From a systems perspective, anxiety, in particular, is a function of groups. Anxiety is the most contagious of emotions, and as anxiety goes up, the emotional connectedness of family members becomes more stressful than comforting. Eventually, if the anxiety persists, one or more family members feel overwhelmed, isolated, or out of control, and the system begins to respond.

Over Functioning

One member of the family takes on too much responsibility, becomes controlling, knows what is best for everyone, often seeks solutions without perspective, and becomes highly active, anxious, and agitated.

Under Functioning

In response to anxiety, a person lets go of responsibility, which can be observed in chronic lateness, neglecting responsibilities, addiction, and disconnection.

Triangles

A triangle is a system of relationships between three people. As the strain shifts across the three connections, a triangle can have far more tension than a two-person relationship. Tension might spread to other interlocking triangles if it is too high. A person's behaviour in a triangle show how hard they are working to maintain their emotional ties to other people. Triangles can exert social control by putting one on the outside or bringing in an outsider when tension escalates between the two. Increasing the number of triangles can help stabilise the spreading tension.

Differentiation of Self

Individuals who lack self-differentiation rely on other people's acceptance and approval. To live up to others' expectations, they immediately modify their thoughts and words. When faced with disagreement, criticism, or rejection, those who have a well-differentiated self can remain composed and unflappable despite acknowledging their need for others.

Nuclear Family Processes

Systems theory purports that extended or heightened family strife may contribute to the emergence of clinical problems or symptoms. The more anxiety one person or one relationship absorbs, the less anxiety other individuals need to absorb.

There are four basic relationship patterns

• Marital conflict

• Dysfunction in one spouse

• Impairment of one or more children

• Emotional distance

Family Projection Processes

A projection process may affect a child or children's functioning and make them more susceptible to clinical symptoms.

• Parents focus on a child out of fear that something is wrong with the child.
• Parents interpret the child's behaviour as confirming the fear.
• Parents treat the child as if something is wrong with the child.

Multigenerational Processes

It explains how minute variations in the degree of distinction between parents and children create patterns of responding among members of a multigenerational family. Levels of differentiation can affect longevity, marital stability, reproduction, health, educational accomplishments, and success. Highly differentiated people generally have stable nuclear families. People who are poorly differentiated typically lead more chaotic or turbulent personal lives and rely more on others to support them.

Emotional Cut-off

Family members may manage unresolved issues by cutting off emotional contact. In this case, problems remain dormant and unresolved.

Examples Unresolved Attachments

• When at home, the person feels more like a child and seeks his parents to make choices for him that he is capable of making on his own.
• When interacting with parents, the person experiences shame and feels obligated to resolve their problems or disagreements.
• The person feels aggrieved that his parents or peers do not seem to comprehend or approve of him.

Sibling Position

Sibling order is associated with specific characteristics. Oldest children gravitate toward leadership positions and assume more responsibility. The youngest children like to follow. Children in the middle age group acquire traits from both positions. Some traits are complementing rather than "better" than others.

Societal Emotional Process

Every idea in Bowen's theory is relevant to nonfamily groups as well as organisations. Individuals respond within groups to anxiety in the environment, and this can lead to a regression of functioning. Anxiety in one member can overwhelm the entire system.

How does Family Therapy work?

In cases when members of a family structure are emotionally entwined, altering the family structure will also need altering the associated mental and emotional processes. According to a behaviorist viewpoint, each family member's behaviors either facilitate or obstruct the others', and each person's actions ultimately impact the homeostasis of the family. In family therapy, the therapist plays an impartial role in helping the family come to a decision on their own by posing open-ended questions and promoting candid conversation that results in solutions.

Case Study

Manu, a 24-year-old woman, goes to her family therapist for help because her family is still dysfunctional. Her father's drinking and abuse during her childhood created an abusive home environment that had a lasting effect on her and her family's relationships. The complexity of Manu's familial relationships is explored in this case study, which also looks at family triangles, sibling positions, and family process concerns.

Background: Her father's drunkenness and violent conduct cast a shadow over Manu's upbringing. The ramifications of her father's actions are evident, even if it is unknown how much abuse Manu and her mother, Lilian, endured. In reaction to her father's actions, Manu and her mother created an alliance triangle. The family dynamics were further shaped by this partnership, which was used as a coping mechanism to deal with the difficulties her father's actions presented.

Case Study Analysis

A number of dysfunctions arise in Manu's family as a result of the family triangle and multigenerational elements. Relationship tensions and complex power relations resulted from the family's rift caused by George, the abusive dad. Manu's coalition building within the family system, which affects communication styles and conflict resolution techniques, is exemplified by her alliance with her mother against her father.

In this case study, Manu does not have siblings; however, the relationships would have been made more complex by the placement of siblings inside the family. Because of how each of her siblings would have responded differently to their father's actions, Manu's relationship with her siblings will be characterised by differing degrees of intimacy and rivalry. These sibling dynamics will then contribute to the complexity of family interactions and impact Manu's sense of belonging and support within the family unit.

Intervention

A thorough therapy strategy is necessary to address the complex issues that Manu and her family are facing. A framework for investigating and comprehending the fundamental dynamics of the dysfunctions in the family system is provided by family therapy. Family therapy seeks to improve coping mechanisms, address Gorge's alcoholism and related emotional dysregulation, and encourage healthier relational patterns through psychoeducation, training in communication skills, and examination of family roles and limits.

Consequent to family therapy, the following parallel processes are encouraged: Manu is recommended individual therapy as it gives her a place to go through her experiences, deal with symptoms associated with trauma, and strengthen her resilience. Her early traumas may lead to dysfunctional thought patterns and coping methods that cognitive behavioural therapy (CBT) may help her with. George is recommended an alcohol rehabilitation programme to assist him with a range of skills needed to maintain a sober lifestyle and improve interpersonal skills.

CONCLUSION

In conclusion, this chapter offers a comprehensive exploration of psychosocial therapies within the framework of occupational therapy, focusing on key modalities such as cognitive behavioral therapy (CBT), acceptance and commitment therapy (ACT), and family therapy. Readers are given an understanding of the adaptability and effectiveness of these interventions in addressing a range of psychological difficulties through a blend of theoretical underpinnings, guiding principles, and practical implementations. Integrating theory with practical application empowers practitioners to deliver holistic, client-centered care that promotes optimal functioning and quality of life.

REFERENCES

Arbesman, M., Bazyk, S., Nochajski, S.M. (2013). Systematic review of occupational therapy and mental health promotion, prevention, and intervention for children and youth. *Am. J. Occup. Ther., 67*(6), e120-e130.
[http://dx.doi.org/10.5014/ajot.2013.008359] [PMID: 24195907]

Barrowclough, C., Tarrier, N., Lewis, S., Sellwood, W., Mainwaring, J., Quinn, J., Hamlin, C. (1999). Randomised controlled effectiveness trial of a needs-based psychosocial intervention service for carers of people with schizophrenia. *Br. J. Psychiatry, 174*(6), 505-511.
[http://dx.doi.org/10.1192/bjp.174.6.505] [PMID: 10616628]

Barrowclough, C., Johnston, M., Tarrier, N. (1994). Attributions, expressed emotion, and patient relapse: An attributional model of relatives' response to schizophrenic illness. *Behav. Ther., 25*(1), 67-88.
[http://dx.doi.org/10.1016/S0005-7894(05)80146-7]

Barrowclough, C., Parle, M. (1997). Appraisal, psychological adjustment and expressed emotion in relatives of patients suffering from schizophrenia. *Br. J. Psychiatry, 171*(1), 26-30.
[http://dx.doi.org/10.1192/bjp.171.1.26] [PMID: 9328490]

Brown, J. (2020). Engaging with Parents in Child and Adolescent Mental Health Services. *Aust. N. Z. J. Fam. Ther., 41*(2), 145-160.
[http://dx.doi.org/10.1002/anzf.1409]

Cottrell, D., Boston, P. (2002). Practitioner Review: The effectiveness of systemic family therapy for children and adolescents. *J. Child Psychol. Psychiatry, 43*(5), 573-586.
[http://dx.doi.org/10.1111/1469-7610.00047] [PMID: 12120854]

Falkov, A. (2004). Talking with children whose parents experience mental illness. *Children of Parents With A Mental Illness: Personal And Clinical Perspectives.* Cowling V, editors. Camberwell, Vic: The Australian Council For Educational Research Ltd (ACER);.

Falloon, I. R., McGill, C. W., Boyd, J. L., & Pederson, J. (1987). Family management in the prevention of morbidity of schizophrenia: social outcome of a two-year longitudinal study. Psychological medicine, 17(1), 59-66.

Gajecki, M., Berman, A.H., Sinadinovic, K., Andersson, C., Ljótsson, B., Hedman, E., Rück, C., Lindefors, N. (2014). Effects of baseline problematic alcohol and drug use on internet-based cognitive behavioral therapy outcomes for depression, panic disorder and social anxiety disorder. *PLoS One, 9*(8), e104615.
[http://dx.doi.org/10.1371/journal.pone.0104615] [PMID: 25122509]

Haine-Schlagel, R., Walsh, N.E. (2015). A review of parent participation engagement in child and family mental health treatment. *Clin. Child Fam. Psychol. Rev., 18*(2), 133-150.
[http://dx.doi.org/10.1007/s10567-015-0182-x] [PMID: 25726421]

Healthdirect. (2021). Mental Health and Wellbeing. Available from: https://www.healthdirect.gov.au/mental-health-and-wellbeing.

Hosman, C. (2005). Prevention of Mental Disorders: Effective Interventions And Policy Options. *The Prevention of Mental Disorders: Effective Interventions And Policy Options, 2004..* Oxford: Oxford University Press.

Kieling, C., Baker-Henningham, H., Belfer, M., Conti, G., Ertem, I., Omigbodun, O., Rohde, L.A., Srinath, S., Ulkuer, N., Rahman, A. (2011). Child and adolescent mental health worldwide: evidence for action. *Lancet, 378*(9801), 1515-1525.
[http://dx.doi.org/10.1016/S0140-6736(11)60827-1] [PMID: 22008427]

Levin, M.E., Krafft, J., Hicks, E.T., Pierce, B., Twohig, M.P. (2020). A randomized dismantling trial of the open and engaged components of acceptance and commitment therapy in an online intervention for distressed college students. *Behav. Res. Ther., 126*, 103557.
[http://dx.doi.org/10.1016/j.brat.2020.103557] [PMID: 32014692]

MacDonald, K., Fainman-Adelman, N., Anderson, K.K., Iyer, S.N. (2018). Pathways to mental health services for young people: a systematic review. *Soc. Psychiatry Psychiatr. Epidemiol., 53*(10), 1005-1038. [http://dx.doi.org/10.1007/s00127-018-1578-y] [PMID: 30136192]

Nardella, M. S., Carson, N. E., Colucci, C. N., Corsilles-Sy, C., Hissong, A. N., Simmons, D., Taff, S. D., Amin-Arsala, T., DeAngelis, T., Fitzcharles, D., Grajo, L. C., Higgins, S., Gray, J. M., Stoll, M., Harvison, N. (2018). Importance of collaborative occupational therapist-occupational therapy assistant intraprofessional education in occupational therapy curricula. *The American Journal of Occupational Therapy, 72*((Supplement_2)) [http://dx.doi.org/10.5014/ajot.2018.72S207]

Queensland Government, (2021). *Children's Health Queensland Hospital and Health Service.* Available from: https://www.childrens.health.qld.gov.au/service-mental-health-community-clinics/.

Reardon, T., Harvey, K., Baranowska, M., O'Brien, D., Smith, L., Creswell, C. (2017). What do parents perceive are the barriers and facilitators to accessing psychological treatment for mental health problems in children and adolescents? A systematic review of qualitative and quantitative studies. *Eur. Child Adolesc. Psychiatry, 26*(6), 623-647. [http://dx.doi.org/10.1007/s00787-016-0930-6] [PMID: 28054223]

Remschmidt, H., Belfer, M. (2005). Mental health care for children and adolescents worldwide: a review. *World Psychiatry, 4*(3), 147-153. [PMID: 16633533]

Tarrier, N., Barrowclough, C., Porceddu, K., Fitzpatrick, E. (1994). The Salford Family Intervention Project: relapse rates of schizophrenia at five and eight years. *Br. J. Psychiatry, 165*(6), 829-832. [http://dx.doi.org/10.1192/bjp.165.6.829] [PMID: 7881788]

Tarrier, N., Barrowclough, C., Vaughn, C., Bamrah, J.S., Porceddu, K., Watts, S., Freeman, H. (1988). The community management of schizophrenia. A controlled trial of a behavioural intervention with families to reduce relapse. *Br. J. Psychiatry, 153*(4), 532-542. [http://dx.doi.org/10.1192/bjp.153.4.532] [PMID: 3074860]

Victorian Dept of Human services (2008). *Working Together with Families and carers.* Available from: http://www.health.vic.gov.au/mentalhealth/cpg.

Waid, J., Kelly, M. (2020). Supporting family engagement with child and adolescent mental health services: A scoping review. *Health Soc. Care Community, 28*(5), 1333-1342. [http://dx.doi.org/10.1111/hsc.12947] [PMID: 31951087]

World Health Organisation (WHO), (2021). *Adolescent Mental Health.* Available from: https://www.who.int/news-room/fact-sheets/detail/adolescent-mental-health.

Young, E., Green, L., Goldfarb, R., Hollamby, K., Milligan, K. (2020). Caring for children with mental health or developmental and behavioural disorders: Perspectives of family health teams on roles and barriers to care. *Can. Fam. Physician, 66*(10), 750-757. [PMID: 33077456]

CHAPTER 11

Leisure

Jessica Levick[1,*] and **Stewart Alford**[1]

[1] *School of Health Sciences, University of Southern Queensland, Occupational Therapy Program Ipswich, Queensland, Australia*

Abstract: Leisure is a powerful therapeutic modality that can build meaning and purpose for consumers, particularly those who have mental health issues. When acutely unwell, it can be challenging to engage in productive activities or understand cognitive-based interventions; therefore, leisure is an opportunity to build graded engagement. This chapter explores leisure as an evidence-based therapeutic modality in occupational therapy.

A brief history of leisure and how this has been incorporated in leisure or recreation settings is explored to provide context for Australia's current mental health system. A number of leisure theories are explored and applied to a mental health context, including the flourishing model, salutogenesis, serious leisure, and resilience. Furthermore, prominent leisure theory is then applied to occupational therapy theory to provide an occupational therapy focussed lens to the broader scope of leisure that could be utilised by multiple disciplines.

With the consideration of theory and occupational therapy, a number of informal and formal assessment strategies are explored with a specific spotlight on participation, satisfaction, and boredom in leisure. Utilisation of leisure as a therapeutic intervention is explored based on mental health contexts such as inpatient, rehabilitation, and community settings.

Finally, evidence-based recommendations are suggested to implement leisure in therapeutic services, such as inpatient and community settings. Occupational therapists can improve occupational engagement and performance by using occupation as an opportunity to explore, assess, and build meaningful engagement.

Keywords: Activity, Assessment, Community, Diversional therapy, Inpatient, Intervention, Hope, Leisure, Meaningful occupation, Multidisciplinary team, Occupational enrichment, Recovery, Recreation therapy, Salutogenesis, Therapeutic recreation, Volition.

* **Corresponding author Jessica Levick:** School of Health Sciences, University of Southern Queensland, Occupational Therapy Program Ipswich, Queensland, Australia; E-mail: Jessica.Levick@unisq.edu.au

Tawanda Machingura (Ed.)

INTRODUCTION

Leisure is one of the four key domains of occupation (including rest, self-care, and productivity) (American Occupational Therapy Association, 2020). Leisure is an important part of a person's occupational profile, which can provide meaning and purpose to life. In mental health, leisure can be harnessed as a powerful therapeutic modality that facilitates meaningful engagement in an occupation that is conducive to recovery from severe and complex mental health issues. At times, engagement in occupation can be challenging for those with mental health conditions such as schizophrenia. There are a number of complexities that impact someone's ability to participate in an occupation, such as medication side effects (sedation and metabolic issues), volition, and reduced occupational opportunity. In occupational therapy, the core focus of therapy is to enhance occupational performance.

Leisure engagement should be carefully considered an important aspect of an individual's occupational profile (Townsend & Stanton, 2002). As part of the occupational therapy process, a person's daily activities, including leisure, should be considered (Townsend & Stanton, 2002). This starts with understanding their occupational profile, assessing their current skills or abilities through task analysis, and exploring their occupational performance issues (Townsend & Stanton, 2002). Each domain of occupation can then be considered when planning interventions, providing an intervention, and exploring outcome measures to effectively understand improvement in occupational performance. By identifying meaningful occupations, interventions can be tailored to the individual making the approach to therapy truly person-centred (Townsend & Stanton, 2002).

Understanding the link between participation, engagement, and interests is more predictive of subjective well-being compared to purely considering the number of leisure activities people choose to engage in (Schulz *et al.*, 2018). This consideration is reminiscent of core occupational therapy practice and particular models such as the Canadian Model of Occupational Performance and Engagement (CMOP-E) and the Model of Human Occupation (MOHO) (Craik, 2009; Forsyth & Kielhofner, 2003). There are several reasons that people choose to participate in leisure activities, which include support for mental health, balance between occupations, improved physical health (such as strength and fitness), increased social connections, and support for self-esteem and confidence (Caldwell, 2005).

In mental health settings, leisure can be used as a powerful therapeutic modality to support meaningful engagement and build a sense of purpose. Leisure can also support the facilitation of treatment goals, assessment of function and cognition, and building a therapeutic alliance. Particularly in mental health settings, consumers are often found to be bored and sedentary. In public health settings, there are limited leisure activities offered, and often, consumers have limited occupational opportunities to engage in activities that form part of their occupational profile.

This chapter will explore the use of leisure and recreation as an evidence-based therapeutic modality. Furthermore, this chapter will explore shared ideas about the use of leisure and recreation in mental health settings by an occupational therapist and recreation therapist.

This chapter will define leisure and provide context to the application of leisure in mental health settings and a brief overview of the history of occupational therapy and mental health. It will discuss the key stakeholders involved in leisure participation, evidence-informed ways to assess leisure participation, and the contexts leisure can be used in.

History of Leisure

Leisure activity has always been a key domain of occupational therapy practice (Craik & Pieris, 2006; Iwasaki *et al.*, 2014; Shaw, 1985; Suto, 1998). Humans innately participate in activities and find opportunities to bring meaning or purpose to their engagement (Wilcock, 1995). Over time, occupations have been classed into categories, which provides a dearth of understanding of how individuals participate in activity (Wilcock, 1995). As society evolves and changes, our engagement in occupations does as well.

Over the past 100 years, there has been a paradigm shift in the way leisure is viewed by the general population and how people engage in leisure activities. In modern society, there is a higher emphasis on the importance of participating in leisure activities for 'self-care' or well-being, making activity prioritised as part of regular routine and self-identity (Christiansen, 1999). Leisure can also be considered salutogenic, a concept where participation in an activity is health-creating and health-promoting (Caldwell, 2005). Previously, leisure was defined as any activity that was not productivity (work) or rest (sleeping), grouping **instrumental activities of daily living (IADL)** such as laundry or meal preparation and leisure (or play) together. In the 1850s, during the gold rush in Australia, the average workday shifted from 12 hours per day, 6 days per week, with a strong emphasis on productivity, IDAL, and self-care to the '8-8-8' campaign, which introduced unionism and the importance of **occupational balance** (Christiansen & Matuska, 2006; Whiteford, 2000).

In the last 50 years, there has been significant technological advancement that has changed the way in which people participate in occupation and improved efficiencies for IADL. Some examples of these technological advancements include the washing machine, which has reduced the time taken to hand wash garments, and the dishwasher, which has increased individuals' ability to participate in more meaningful occupations such as leisure or recreation (Aguiar & Hurst, 2007). Another technological advancement that has contributed to an increase in engagement is the development of smartphones, which has imprinted new demands on our time and blurred the classic distinctionbetween work and leisure (Wijesinghe, 2017). On the other hand, new activities, such as video games or social media, may be a trending or prominent activity in a person's occupational profile, whilst others, such as hand embroidery, may become more niche due to industrialism and advancement in technology.

Leisure

The term leisure is a common term used in occupational therapy jargon. Within occupational therapy, a core belief held by the profession is that human beings are occupational beings (Farnworth, 1998; Wilcock, 1998). **Leisure** can be defined as *a chosen activity, conducted individually or as a group in the spare time that is not work-related, which can be enjoyable, relaxing, and/or fun and can support the creation of personal health and well-being* (Levick *et al.*, 2022).

Leisure activity will change over the lifetime and will look different in each category (Fig. **1**). An activity that an infant will participate in may evolve through childhood and adolescence into adulthood; however, this is not always the case. Some leisure activities may cease during childhood and adolescence, such as team sports or computer games, as an individual's interests evolve and they do not have the same occupational opportunities, or they are no longer motivated to participate. Regardless of the length of participation, leisure activities can be enjoyable to participate in and can build a sense of accomplishment, which assists in forming an identity. Often, people will associate their sense of self or spirituality with their occupational engagement. An example of this could be an individual who has participated in long-distance running throughout childhood and adolescence and now identifies themselves as a 'runner' in adulthood.

The form of an occupation, such as leisure, can be changed based on who is participating in the activity. For example, reading in solitude in your living room is different from reading to a group of small children. The level of engagement, interest, and satisfaction may be different. Similarly, having a coffee quietly on your patio on a Sunday morning by yourself is different from drinking a coffee with a friend socially at a busy café. This is an important consideration when contextualising an individual's interest in participating in an activity and the social networks that are available to engage in the occupation with them. For someone who has a high level of internal stimuli (such as auditory hallucinations), a busy café environment may be distressing and overstimulating.

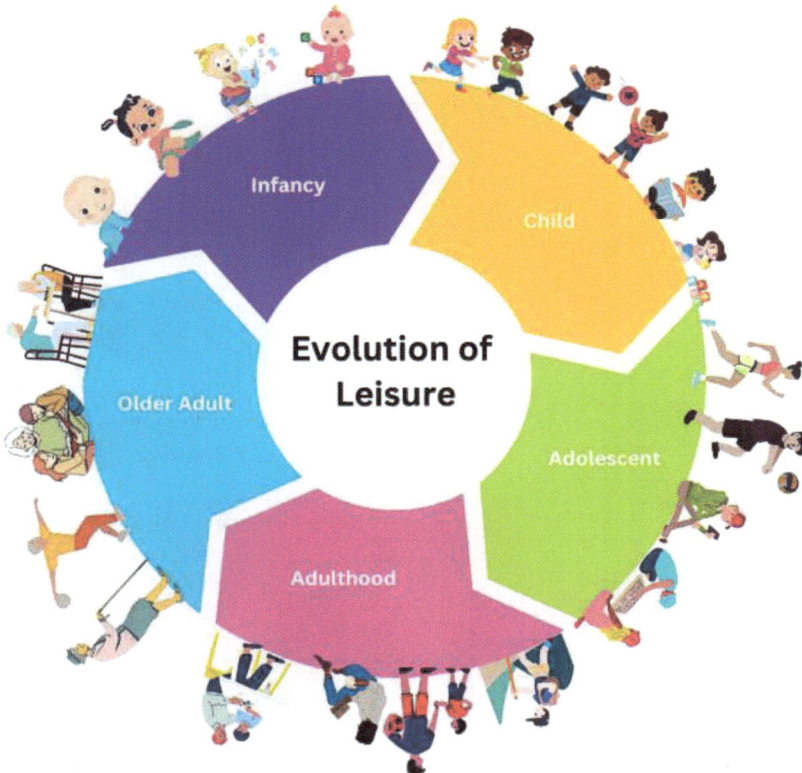

Fig. (1). The evolution of leisure activity across the lifespan.

The Mental Health Context

A Brief History

To understand how to utilise leisure as a therapeutic modality in contemporary mental health practice, it is important to understand the evolution of occupational therapists over the past 100 years (Fig. **2**). Mental health institutions or asylums were locked clinical settings where people were incarcerated for issues or conditions that impacted their ability to function in society (Cusick & Bye, 2021). The first asylum in Australia was founded in 1811, called Castle Hill in Victoria (Parkinson, 1981). It was created to accommodate Irish convicts who arrived by boat during the European settlement (Parkinson, 1981). These conditions included mental health and behavioural, physical, or emotional issues. People who were admitted to institutions in Australia had varied physical health issues, including infectious diseases such as tuberculosis or measles, developmental delays including intellectual impairment, brain injury, and alcohol and drug issues. Mental health issues commonly include hysteria or grief, homosexuality, psychotic disorders, delusions, depression, and mania (Brunton & McGeorge, 2017; Lewis & Garton, 2017).

Timeline of Occupational Therapy in Australia

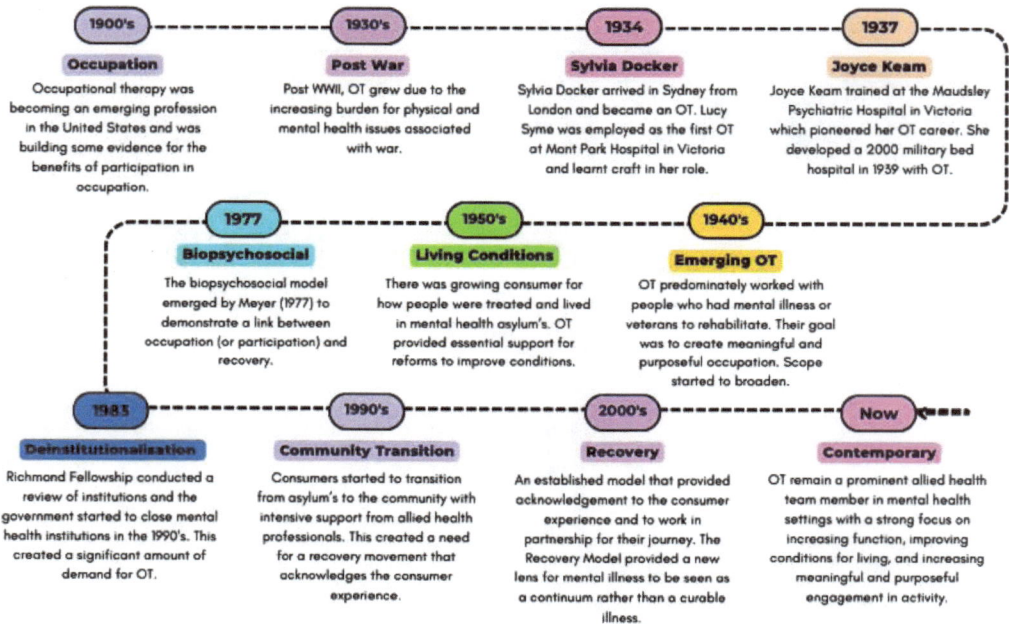

1900's — Occupation
Occupational therapy was becoming an emerging profession in the United States and was building some evidence for the benefits of participation in occupation.

1930's — Post War
Post WWII, OT grew due to the increasing burden for physical and mental health issues associated with war.

1934 — Sylvia Docker
Sylvia Docker arrived in Sydney from London and became an OT. Lucy Syme was employed as the first OT at Mont Park Hospital in Victoria and learnt craft in her role.

1937 — Joyce Keam
Joyce Keam trained at the Maudsley Psychiatric Hospital in Victoria which pioneered her OT career. She developed a 2000 military bed hospital in 1939 with OT.

1977 — Biopsychosocial
The biopsychosocial model emerged by Meyer (1977) to demonstrate a link between occupation (or participation) and recovery.

1950's — Living Conditions
There was growing consumer for how people were treated and lived in mental health asylum's. OT provided essential support for reforms to improve conditions.

1940's — Emerging OT
OT predominately worked with people who had mental illness or veterans to rehabilitate. Their goal was to create meaningful and purposeful occupation. Scope started to broaden.

1985 — Deinstitutionalisation
Richmond Fellowship conducted a review of institutions and the government started to close mental health institutions in the 1990's. This created a significant amount of demand for OT.

1990's — Community Transition
Consumers started to transition from asylum's to the community with intensive support from allied health professionals. This created a need for a recovery movement that acknowledges the consumer experience.

2000's — Recovery
An established model that provided acknowledgement to the consumer experience and to work in partnership for their journey. The Recovery Model provided a new lens for mental illness to be seen as a continuum rather than a curable illness.

Now — Contemporary
OT remain a prominent allied health team member in mental health settings with a strong focus on increasing function, improving conditions for living, and increasing meaningful and purposeful engagement in activity.

Fig. (2). A brief timeline of occupational therapy in Australia within mental health settings.

Mental health asylums, which were renamed to mental health institutions and then later hospitals, were typically simple environments with limited visual stimulation. Most institutions had set routines for consumers to participate in, including self-care, laundry, cleaning, and meals (Cusick & Bye, 2021). A combination of leisure and productive occupations was used to fill most consumer's days with activities such as farming, handicrafts, basket weaving, leather work, building, gardening, and sewing (Fig. **3**).

(Cusick & Bye, 2021).

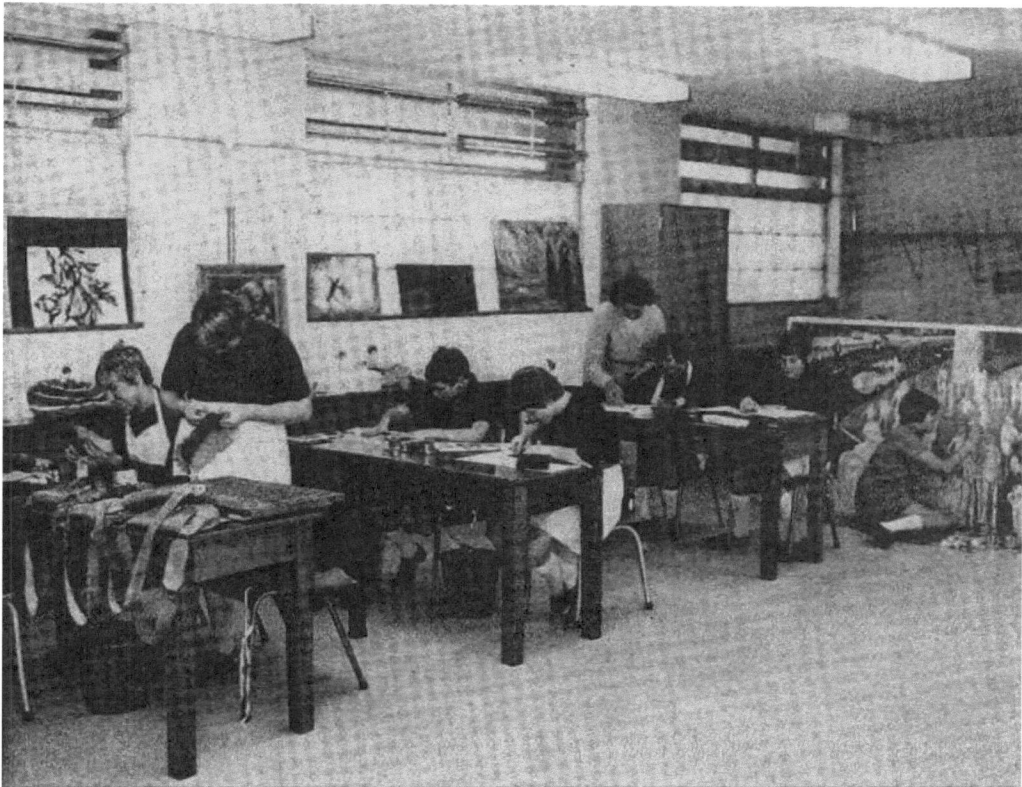

Creative art and craft activities have been expanded following the opening of the new instruction block at the Training School for Girls, Parramatta

Fig. (3). Image of girls engaging in arts and crafts, Training School for Girls, Parramatta (State of New South Wales, 1970). Image sourced from Find and Connect and is free for sharing under creative commons.

Occupational therapy emerged as a profession in the early 1940's post World War II, after there was an increased need for physical and mental health rehabilitation. Occupational therapists typically worked with veterans or mental health consumers in asylums during this time. In the 1950s-1960s, the treatment of consumers in asylums was spotlighted, and there was a growing concern for the conditions people were living under. Some of the concerns included understaffing, overworking, overcrowding, poor treatment of consumers that was considered inhumane, and a lack of adequate facilities. Occupational therapy provided an essential role in the reforms to introduce a change in conditions for consumers who were living in such institutions. During this time, occupational therapists were planning treatment, understanding how to interpret evidence and research, and implementing occupations that consumers could use, such as arts, crafts, and trades.

Deinstitutionalisation started to occur across Australia in the 1960s due to the growing concern for the conditions people were living under. There were a number of private organisations that attempted to support people leaving the institutions with shared accommodation and additional support from members of the community. Governments started to look into the claims that there was a concern for the treatment of the mentally ill and intellectually disabled, which resulted in a report from Richmond Fellowship (Dunlop & Pols, 2022). The theory emerged from Meyer (1977) on the use of a biopsychosocial model, which is still used today, to demonstrate a link between occupation and recovery. Following the Richmond Report published in 1983, institutions started to close in the 1990s, and community-based treatment became the priority for the care of people with mental and emotional issues (Dunlop & Pols, 2022).

Since the 1990s, consumers have started to transition into community settings and required intensive support to adjust to their new living circumstances. This created cause for the need to acknowledge consumer's experience of mental illness and work in partnership with their experience. The recovery model provided a needed framework that is used in Australia to explore consumers' experience of their mental illness as a continuum and journey rather than a permanent and incurable illness as previously viewed (Bonney & Stickley, 2008). Occupational therapists have remained key members of multidisciplinary teams in mental health contexts to this day.

Recovery

Mental health and mental illness throughout the ages have been quite perplexing to greater society, as has been the treatment of mental illness. Historically, mental illness was treated in institutions that were purpose-built to provide treatment and accommodation to individuals with a lived experience of mental illness (Cusick & Bye, 2021). Stigma surrounding mental illness in the greater community, however, facilitated high levels of growth in these facilities, becoming the normal treatment environment for a range of developmental, psychological, and neurodegenerative illnesses, as well as many cases of purposeful misdiagnosis related to any range of interpersonal and familiar issues (unwanted pregnancy, rebellious attitude, *etc.*). Society at the time subscribed to the ideology of out of sight, out of mind.

Leisure in these facilities was a key element of the care provided with a range of other activities. The ideology is that growth can and will occur through a range of mediums. Historically, in these bigger institutions, individuals with a lived experience of mental illness had an array of leisure and recreational options that they could engage in, from sports such as cricket and rugby to occupational pursuits such as farming, cooking, and woodwork. These facilities often played host to community dances, trivia, and movie nights.

More recently, there have been efforts to deinstitutionalise the care of individuals with a lived experience of mental illness due to the poor treatment outcomes and inhumane treatment of the individuals with a lived experience who resided in these facilities instead of treating these individuals in the community (Dunlop & Pols, 2022). Whilst many benefits have been seen from this move to deinstitutionalisation, one negative aspect is the lack of therapeutic opportunity now afforded to individuals in the community with their lives somewhat void of supported leisure opportunities.

Leisure can be used as a therapeutic modality for meaningful engagement, fostering hope, improving motivation, encouraging participation, and providing an opportunity for recovery. In Australia, the National Recovery Framework is used to guide practice (Commonwealth of Australia, 2013).

Leisure Theory

There are several theories in leisure that provide a unique perspective. Theories about leisure have been generated from several professions, including occupational therapy and occupational science, recreation theory, diversional therapy, tourism and recreation, public health, and academia, to name a few. Occupational therapy has historically explored other theories and incorporated relevant and supporting theories into our practice. Theories external to occupational therapy have been further explored. These theorems include the Flourishing Model, Salutogenesis, Serious Leisure, Self-determination, and Resilience.

Flourishing Model

Anderson and Heyne (2012) extended the earlier established leisure wellbeing model of therapeutic recreation practice initially theorised by Carruthers and Hood (2007). This model emphasises the importance of leisure activities in promoting personal well-being, happiness, and overall flourishing in an individual's life, with Anderson and Heyne (2012) extending this to more holistically include the array of environmental or contextual factors that contribute to an individual's wellbeing and also impact on an individual's leisure participation, leisure choices, and previous leisure exposure.

The premiss of this theory is that leisure activities, when approached intentionally and meaningfully, can significantly contribute to an individual's overall well-being and flourishing (Anderson & Heyne, 2012; Carruthers & Hood, 2007). Specifically, leisure activities have inherent benefits to each individual who participates. These benefits can be categorised in one or more of the following well-being domains: leisure, cognitive, physical, spiritual, social, psychological, and emotional. Flourishing here refers to a state of optimal well-being and life satisfaction, encompassing more than just the absence of negative experiences; rather, it represents a positive and fulfilling life punctuated by the various domains of well-being (Carruthers & Hood, 2007). Importantly within this theory is the identification of the role of the therapist -to support the individual in developing strengths and resources in these leisure-well-being domains through leisure activities that will ultimately enhance the individual's experience of leisure and the benefits of well-being (Carruthers & Hood, 2007).

Salutogenesis

Salutogenesis has been used as a predominant theoretical framework in public health, which suggests that engagement in occupation can be health-promoting and health-creating, which enhances overall well-being (Lindström & Eriksson, 2005; World Health Organization, 1986). It is suggested that health should be viewed along a continuum with multiple factors that contribute to well-being, not only the incidence of disease. The application of the movement to leisure is understood that it is a deliberate and planned activity that is purposeful and beneficial to overall health and well-being.

Occupational science supports the notion that engagement in meaningful and purposeful occupation can be health-promoting (Tinsley & Eldredge, 1995). In more recent times, there has been a large social movement through social media to promote 'self-care', which typically refers to engaging in activities that improve your well-being, such as journalling, meditation, and exercise (World Health Organization, 2020). The recent global pandemic of COVID-19 has urged people to consider their own sense of well-being and explore their **occupational balance.** From an occupational therapy perspective, this is the act of participating in a meaningful leisure activity that can contribute to your well-being (or a salutogenic activity) (Caldwell, 2005). There are a number of occupations that people can participate in to relax that do not necessarily promote health and well-being, such as substance abuse; this would not be considered a salutogenic activity (Twinley, 2012).

Serious Leisure

A leisure theory with controversial perspectives is called 'Serious Leisure'. **Serious Leisure** can be defined as a methodical pursuit of a hobbyist or amateur or a volunteer activity that individuals find so meaningful and interesting that they pursue a walk of life centred on acquiring and expressing the specific skills, knowledge, and experience associated with the leisure medium (Stebbins, 2020). Serious leisure can be broken into three categories: serious, project-based, and casual leisure. Serious leisure originally emerged decades ago by Robert Stebbins (Stebbins, 1982). This theory does not belong to occupational therapy but will be explored from an occupational therapy lens.

Serious leisure has multiple differentiating factors from the traditional views of occupational therapy, which suggest that engagement in occupation promotes meaning, contributes to identity, and builds a sense of purpose for individuals. Participation in leisure activities, regardless of how frequent, contributes to an individual's occupational performance and function. The notion of serious leisure leading to wilful employment or a career prospect can be viewed in the category of productivity, where an occupation is participating for the sake of employment.

Table 1. The key categories of serious leisure

Category	Types of Leisure		Differentiating Qualities
Casual	Play Relaxation / Mindfulness Entertainment (passive and active) Socialising Sensory stimulation Volunteering Enjoyable aerobic activity		1. Not substantial engagement 2. Does not lead to a potential career or employability. 3. Does not require training or education to participate. 4. Immediate satisfaction and perceived reward 5. Hedonic in nature 6. Brief or short-lived 7. Can be sporadic or dull
Project-based			
Serious	Amateur	Science Sport Arts Entertaining	1. Have the prospect of a career or monetary income. 2. Requires perseverance and dedication. 3.
	Volunteering		
	Hobbyist	Collecting Handy-crafts or self-made Not competitive	

Self-determination

Self-determination is viewed as one of the most essential rights related to health outcomes (La Guardia & La Guardia, 2017). In particular, individuals with a lived experience of mental illness experience a level of restriction on their levels of self-determination and autonomy that has huge implications for their ongoing recovery and entrenches elements of learned helplessness, service dependency, and overall disadvantage. **Self-determination** can be defined as both the power and act of making a decision free from influence or coercion (Ryan & Deci, 2017). Self-determined individuals have authorship over their thoughts, behaviour, actions, and choices. This contrasts with the thwarting environments individuals with mental illness find themselves in, with pressures to conform to social norms, comply with treatment directives, and agree to therapeutic interventions they may not agree with.

Self-determination theory, proposed by Deci & Ryan (1985), is a theory that highlights how individuals experience self-determination and, importantly, what elements influence self-determination, self-determined motivation, and autonomy within an individual's life. These elements, termed 'basic psychological needs', are proposed to be moderators in how an individual experiences self-determination. The specifics of a leisure intervention can influence an individual's basic psychological needs and, in turn, self-determination. The therapist is able to titrate the specific elements of the leisure intervention to support the individual's experience and potential outcomes. For example, in a recreation camp context, basic psychological needs support has been seen to influence self-determination among a range of other inherent benefits (Alford *et al.*, 2021).

Table 2. Table. of elements for 'basic psychological terms' adapted from Ryan & Deci (2017)

Autonomy	Autonomy relates to the aspects of choice and perceived control within an individual's behaviour
Competence	Competence relates to the feeling of or ability to complete something efficiently
Relatedness	Relatedness is defined as a need to feel connected to others

There have been various studies that have affirmed basic psychological needs support within healthcare environments. Important for occupational therapists is the understanding of these basic psychological needs and how they interplay with an individual's self-determination and how both environments and interventions can be modified to enhance the support of an individual's basic psychological needs. In mental health cohorts, enhanced self-determination through basic psychological needs support has been linked to recovery outcomes such as resilience (Alford *et al.*, 2021; Perlman *et al.*, 2018), improved mood (Ng *et al.*, 2012), and quality of life (La Guardia & La Guardia, 2017; Ng *et al.*, 2012).

Resilience

Resilience has gained contemporary status recently due to its versatility as an umbrella term aligning with many of the outcomes of value within the well-being industry. However, its most basic premise is that individuals experience stress and adversity (disruption) and respond (reintegrate) in various ways: dysfunctional, with loss, back to homeostasis, and resiliently (*i.e.*, having grown in some way, shape, or form due to the experience) (Richardson *et al.*, 1990).

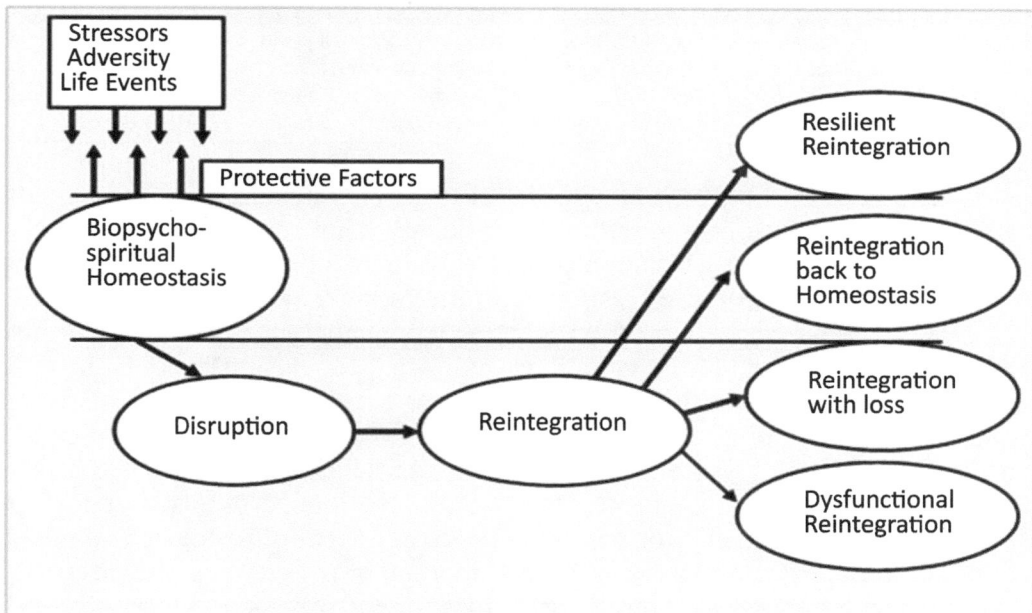

Fig. (3). A diagram of the Resiliency Model from Richardson, Neiger, and Jensen (1990).

Resilience is defined as an individual's ability to cope with significant challenge/s and adversity in life (Rutter, 2000). Resilience theory, over time, has become more complex and is seen as a skill, energy, and outcome. Resilience is considered a standard human response that matures within many of the typical developmental processes throughout life (Lopez & Snyder, 2009). Many of these developmental processes, however, are lacking or inherently challenging within the lives of individuals with a lived experience of mental illness (*i.e.*, experiences of schooling, family life, puberty, and leisure). The viewpoint of resilience presented below aligns with the three waves of intellectual inquiry within resilience research (Richardson, 2002).

Table 3. Key terms associated with resilience

Skill - traits and environmental characteristics that allow individuals to overcome adversity.	Resilience can be considered a specific skill or skillset used and/or refined within the process of responding to significant stress/adversity (Patterson, 2002).
Energy - the internal processes related to stress, adversity, and coping.	A resilient response requires the innate energy to achieve a result that surpasses the pre-adversity state of biopsycho-spiritual homeostasis with growth. This energy is supported and thwarted by life's pressures and supporters influencing an individual's ability to cope (Masten & Obradović, 2006).
Outcome - how individuals grow and are transformed following adverse events.	The capacity to respond to adversity in a positive manner and to experience growth and other outcomes, such as skills development, improved coping, and development of mental resolve/toughness, is understood to be within every individual (Rutter, 2023).

A key moderator in the development of resilience is exposure to an individually challenging experience or a variety of individually challenging experiences that can cultivate resilience. Leisure provides this level of individual challenging essential for the cultivation of resilience in a relatively safe way (Alford *et al.*, 2021). These experiences in a leisure context can challenge an individual with a lived experience of mental illness with learnings that can be applied outside of the leisure context; for example, exposure to a pro-social leisure activity such as tenpin bowling may promote the development of social skills and social coping that can be utilised in subsequent social environments that many with a lived experience find challenging in day to day life. Resilience, whilst not focused within occupational therapy, offers much in terms of the influence environments individuals come from, and their individual journey of recovery can be influenced by occupational therapists in their interventions.

Within OT, different theoretical perspectives can be taken to support individuals with their recovery journey. Working in multidisciplinary teams, different key players can support individuals to participate in leisure activities.

Key Players in Leisure

There are a number of disciplines that are involved in healthcare teams. Whether they are described as a multidisciplinary team or an allied health team, the key stakeholders all play an important part in delivering recovery-oriented care. This includes the delivery of leisure activities (Levick *et al.*, 2022). Members of the multidisciplinary team include nurses, recreation therapists, occupational therapists, social workers, psychologists, psychiatrists, peer-support workers, and sometimes speech pathologists (paediatric settings). Each member of the team provides a unique lens to providing care, but all should be responsible for the delivery of leisure activities to provide evidence-based care (Levick *et al.*, 2022).

Some health professionals believe that leisure activity is the responsibility of a recreational therapist or diversional therapist. Others suggest that leisure is the responsibility of the occupational therapist.

There are multiple key members of the multidisciplinary team who are responsible for the facilitation of activity in mental health inpatient units and in the community. A key aspect of improving mental health for consumers is engaging in activity that is salutogenic. This is a shared perspective in health and is typically adopted by the entire team. Typically, members of the multidisciplinary team will attribute participation in any occupation as the occupational therapists or recreation/diversional therapists' role. This is a false assumption but is very common. At times, there can be challenges in the multidisciplinary team to bring the individual theories and perspectives of professions together. Particularly in inpatient settings, all members of the multidisciplinary team can use leisure as a therapeutic means to increase motivation, build interest, and build a therapeutic alliance. The differentiation for occupational therapists is harnessing leisure as a means to assess and utilise as a key means of therapy to support or facilitate engagement.

Assessing Leisure Interests

Occupation is at the centre of occupational therapy practice. This is often lost with prescriptive modalities rather than recovery-oriented care (Coffey *et al.*, 2019). Even though each client may not achieve occupational balance, leisure is an important consideration within therapeutic modalities. Leisure activity can be utilised in any therapeutic context as an opportunity to discuss lifestyle choices, balance, roles, and habits. Leisure activity can be assessed through informal discussion, standardised assessment tools, or semi-structured interviews. An **informal discussion**is where a therapist may explore a consumer's engagement, interests, and current participation in leisure activity. Naturally, assessing and understanding leisure engagement lead to leisure education. To support the facilitation of leisure, therapists can ask leisure-focussed questions to expand on this area of occupation, such as:

- What does a typical weekday look like for you from the time you wake up to the time you go to bed? What does a typical weekend day look like?
- What do you typically like to do in your free or spare time?

- What activities do you like to do to enjoy yourself?
- What activities do you like to do that are relaxing?
- What do you like to do to unwind or take your mind off of things that worry you?
- Have you done activities in the past that you enjoyed but do not do anymore? What are those activities? Why do you not engage in these activities anymore?
- How much of your day do you relax or do activities you enjoy versus working or spending time doing chores? Are you happy with this, or would you like to change this?
- What activities do you do regularly that contribute to improving your health and wellbeing? Tell me about them.

Another way of exploring a consumer's leisure interest is through **standardised assessment tools**. A standardised assessment is an evidence-based formal tool that has evidence of validity and reliability with a particular cohort. Standardised tools are a repeatable measure that aims to assess a person's function and ability to participate in occupations. Within the profession of occupational therapy, there are several discipline-specific and generic assessments that therapists can utilise in their assessment and formulation.

There are several evidence-based tools that can assess leisure engagement. Some of the sub-domains that are assessed in these tools include boredom, satisfaction, leisure preferences, and performance capacities (see Table **4**). Tools can be an effective way to measure a person's volition, skills, and abilities to participate in a desired occupation and to explore new interests that can assist with the development of goals. Some tools require specialised training to conduct with a consumer.

The importance of assessing leisure interests can be to provide a baseline of understanding for the person's current function, participation, satisfaction, and interests in their current occupational profile. This can support to develop goals and provide essential information to the multidisciplinary team about a person's ability to cope within the community.

Leisure as an Intervention

Engaging in leisure for specific outcome/s has only recently developed recognition for its potential health-related benefits (Stumbo *et al.*, 2015; Thomsen *et al.*, 2018). Leisure is being modified and implemented within various clinical and semi-clinical environments with varying impacts internationally (Békési *et al.*, 2011; Hildebrand & Smith, 2017; Litwiller *et al.*, 2016; Thomsen *et al.*, 2018). In North America and Canada, the clinical/professional identity of purposeful leisure is called Therapeutic Recreation [TR], which encompasses the concept, modality, and profession (American Therapeutic Recreation Association, 2023; Canadian Therapeutic Recreation Association, 2023). **Therapeutic Recreation** is defined as a systematic process that employs leisure and other activity-based interventions to address the assessed needs of individuals with illnesses and/or disabling conditions, as a means to enhance psychological and physical health, recovery, and well-being (American Therapeutic Recreation Association, 2023).

Table 4. Standardised and non-standardised tools that assess performance capacities and interests in leisure

Name of Tool	Purpose	Target Population	Format / Testing Area	Duration	Completed by
Participation					
Children's Assessment of Participation and Enjoyment (CAPE) (King *et al.*, 2000)	To understand a child or adolescent's level of participation and enjoyment in selected typical daily activities (this does not include productivity).	Children and adolescents between the ages of 6 to 21 years of age. Participants are cognitively required to sort and categorise/organise.	Self-administered: Children review 55 images of activities and are asked to identify their participation level on a 5-point Likert scale in the past 4 months (this includes have you engaged in this activity, how often, level of enjoyment, with who). Interview-assisted: Children sort and rate activities based on the 5-point Likert scale with a parent or carer. The therapist will then ask the same questions as above.	Typically takes 25 to 30 minutes to complete.	Completed during an interview with a child or independently by the adolescent.
Leisure Participation Assessment Tool for the Elderly (Jeong *et al.*, 2020)	To explore leisure participation, which will support treatment planning for community-based activities.	Older adults (65 years and above) for people with Korean heritage.	81 items with 8 major categories of occupation. Satisfaction and interest are rated based on a 10-point Likert scale. Participation is measured on a 5-point Likert scale.	Not specified.	Self-reported questionnaire.

(Table 4) cont.....

Name of Tool	Purpose	Target Population	Format / Testing Area	Duration	Completed by
Idyll Arbor Leisure Battery (LIM, LAM, LMS, LSM) (Botner-Marigold & Miller, 2007)	To assess a broad range of an individual's leisure abilities. These tools can be used to understand barriers to engagement and support the development of treatment goals.	For adolescents and adults over the age of 12. Also suitable for those with an IQ above 80.	LAM includes 36 items. LIM includes 29 items. LMS includes 48 items. LSM includes 24 items.	LAM, LIM, LSM, and LMS typically take between 5 to 25 minutes to complete.	Self-reported questionnaire.
Leisure Boredom Scale (Iso-Ahola & Weissinger, 1990)	To assess and understand individuals' perspective of boredom they experience based on their leisure opportunities.	Youth and young adults	16 items that include a 5-point Likert scale. 1 indicates no boredom, and 5 indicates a high level of boredom.	Typically takes 10-15 minutes to complete.	Self-reported questionnaire.
Leisure Competence Measure (Kloseck *et al.*, 1996)	Supports to evaluate an individual's leisure function or ability to participate and the changes that occur over time.	Adults and Older Adults	Eight subscales, including leisure awareness, leisure attitude, leisure skills, cultural/social behaviours, interpersonal skills, community integration skills, social contact, and community participation. It includes observation, interviews, and consumer records.	Typically takes 1 hour to complete. There is a manual available.	Completed by therapist.
Satisfaction					
Leisure Satisfaction Scale (Di Bona, 2000)	To understand if an individual is satisfied in their current participation in leisure activities.	General population	Two types of tests: Original version is 51 items with a 5-point Likert scale. Short form is 24 items with 6 subscales.	Short form: Typically takes 10-15 minutes to complete.	Self-reported questionnaire.
Interests					

Name of Tool	Purpose	Target Population	Format / Testing Area	Duration	Completed by
Activity Card Sort (ACS) (Katz *et al.*, 2003)	To provide a range of activity options to adults to support with treatment planning and goal development.	Adults and older adults with or without cognitive issues. Originally targeted at older adults with Alzheimer's.	80 instrumental, leisure, and social activity cards with pictures or photographs. The client is required to place the cards into 5 groups (1. I have never done, 2. I have not done as an adult, 3. I do this now, 4. I don't do this as much, 5. I don't do this now or I gave up).	Typically takes 20 minutes to complete.	Completed by the consumer.
Paediatric Card Sort (PACS) (Mandich *et al.*, 2004)	To explore a child's current interest and engagement in activities. This tool can also be used to develop goals and target interventions.	Children between 6-12 years of age.	75 activity cards (including self-care, productivity/school, leisure (hobbies and sports), and social activities). There are 8 blank cards for other activities children may identify. Children select the five most important activities they currently do and five they would like to do.	Typically takes 15 minutes or longer, depending on the age of the child.	Completed by an occupational therapist with the child and carer.
Preferences for Activities for Children (PAC) (King *et al.*, 2000)	To explore the activity preferences of children.	Children and adolescents between the ages of 6 to 21 years of age.	55 activities that children rate based on a 3-point Likert scale with emoticons to express their interest.	Typically takes 10 to 15 minutes to complete.	Completed during an interview with a child or independently by the adolescent.
Modified Interest Checklist (Kielhofner *et al.*, 1980)	To provide a range of activity options to adults to support treatment planning and goal development.	Adult	68 activities exploring past, current, and future interests.	Typically takes 15 to 20 minutes to complete.	Self-reported questionnaire.

(Table 4) cont.....

Name of Tool	Purpose	Target Population	Format / Testing Area	Duration	Completed by
Checklist of Leisure, Interests and Participation (CLIP) (Levick *et al.*, 2022)	To provide a range of activity options to adults to support treatment planning and goal development.	Adult and Mental Health consumers.	70 activities exploring current and future leisure interests indicated by a 5-point Likert scale.	Typically takes 10 to 15 minutes to complete.	Self-reported questionnaire.

Many components of leisure (*i.e.*, participation, planning, learning, skills development) are also considered to be components of TR (Van Andel, 1998). The American Therapeutic Recreation Association (ATRA) (2018) defines TR as any leisure or activity-based intervention that is utilised to address the assessed needs of individuals caused by a specific illness (American Therapeutic Recreation Association, 2023). Although there is no agreed model of practice within TR, there is general consensus between components of TR being (a) functional intervention/treatment, (b) recreation participation, and (c) leisure education (Stumbo & Pegg, 2004; Stumbo & Peterson, 1998).

Particularly for mental ill-health, there are benefits associated with engaging in leisure due to leisure being a protective factor for the adverse effects of psychosocial stressors and providing physical benefits related to metabolic syndrome (Pondé *et al.*, 2009; Ponde & Santana, 2000). Wankel (1994) discussed that leisure has the potential to benefit an individual's self-actualisation, personal development, and prevention of ill health. In contrast, Craik & Pieris (2006) proposed the idea that 'leisure time' can be just as damaging to an individual with a mental illness's life as a poor occupation, specifically if individual strengths and weaknesses and personal circumstances are not considered. 'Leisure time' can be detrimental due to the potential for harm, such as physical and social injury and damage to interpersonal relationships. However, these same risks are seen as important and essential to the individual's autonomy, self-determination, and dignity of risk (Craik & Pieris, 2006; Iwasaki *et al.*, 2014).

It is widely accepted that the benefits of leisure are very much individual and depend significantly on the individual's contextual factors, such as ethnicity, age, socioeconomic status (Carter & Van Andel, 2019; Hildebrand & Smith, 2017; Veal, 2013), mental state, and health status (Iwasaki *et al.*, 2010; McCormick *et al.*, 2012). Leisure has an identified link to health, in particular, attaining a high level of wellness (Heo *et al.*, 2008; Stumbo *et al.*, 2015). In the context of mental illness, there is an abundance of benefits that have therapeutic implications in a variety of mental ill-health contexts. Most relevant is the use of leisure in health prevention, skills development, health promotion, social connection (Iwasaki *et al.*, 2014), behaviour change (Iwasaki *et al.*, 2010; McCormick *et al.*, 2012), and reduction of leisure boredom (Alford *et al.*, 2017). In contrast, Iwasaki *et al.* (2014) highlight the importance of active living and the notion of thriving, not just surviving within recovery (Bonney & Stickley, 2008).

Leisure has a strong presence in the notion of active living or active recreation. In this line of inquiry and thought, individuals actively engage in life, in particular with activities of interest. Leisure can be seen as the conduit to accessing the health and/or social benefits related to active engagement, with the intrinsic motivation to partake, personal preference, and relevance to the individual fundamental to see these benefits (Craik & Pieris, 2006; McCormick *et al.*, 2012). Other research, depending on the field of thought, identifies skills development, social connections, forming and maintaining peer relationships, emotional and psychological development, as well as generally positive experiences and enjoyment as outcomes of leisure experience (Fullagar, 2008; Goldberg *et al.*, 2002; Heo *et al.*, 2008; Iwasaki *et al.*, 2014). The positive, prosocial experience of leisure is very important for an individual with a lived experience of mental illness as for most, it is a rare or infrequent occurrence (Iwasaki *et al.*, 2014; Iwasaki *et al.*, 2010; Litwiller *et al.*, 2016).

Within the ideologies surrounding leisure, it is widely accepted that without a sense of autonomy or freedom, there is no true leisure (Roberts, 2006). Mental health services are large institution-type organisations that operate under very controlled conditions that need to deal with people in recovery in a very risk-averse manner (Davidson *et al.*, 2016; Slemon *et al.*, 2017). This risk aversion and the freedom that is a necessary part of leisure do not operate easily together, severely limiting the desired outcomes of leisure intervention. The growing area of TR offers the potential for incorporating measured risk-taking activities that increase active engagement in leisure and recreation and promote self-determination and motivation within recovery (Dattilo *et al.*, 1998).

Leisure Education

Leisure education is both learning through leisure and learning about leisure deployed as a modality in varying contexts where either an increased appreciation for leisure can be beneficial or where a level of skill or learning can occur within a leisure medium (Dattilo & Williams, 2012). In its prescriptive nature, leisure education can provide opportunities to develop an individual's knowledge of and capacity for leisure, *i.e.*, new interests, revisiting old interests, etc. For those with a lived experience of mental illness, many may not have been exposed to a variety of leisure activities, and the leisure that they have been exposed to may be quite passive, un-social, and sedentary (Austin, 2009; Stebbins, 2020). The vast majority of individuals with a lived experience of mental illness would benefit from an array of dynamic, social, and physically active leisure experiences regularly in their lives for the inherent health benefits (physical activity/social supports) as well as their moderating ability on an individual's quality of life (Stumbo, 2015), As such, learning about leisure and developing a functioning relationship with leisure is deeply important for them.

Leisure education in the context of learning through leisure is obvious across the lifespan and developmental phases, *i.e.*, puberty, middle age, and retirement. Leisure education often occurs as a natural part of an individual's life through these stages (Kelly, 2019). However, for individuals with a lived experience of mental illness, this natural or normal developmental process is thwarted by the inherent challenges associated with their mental illness and social construct due to their mental illness, *i.e.*, group living environment, risk-averse social supports, and side-effects to treatment. As such, leisure can be deployed to assist in growth and development that may have been lost due to their mental illness.

Inpatient Leisure

Leisure as therapy in Australia is practised predominantly in aged care services due to the growing population represented within this category (Pegg & Lord, 2008). Within mental health settings in Australia, there is limited and varied uptake of leisure as a form of therapy at all levels across states and territories (Pegg & Lord, 2008). Leisure as a form of therapy is generally practised in acute and subacute hospital environments in group and individual type interventions (*e.g.*, group gardening program, individual outings to pro-social environments) (Chimango *et al.*, 2009; Foye *et al.*, 2020; Lim *et al.*, 2007).

Group inpatient leisure programs are tailored to alleviate an element of boredom whilst also providing functional benefits related to the patients involved (Tyler *et al.*, 2019). For example, walking groups, cooking groups, and Karaoke would be diversional in nature; however, for some of the individuals who participate, they would undoubtably be functional benefits in weight management, skills refinement, and social development.

In addition to group programming, leisure is often offered individually to individuals with a lived experience of mental illness specific to their recovery goals (Tyler *et al.*, 2019). In this, the therapist may take the role of coach/mentor or co-participant. For example, attending a local gym to support an individual's confidence in undertaking this activity post-discharge or engaging in a social environment like a coffee shop to support the purchase of coffee and tolerance of the social environment.

Table 5. An example of an idea of an inpatient group activity plan

Monday	Tuesday	Wednesday	Thursday	Friday	Saturday	Sunday
Morning Walk	Morning Walk	Ward Rounds	Morning Walk	Morning Walk	Yoga	Yoga
Cooking	Education Session – Navigating social services	Art	Education Session – Wellness Recovery Action Plan	Cooking	Family Visits	Family Visits
Lunch	Lunch	Lunch	Lunch	Lunch	Lunch	Lunch
Art	Outing: Shopping Centre	Gym – Exercise Physiology	Outing: Library/ Coffee Shop	Art	Family Visits	Family Visits
Movie Afternoon	Wii Games	Karaoke	Wii Games	Movie Afternoon	Movie Afternoon	Sunday Sport

It is essential within these types of interventions that the approach and leisure medium are tailored to the context. For example, in an acute inpatient setting where the most restrictions are placed on the patient (*i.e.*, locked ward, limited social contact), the leisure medium should not add elements of risk or disruption to the individual's mental state with much more passive or low-risk tasks being of benefit here (*i.e.*, dominos, puzzles, arts/crafts). As an individual further their journey of recovery, they benefit from a reduction of contextual restrictions and can be exposed to more variety of leisure activities (*i.e.*, outings, cooking, psychoeducation).

Outpatient and community mental health contexts present the greatest opportunity to utilise leisure to further mental health recovery through either individual or group interventions (Chimango *et al.*, 2009; Foye *et al.*, 2020; Lim *et al.*, 2007). However, the uptake is low due to the namely case management focus of community mental health services (Pegg & Lord, 2008). Instead, the consumer experience of mental illness may be recommended with an array of community supports, both informal (*i.e.*, library, church groups, bowls clubs) and formal (*i.e.*, clubhouse, stepped care, and recovery colleges).

The use of clubhouses as a psychosocial intervention has demonstrated a range of benefits to individuals with a lived experience of mental illness living in the community that is normally distinctive from health and social services (Raeburn *et al.*, 2015). Psychosocial clubhouses provide stable social support, which addresses many of the social issues people face, as well as facilitates supported employment, leisure, and education opportunities that would otherwise be unavailable within treatment as usual (Boyd & Bentley, 2006; Raeburn *et al*., 2015). The clubhouse model has origins in North America and has been shown to support personal empowerment (Boyd & Bentley, 2006), enhanced self-determination and autonomy (Raeburn *et al*., 2017), treatment adherence and service utilisation (Warner *et al*., 1999), related quality of life improvements (Boyd & Bentley, 2006; McGurk *et al*., 2010; Raeburn *et al*., 2017; Warner *et al*., 1999), and skills development and employment opportunities for individuals with a lived experience of mental illness who regularly access these services (McGurk *et al*., 2010).

A natural extension to the clubhouse model more recently adopted is stepped care. Stepped care is fundamentally a supported short-term accommodation service. However, when stepped care is attached to other community supports, it is seen to be most effective. This offers a short-term semi-restrictive environment to support ongoing recovery.

Recovery college is essentially taking the concept of recovery and applying an educative lens (Perkins *et al*., 2012). Recovery colleges are services offered in the community, providing a variety of educational and skills-based classes and workshops focused on the development of competence surrounding recovery and, in addition, competence related to gaining supported employment. Much like a school or collegiate setting, classes run for an extended period (10-12 weeks), with students gaining qualifications related to recovery as a result of the successful completion of multiple classes/courses.

Recovery Camps are gaining acceptance as a therapeutic intervention for individuals with an array of ill health, such as addiction, mental health, and specific disease contexts (*i.e*., craniofacial injury) (Alford *et al*., 2021; Devine & Dawson, 2010). These Recovery Camps are a leisure-based medium developed for a variety or reasons, specifically the provision of supported respite for carers but also opportunities to further an individual's recovery journey through experiential leisure activities. Recovery camps often serve as a reset button for individuals with a lived experience of mental illness who have many contextual stressors (Alford *et al*., 2021). Moreover, dependant on the specific camp, there are often elements present to further individual recovery goals, such as exploring past trauma, developing wellbeing skills and illness-specific skills (*i.e*., body image in the context of eating disorders), as well as the dignity of risk-taking within a supportive environment.

Furthermore, additional forms of treatment and or social support are normally non-government, charity-based organisations with limited income, relying heavily on grants and donations to support individuals with a lived experience of mental illness.

Pro Leisure Culture

Within mental health environments, leisure is not seen as a fundamental tool in recovery; as such, there is a cultural bias from the majority of health staff toward interventions of that nature. Often, therapists who opt for leisure-based modalities need to consider the cultural challenges and barriers toward these types of interventions and work to break them down over time.

The Following Case Studies Detail Common Experiences of a Therapist Using Leisure as a Therapeutic Modality

Case Study 1

James was a new graduate occupational therapist in a rural mental health inpatient facility. Within his assessment of the patient body, he noticed that the current cohort was older (average of 62y.o), with depressive disorders or symptoms impacting a strong proportion of the patient cohort. On deeper exploration, he noted that many of the patients had poor social skills and low numbers of social connections external to the hospital.

Over the course of the week, he spoke with many of the patients who were older and had depressive disorders and noted a general willingness to try something new, such as bowling. On Friday afternoon, James engaged the group of patients in a game of Wii bowling; to great effect, the patients engaged well and developed a competition between one another over the hour-long session. James made the Wii system available in the activity rooms for use over the weekend. On Monday morning, James noticed the Wii system had been left on his desk with a note, "Please return this to your storage, it is not to be left on the ward."

James quizzed patients on if they had used the system over the weekend, and one of the patients mentioned they had enjoyed a session on Saturday morning; however, it was cut short when one of the hospital assistants asked the group to get ready for lunch and after lunch, the system was gone. At the ward meeting on Tuesday, James brought the incident up with the weekend nursing manager, reporting that the patients were having a great game of Wii bowling on Saturday morning, with one of the RNs noting the buzz it gave the ward that was quite pleasant compared to normal. One of the hospital assistants highlighted that they felt it was a risk to the patients. On further probing, the hospital assistant said, 'They might fly of the handle, aren't we trying to keep them calm?', with another adding, 'They are here to get better, not have fun'.

James organised three more sessions of Wii bowling across the week; with many of the intended patients being discharged that week, there was not the need to support the group for the following weekend. James, noting the impact of the activity, spoke with the community rehabilitation team, and a pilot regular ten-pin bowling activity was organised for all service users fortnightly. Surprisingly, after a 3-month trial, there was a general cohort of 9 service users who attended the activity, with 4 from the inpatient group. It was agreed the activity would continue to be supported fortnightly, allowing for the efficient and regular follow-up of these 9 service users.

Reflection Questions

1. What benefits could be gained from the Wii bowling for the intended cohort?
2. What barriers were experienced by the patients and therapist?
3. What strategies could be used to educate staff on the use of leisure as a therapeutic modality?

Case Study 2

Gary is a 54-year-old single man who lives independently in a 1-bedroom unit in the CBD. He is currently receiving a disability support pension, which is approximately $942 per fortnight.

Gary has a confirmed diagnosis of paranoid schizophrenia and is currently managed by a Treatment Authority (community) (under the Mental Health Act 2016 – QLD). He was diagnosed with schizophrenia at the age of 22 with a family history of psychotic disorders. Gary has been trialled on multiple anti-psychotic medications over the past 32 years and has been on clozapine for the past 9 years. Gary's last admission was 3 years ago.

Occupational Profile

Gary is able to perform all tasks independently. He does not enjoy cooking and was never taught, so he tends to cook simple meals or purchase microwave meals. Gary has worked sporadically for the past 30 years as a labourer on construction sites. He currently works casually 20 hours per week. He finds it difficult to get to work as he often wakes up still feeling very drowsy.

He enjoys being outside and meeting new people. He has a few close friends that he typically spends his spare time with. He enjoys going to the men's shed and attending a soccer group on a Monday with his community case manager. Gary previously competed in soccer during high school and has enjoyed being able to participate in this activity again. Gary spends a lot of his time in his home. He enjoys reading and spending time with his dog. He does not enjoy watching the television because, at times, he has ideas of reference that are distressing.

Gary would like to do more with his time and find some new interests. His new case manager would like to develop some treatment goals for their weekly 1-hour session.

Reflection Questions

1. How can Gary's case manager assess his engagement and function in the community based on the information provided?
2. How would you assess Gary's current satisfaction with his leisure occupations?
3. Gary is looking to find some new hobbies and make some new social connections. What are some approaches you could utilise to support Gary in making some more social connections?
4. Consider and reflect on why leisure activities would be a useful tool to incorporate into Gary's treatment goals.

Case Study 3

Stephanie (who prefers to be called 'Steph') is an 18-year-old female who is currently living with her parents. Steph has a younger brother who is in 10th grade. Steph is currently a voluntary consumer and receiving treatment in an acute mental health inpatient unit. Steph has a diagnosis of anorexia nervosa and anxiety. Steph was bullied during high school for being overweight and, since leaving school, has engaged in disordered eating. Steph has reduced her calories to 600 calories per day and will not drink more than 500mls of water per day. Steph has lost 20 kilograms in the past 6 months, and her family is very concerned about her.

Occupational Profile

Stephanie graduated from school last year and has not found a new productive occupation since. She applied for university but declined any offers as she could not decide what she wanted to study. She decided to have a gap year this year but has not found employment. Steph has been in hospital for the past 6 weeks, and she does not yet have a discharge date.

Steph has very limited adaptive coping strategies and has been finding it difficult to engage in cognitive behavioural therapy due to fatigue and lack of concentration. Steph typically spends her time speaking to other women on the inpatient unit and playing board games. Steph often complains to the nurses that she is bored and looks forward to going on day leave with her family. Steph has very few friends and does not talk to anyone from high school.

Reflection Questions

1. As the occupational therapist on the inpatient unit, how would you assess Steph's current occupational profile?
2. How would you assess or explore Steph's current interests?
3. How could you use leisure as a therapeutic modality for Steph's discharge planning?

RECOMMENDATIONS

The field of occupational therapy is progressive in nature and constantly emerging with evidence to support what is known to be effective in clinical practice. Leisure is one of the occupational areas that is an emerging area of research and evidence. Some considerations for delivering leisure as a therapeutic modality were consolidated by Levick *et al.* (2022). In total, 10 leisure principles were developed for mental health inpatient units to interpret, adapt, and implement in their services (Levick *et al.*, 2022). The principles draw from the occupational theory, national standards of mental health (Australian Government, 2010), and the recovery model (Commonwealth of Australia, 2013). These principles allow any allied health or medical professional to consider an occupation-focussed and evidence-based lens. The principles were initially created based on an inpatient setting but can be applied to any practice area, such as non-government organisations, community practice, and rehabilitation settings.

The practice principles include the following:

1. Leisure is a health-creating and health-promoting activity that brings meaning and purpose to life. Engagement in activity assists with recovery. Leisure is an important therapeutic modality.
2. A variety of activities should always be on offer and beyond business hours. Activity should be as readily available as it would be in the community.
3. A positive amount of risk should be taken to allow participation. Activities should be freely available to consumers to provide opportunities to engage in meaningful leisure activities that they would typically have in their home environment.
4. Scheduled activities, including individual and group programs, should be offered every day. The responsibility of engagement should be shared amongst the entire multi-disciplinary team to provide optimal care. A champion from each discipline should support the facilitation of leisure.
5. Social engagement and meaningful conversation with consumers are invaluable. This should be considered a necessary part of staff's roles.
6. The governance structure should reflect these leisure-related principles as

necessary and important evidence-based care. Some of the areas this could be reflected include policy, strategic and operational plans, and role descriptions.

7. A monotonous and uninviting built environment inhibits engagement, fosters boredom, and delays recovery. The built environment should be inviting and 'home-like' to promote recovery.

8. Consumers should be involved in developing their treatment goals. A consideration of consumers' interests, likes, and ambitions should be included to motivate and encourage participation.

9. Documentation needs to reflect meaningful engagement and leisure preferences to support treatment. Leisure-related standardised tools and checklists should be used at intake and discharge as best practice.

10. Acute environments need to have the necessary resources to provide genuine participation. Resources should include physical materials and staff to support the facilitation of leisure activity.

At the core of the occupational therapy profession is to engage in meaningful and purposeful occupation. The aforementioned recommendations provide the evidence-base to support the use of leisure as a valid and therapeutic modality as one of the many tools that an occupational therapist can use to assess and facilitate engagement in occupation.

SUMMARY

Leisure is a broad term that can be used by many professions. Leisure can be defined as an activity that is health-promoting or health-creating, which enables activity to be used as an adaptive coping strategy for people having difficulty with their mental health. It can also promote health, build a sense of community, and provide enjoyment. In modern society, leisure has become an important and established category of occupation that all individuals participate in.

Leisure is a valid, evidence-based therapeutic modality with a powerful ability to promote engagement and a sense of purpose. Therefore, participating in leisure can foster a strong therapeutic alliance and appreciation in occupational therapy. Leisure is an underrated use of an occupational therapist's time that should be considered equally important to other therapeutic modality choices. Participation in leisure activities is the responsibility of all staff in the multidisciplinary team.

Key Learning objectives

1. To understand the benefit of leisure as a therapeutic modality in mental health settings.
2. To provide occupational therapists a lens to integrate leisure as an evidence-based therapy within practice.

3. To understand the multiple methods of assessing leisure (standardised and informal) engagement in occupational therapy practice and how OTs can integrate leisure within the practice.
4. To understand the theoretical underpinnings and evidence-base of leisure engagement in mental health recovery.
5. To explore the concept that not all engagement in leisure engagement is health promoting or health creating, in turn, potentially causing harm to the individual.

ACKNOWLEDGEMENTS

• Both authors have substantially contributed to the design, performance, analysis, and reporting of the work.

CONFLICT OF INTEREST

• There are no conflicts of interest to declare for this work.

• JL completed the chapter as part of her paid role as an academic at the University of Southern Queensland.

• SA did not receive financial contributions for his involvement in the chapter.

• No other financial contributions have been awarded.

REFERENCES

Aguiar, M., Hurst, E. (2007). Measuring trends in leisure: the allocation of time over five decades. *Q. J. Econ., 122*(3), 969-1006.
[http://dx.doi.org/10.1162/qjec.122.3.969]

Alford, S., Perlman, D., Sumskis, S., Moxham, L., Patterson, C. (2021). *Leisure as a cutting edge innovation to increase self-determination and personal resilience.*

Alford, S., Perlman, D., Sumskis, S., Moxham, L., Patterson, C., Brighton, R., Taylor, E., Heffernan, T. (2017). What can leisure offer those with a mental illness; diversion, experience or something much richer? *World Leis. J., 59*(3), 218-226.
[http://dx.doi.org/10.1080/16078055.2017.1345486]

American Occupational Therapy Association. (2020). *Occupational Therapy Practice Framework: Domain Et Process.*
[http://dx.doi.org/10.5014/ajot.2020.74S2001]

American Therapeutic Recreation Association. (2023). *American Therapeutic Recreation Association.*Available from: https://www.atra-online.com/.

Anderson, L.S., Heyne, L.A. (2012). Flourishing through leisure: An ecological extension of the leisure and well-being model in therapeutic recreation strengths-based practice. *Ther. Recreation J., 46*(2), 129.

Australian Government. (2010). *National Standards for Mental Health Services.*

Békési, A., Török, S., Kökönyei, G., Bokrétás, I., Szentes, A., Telepóczki, G. (2011). Health-related quality of life changes of children and adolescents with chronic disease after participation in therapeutic recreation camping program. *Health Qual. Life Outcomes, 9*(1), 43.

[http://dx.doi.org/10.1186/1477-7525-9-43] [PMID: 21672254]

Bonney, S., Stickley, T. (2008). Recovery and mental health: a review of the British Literature. *J. Psychiatr. Ment. Health Nurs., 15*(2), 140-153.
[http://dx.doi.org/10.1111/j.1365-2850.2007.01185.x] [PMID: 18211561]

Botner-Marigold, E.M., Miller, W.C. (2007). A qualitative evaluation of the Idyll Arbor Leisure Battery for individuals with spinal cord injury. *Ther. Recreation J., 41*(3), 244.

Boyd, A.S., Bentley, K.J. (2006). The relationship between the level of personal empowerment and quality of life among psychosocial clubhouse members and consumer-operated drop-in center participants. *Soc. Work Ment. Health, 4*(2), 67-93.
[http://dx.doi.org/10.1300/J200v04n02_05]

Brunton, W., McGeorge, P. (2017). Grafting and Crafting New Zealand's Mental Health Policy. *Mental health in Asia and the Pacific: Historical and cultural perspectives* In H. Minas & M. Lewis (Eds.), Springer..
[http://dx.doi.org/10.1007/978-1-4899-7999-5_18]

Caldwell, L.L. (2005). Leisure and health: why is leisure therapeutic? *Br. J. Guid. Counc., 33*(1), 7-26.
[http://dx.doi.org/10.1080/03069880412331335939]

Canadian Therapeutic Recreation Association. (2023). *Canadian Therapeutic Recreation Association.* Available from: http://canadian-tr.org/.

Carruthers, C.P., Hood, C.D. (2007). Building a life of meaning through therapeutic recreation: The leisure and well-being model, part I. *Ther. Recreation J., 41*(4), 276.

Carter, M.J., Van Andel, G.E. (2019). *Therapeutic recreation: A practical approach..* Waveland press.

Chimango, J.L., Kaponda, C.N., Jere, D.L., Chimwaza, A., Crittenden, K.S., Kachingwe, S.I., Norr, K.F., Norr, J.L. (2009). Impact of a peer-group intervention on occupation-related behaviors for urban hospital workers in Malawi. *J. Assoc. Nurses AIDS Care, 20*(4), 293-307.
[http://dx.doi.org/10.1016/j.jana.2009.03.005] [PMID: 19576546]

Christiansen, C.H. (1999). The 1999 Eleanor Clarke Slagle Lecture. Defining lives: occupation as identity: an essay on competence, coherence, and the creation of meaning. *Am. J. Occup. Ther., 53*(6), 547-558.
[http://dx.doi.org/10.5014/ajot.53.6.547] [PMID: 10578432]

Christiansen, C.H., Matuska, K.M. (2006). Lifestyle balance: A review of concepts and research. *J. Occup. Sci., 13*(1), 49-61.
[http://dx.doi.org/10.1080/14427591.2006.9686570]

Coffey, M., Hannigan, B., Barlow, S., Cartwright, M., Cohen, R., Faulkner, A., Jones, A., Simpson, A. (2019). Recovery-focused mental health care planning and co-ordination in acute inpatient mental health settings: a cross national comparative mixed methods study. *BMC Psychiatry, 19*(1), 115.
[http://dx.doi.org/10.1186/s12888-019-2094-7] [PMID: 30991971]

Commonwealth of Australia. (2013). *A National Framework For Recovery-Oriented Mental Health Services.*

Craik, C., Pieris, Y. (2006). Without leisure…'it wouldn't be much of a life': The meaning of leisure for people with mental health problems. *Br. J. Occup. Ther., 69*(5), 209-216.
[http://dx.doi.org/10.1177/030802260606900503]

Craik, J.M. (2009). Canadian model of occupational performance. *Br. J. Occup. Ther., 72*(3), 138-139.

Cusick, A., Bye, R. (2021). Chapter 3: History of Australian Occupational Therapy *Occupational therapy in Australia : professional and practice issues* In T. Brown, H. Bourke-Taylor, S. Isbel, R. Cordier, & L. Gustafsson (Eds.), Routledge, Taylor & Francis Group..

Dattilo, J., Kleiber, D., Williams, R. (1998). Self-determination and enjoyment enhancement: A psychologically-based service delivery model for therapeutic recreation. *Ther. Recreation J., 32*, 258-271.

Davidson, G., Brophy, L., Campbell, J. (2016). Risk, recovery and capacity: Competing or complementary

approaches to mental health social work. *Aust. Soc. Work, 69*(2), 158-168.
[http://dx.doi.org/10.1080/0312407X.2015.1126752]

Deci, E., Ryan, R.M. (1985). *Intrinsic motivation and self-determination in human behavior Plenum Press..*
New York.
[http://dx.doi.org/10.1007/978-1-4899-2271-7]

Devine, M.A., Dawson, S. (2010). The effect of a residential camp experience on self esteem and social
acceptance of youth with craniofacial differences. *Ther. Recreation J., 44*(2), 105-120.

Di Bona, L. (2000). What are the benefits of leisure? An exploration using the Leisure Satisfaction Scale. *Br.
J. Occup. Ther., 63*(2), 50-58.
[http://dx.doi.org/10.1177/030802260006300202]

Dunlop, R., Pols, H. (2022). Deinstitutionalisation and mental health activism in Australia: emerging voices
of individuals with lived experience of severe mental distress, 1975–1985. *History Australia, 19*(1), 92-114.
[http://dx.doi.org/10.1080/14490854.2022.2028559]

Farnworth, L. (1998). Doing, being, and boredom. *J. Occup. Sci., 5*(3), 140-146.
[http://dx.doi.org/10.1080/14427591.1998.9686442]

Forsyth, K., Kielhofner, G. (2003). Model of Human Occupation. In: Krammer, P., Hinojosa, J., Royeen,
C.B., (Eds.), *Perspectives in Human Occupation.* Lippincott Williams & Wilkins.

Foye, U., Li, Y., Birken, M., Parle, K., Simpson, A. (2020). Activities on acute mental health inpatient wards:
A narrative synthesis of the service users' perspective. *J. Psychiatr. Ment. Health Nurs., 27*(4), 482-493.
[http://dx.doi.org/10.1111/jpm.12595] [PMID: 31957154]

Fullagar, S. (2008). Leisure practices as counter-depressants: Emotion-work and emotion-play within
women's recovery from depression. *Leis. Sci., 30*(1), 35-52.
[http://dx.doi.org/10.1080/01490400701756345]

Goldberg, B., Brintnell, E.S., Goldberg, J. (2002). The Relationship Between Engagement in Meaningful
Activities and Quality of Life in Persons Disabled by Mental Illness. *Occup. Ther. Ment. Health, 18*(2), 17-
44.
[http://dx.doi.org/10.1300/J004v18n02_03]

Heo, J., Lee, Y., Lundberg, N., McCormick, B., Chun, S. (2008). Adaptive sport as serious leisure: Do self-
determination, skill level, and leisure constraints matter. *Annual in Therapeutic Recreation, 16*, 31-38.

Hildebrand, S., Smith, R.E. (2017). *Case studies in therapeutic recreation..* Sagamore-Venture Publishing,
LLC.

Iso-Ahola, S.E., Weissinger, E. (1990). Perceptions of boredom in leisure: Conceptualization, reliability and
validity of the leisure boredom scale. *J. Leis. Res., 22*(1), 1-17.
[http://dx.doi.org/10.1080/00222216.1990.11969811]

Iwasaki, Y., Coyle, C., Shank, J., Messina, E., Porter, H., Salzer, M., Baron, D., Kishbauch, G., Naveiras-
Cabello, R., Mitchell, L., Ryan, A., Koons, G. (2014). Role of leisure in recovery from mental illness. *Am. J.
Psychiatr. Rehabil., 17*(2), 147-165.
[http://dx.doi.org/10.1080/15487768.2014.909683]

Iwasaki, Y., Coyle, C.P., Shank, J.W. (2010). Leisure as a context for active living, recovery, health and life
quality for persons with mental illness in a global context. *Health Promot. Int., 25*(4), 483-494.
[http://dx.doi.org/10.1093/heapro/daq037] [PMID: 20543204]

Katz, N., Karpin, H., Lak, A., Furman, T., Hartman-Maeir, A. (2003). Participation in occupational
performance: Reliability and validity of the Activity Card Sort. *OTJR (Thorofare, N.J.), 23*(1), 10-17.
[http://dx.doi.org/10.1177/153944920302300102]

Kielhofner, G., Burke, J.P., Igi, C.H. (1980). A model of human occupation, Part 4. Assessment and
intervention. *Am. J. Occup. Ther., 34*(12), 777-788.
[http://dx.doi.org/10.5014/ajot.34.12.777] [PMID: 7282839]

King, G.A., Law, M., King, S., Hurley, P., Hanna, S., Kertoy, M., Rosenbaum, P., Young, N. (2000). *Children's assessment of participation and enjoyment (CAPE) and preferences for activities of children (PAC)..* PsychCorp London.

Kloseck, M., Crilly, R.G., Ellis, G.D., Lammers, E. (1996). Leisure Competence Measure: Development and reliability testing of a scale to measure functional outcomes in therapeutic recreation. *Ther. Recreation J., 30,* 13-26.

La Guardia, J. G., La Guardia, J. G. (2017). *Self-determination theory in practice: How to create an optimally supportive health care environment.*éditeur inconnu..

Levick, J., Broome, K., Oprescu, F., Gray, M. (2022). *Investigation of stakeholder perspectives on leisure activity in mental health inpatient units.*

Lewis, M., Garton, S. (2017). Mental Health in Australia, 1788–2015: A History of Responses to Cultural and Social Challenges. *Mental health in Asia and the Pacific: Historical and cultural perspectives* H. Minas & M. Lewis (Eds.), Springer.

Lim, K.H., Morris, J., Craik, C. (2007). Inpatients' perspectives of occupational therapy in acute mental health. *Aust. Occup. Ther. J., 54*(1), 22-32.
[http://dx.doi.org/10.1111/j.1440-1630.2006.00647.x]

Lindström, B., Eriksson, M. (2005). Salutogenesis. *J. Epidemiol. Community Health, 59*(6), 440-442.
[http://dx.doi.org/10.1136/jech.2005.034777] [PMID: 15911636]

Litwiller, F., White, C., Gallant, K., Hutchinson, S., Hamilton-Hinch, B. (2016). Recreation for mental health recovery. *Leisure/Loisir, 40,* 345-365.
[http://dx.doi.org/10.1080/14927713.2016.1252940]

Lopez, S.J., Snyder, C.R. (2009). *The Oxford handbook of positive psychology..* Oxford University Press.
[http://dx.doi.org/10.1093/oxfordhb/9780195187243.001.0001]

Mandich, A., Polatajko, H.J., Miller, L., Baum, C. (2004). *Paediatric Activity Card Sort: PACS..* ON: Canadian Association of Occupational Therapists Ottawa.

Masten, A.S., Obradović, J. (2006). Competence and resilience in development. *Ann. N. Y. Acad. Sci., 1094*(1), 13-27.
[http://dx.doi.org/10.1196/annals.1376.003] [PMID: 17347338]

McCormick, B.P., Snethen, G., Smith, R.L., Lysaker, P.H. (2012). Active leisure in the emotional experience of people with schizophrenia. *Ther. Recreation J., 46*(3), 179.

McGurk, S.R., Schiano, D., Mueser, K.T., Wolfe, R. (2010). Implementation of the thinking skills for work program in a psychosocial clubhouse. *Psychiatr. Rehabil. J., 33*(3), 190-199.
[http://dx.doi.org/10.2975/33.3.2010.190.199] [PMID: 20061255]

Meyer, A. (1977). The philosophy of occupation therapy. Reprinted from the Archives of Occupational Therapy *The American journal of occupational therapy: official publication of the American Occupational Therapy Association, 31*(10), 639-642.

Ng, J.Y.Y., Ntoumanis, N., Thøgersen-Ntoumani, C., Deci, E.L., Ryan, R.M., Duda, J.L., Williams, G.C. (2012). Self-determination theory applied to health contexts: A meta-analysis. *Perspect. Psychol. Sci., 7*(4), 325-340.
[http://dx.doi.org/10.1177/1745691612447309] [PMID: 26168470]

Parkinson, J.P. (1981). The Castle Hill lunatic asylum (1811-1826) and the origins of eclectic pragmatism in Australian psychiatry. *Aust. N. Z. J. Psychiatry, 15*(4), 319-322.
[http://dx.doi.org/10.3109/00048678109159454] [PMID: 7041878]

Patterson, J.M. (2002). Integrating family resilience and family stress theory. *J. Marriage Fam., 64*(2), 349-360.
[http://dx.doi.org/10.1111/j.1741-3737.2002.00349.x]

Pegg, S., Lord, E. (2008). Trials and tribulations of therapeutic recreation provision in the Australian mental health setting. *Annual in Therapeutic Recreation, 16*(1), 181-187.

Perkins, R., Repper, J., Rinaldi, M., Brown, H. (2012). *1. Recovery colleges..* Centre for Mental Health London.

Perlman, D., Taylor, E., Molloy, L., Brighton, R., Patterson, C., Moxham, L. (2018). A path analysis of self-determination and resiliency for consumers living with mental illness. *Community Ment. Health J., 54*(8), 1239-1244.
[http://dx.doi.org/10.1007/s10597-018-0321-1] [PMID: 30121901]

Pondé, M.P., Peireira, C.T.M., Leal, B., Oliveira, S.C. (2009). The role of leisure in the lives of psychotic patients: a qualitative study. *Transcult. Psychiatry, 46*(2), 328-339.
[http://dx.doi.org/10.1177/1363461509105822] [PMID: 19541754]

Pondé, M.P., Santana, V.S. (2000). Participation in leisure activities: Is it a protective factor for women's mental health? *J. Leis. Res., 32*(4), 457-472.
[http://dx.doi.org/10.1080/00222216.2000.11949927]

Raeburn, T., Schmied, V., Hungerford, C., Cleary, M. (2015). Self-determination theory: a framework for clubhouse psychosocial rehabilitation research. *Issues Ment. Health Nurs., 36*(2), 145-151.
[http://dx.doi.org/10.3109/01612840.2014.927544] [PMID: 25325308]

Raeburn, T., Schmied, V., Hungerford, C., Cleary, M. (2017). Autonomy Support and Recovery Practice at a Psychosocial Clubhouse. *Perspect. Psychiatr. Care, 53*(3), 175-182.
[http://dx.doi.org/10.1111/ppc.12149] [PMID: 26813736]

Richardson, G.E. (2002). The metatheory of resilience and resiliency. *J. Clin. Psychol., 58*(3), 307-321.
[http://dx.doi.org/10.1002/jclp.10020] [PMID: 11836712]

Richardson, G.E., Neiger, B.L., Jensen, S., Kumpfer, K.L. (1990). The resiliency model. *Health Educ., 21*(6), 33-39.
[http://dx.doi.org/10.1080/00970050.1990.10614589]

Roberts, K. (2006). *Leisure in contemporary society..* Cabi.
[http://dx.doi.org/10.1079/9781845930691.0000]

Rutter, M. (2000). *Resilience reconsidered: Conceptual considerations, empirical findings, and policy implications.*

Rutter, M. (2023). Resilience: Some conceptual considerations. *Soc. Work,* 122-127.

Ryan, R.M., Deci, E.L. (2017). *Self-determination theory: Basic psychological needs in motivation, development, and wellness..* Guilford publications.
[http://dx.doi.org/10.1521/978.14625/28806]

Schulz, P., Schulte, J., Raube, S., Disouky, H., Kandler, C. (2018). The Role of Leisure Interest and Engagement for Subjective Well-Being. *J Happiness Stud., 19*(4), 1135-1150.
[http://dx.doi.org/10.1007/s10902-017-9863-0]

Shaw, S.M. (1985). The meaning of leisure in everyday life. *Leis. Sci., 7*(1), 1-24.
[http://dx.doi.org/10.1080/01490408509512105]

Slemon, A., Jenkins, E., Bungay, V. (2017). Safety in psychiatric inpatient care: The impact of risk management culture on mental health nursing practice. *Nurs. Inq., 24*(4), e12199.
[http://dx.doi.org/10.1111/nin.12199] [PMID: 28421661]

State of New South Wales. (1970). Creative Art and Craft Activities. In A. R. C. W. D. o. N. S. W. Child Welfare Department, New South Wales government, 1923-1970. (Ed.). Training School for Girls, Parramatta.

Stebbins, R.A. (1982). Serious leisure: A conceptual statement. *Pac. Sociol. Rev., 25*(2), 251-272.
[http://dx.doi.org/10.2307/1388726]

Stebbins, R.A. (2020). *The serious leisure perspective: A synthesis..* Springer Nature.

[http://dx.doi.org/10.1007/978-3-030-48036-3]

Stumbo, N.J., Pegg, S. (2004). Choices and challenges: Physical activity and people with disabilities. *Ann. Leis. Res.,* *7*(2), 104-126.
[http://dx.doi.org/10.1080/11745398.2004.10600945]

Stumbo, N.J., Peterson, C.A. (1998). The leisurability model. *Ther. Recreation J.,* *32*, 82-96.

Stumbo, N.J., Wilder, A., Zahl, M., DeVries, D., Pegg, S., Greenwood, J., Ross, J-E. (2015). Community integration: showcasing the evidence for therapeutic recreation services. *Ther. Recreation J.,* *49*(1)

Suto, M. (1998). Leisure in occupational therapy. *Can. J. Occup. Ther.,* *65*(5), 271-278.
[http://dx.doi.org/10.1177/000841749806500504]

Thomsen, J.M., Powell, R.B., Monz, C. (2018). A systematic review of the physical and mental health benefits of wildland recreation. *J. Park Recreat. Admi.,* *36*(1), 123-148.
[http://dx.doi.org/10.18666/JPRA-2018-V36-I1-8095]

Tinsley, H.E.A., Eldredge, B.D. (1995). Psychological benefits of leisure participation: A taxonomy of leisure activities based on their need-gratifying properties. *J. Couns. Psychol.,* *42*(2), 123-132.
[http://dx.doi.org/10.1037/0022-0167.42.2.123]

Townsend, E., Stanton, S. (2002). *Enabling occupation: An occupational therapy perspective..* Canadian Association of Occupational Therapists.

Twinley, R. (2013). The dark side of occupation: A concept for consideration. *Aust. Occup. Ther. J.,* *60*(4), 301-303.
[http://dx.doi.org/10.1111/1440-1630.12026] [PMID: 23888980]

Tyler, N., Wright, N., Waring, J. (2019). Interventions to improve discharge from acute adult mental health inpatient care to the community: systematic review and narrative synthesis. *BMC Health Serv. Res.,* *19*(1), 833.
[http://dx.doi.org/10.1186/s12913-019-4658-0] [PMID: 31760955]

Van Andel, G.E. (1998). TR service delivery and TR outcome models. *Ther. Recreation J.,* *32*, 180-193.

Veal, A. (2013). Lifestyle and leisure theory. *Routledge handbook of leisure studies.* Routledge.

Wankel, L.M. (1994). Health and leisure: Inextricably linked. *J. Phys. Educ. Recreat. Dance,* *65*(4), 28-31.
[http://dx.doi.org/10.1080/07303084.1994.10606894]

Warner, R., Huxley, P., Berg, T. (1999). An evaluation of the impact of clubhouse membership on quality of life and treatment utilization. *Int. J. Soc. Psychiatry,* *45*(4), 310-320.
[http://dx.doi.org/10.1177/002076409904500410] [PMID: 10689615]

Whiteford, G. (2000). Occupational deprivation: Global challenge in the new millennium. *Br. J. Occup. Ther.,* *63*(5), 200-204.
[http://dx.doi.org/10.1177/030802260006300503]

Wijesinghe, S.N.R. (2017). Of time, work, & leisure. *Ann. Leis. Res.,* *20*(4), 514-517.
[http://dx.doi.org/10.1080/11745398.2017.1350346]

Wilcock, A. (1995). The occupational brain: A theory of human nature. *J. Occup. Sci.,* *2*(2), 68-72.
[http://dx.doi.org/10.1080/14427591.1995.9686397]

Wilcock, A.A. (1998). Reflections on doing, being and becoming. *Can. J. Occup. Ther.,* *65*(5), 248-256.
[http://dx.doi.org/10.1177/000841749806500501]

World Health Organization. (1986). *Ottawa charter for health promotion, 1986..*

World Health Organization. (2020). *Mental health and psychosocial considerations during the COVID-19 outbreak.,* 1-6.

CHAPTER 12

Group Theory and Group Interventions in Occupational Therapy Practice

Shalini Quadros[1,*] and **Smrithi Natanasubramanian**[1]

[1] *Department of Occupational Therapy, Manipal University, Manipal, Karnataka, India*

Abstract: This chapter provides an in-depth exploration of the concepts and characteristics of group therapy and theories that highlight the need for using group therapy in practice. It equips occupational therapists with the tools to substantiate the incorporation of group therapy into their interventions. It also brings into foreground the various stages of conducting development and how it is used in the realm of occupational therapy. Different types of groups that are used in occupational therapy are discussed, supplemented with evidence-based examples. This aids occupational therapists in making informed decisions regarding the selection and timing of group interventions. The advantages of utilizing group therapy in occupational therapy, in contrast to individual therapy, are discussed. The chapter also addresses pertinent challenges and issues faced by therapists when employing group therapy. Lastly, steps in developing group protocols are explained using examples. This comprehensive content aims to assist practitioners in effectively conducting group sessions.

Keywords: Group types, Group therapy, Group concepts, Group theories, Group dynamics, Group protocols, Group characteristics, Occupational therapy.

INTRODUCTION

The importance of groups in occupational therapy practice

This chapter provides a structured approach to understanding the theory, practice, and ethical considerations of group interventions in occupational therapy. Group interventions are defined as planned interventions that use group dynamics provided to a group of three or more individuals together with a common purpose (American Occupational Therapy Association, 2020).

Human behavior is profoundly influenced by the interactions occurring within their social environment. These interactions, taking place within social groups involving two or more individuals, contribute to the development of one's social

---

* **Corresponding author Shalini Quadros:** Department of Occupational Therapy, Manipal University, Manipal, Karnataka, India; E-mail: shalini.quadros@manipal.edu

Tawanda Machingura (Ed.)

identity (McLeish & Oxoby, 2010). Being a part of a group offers essential support for fulfilling occupational roles, fostering confidence, and enhancing self-esteem. In the realm of occupational therapy, groups serve as a crucial treatment modality, leveraging inherent therapeutic factors like universality, altruism, and cohesiveness to help therapists achieve their clients' goals. These therapeutic factors, in conjunction with group features such as cohesiveness, norms, goals, boundaries, roles, and context, work synergistically to enhance clients' knowledge, attitudes, and skills within these group settings (Sousa *et al.*, 2020). Group therapy is a widely employed method by occupational therapists due to its cost-effectiveness and the ability to address multiple goals simultaneously (Bertelsen, 2022).

Moreover, therapeutic groups are applicable not only to children but also to adolescents, adults, and the elderly. Groups can be open or closed and vary in homogeneity or heterogeneity, with group sizes ranging from 3 to 12 participants. These variables can influence the defined goals, the group dynamic, and the approaches employed by the leader during the therapy process.

Group therapy is not exclusively for clients; it can be extended to caregivers as well (Aboulafia-Brakha, 2014; Lapid *et al.*, 2021; Karimi, 2019). Caregiver groups serve as a valuable platform to address specific issues through psychoeducation and foster a sense of closeness among caregivers who share similar experiences. For instance, the Multiple Family Groups (MFG) program, facilitated by a therapist, encompasses the individual (typically a youth, in this case, a juvenile offender), parents/caregivers, and other youth, along with their family members. This group serves to strengthen familial bonds through interaction, the cultivation of empathy, and the instigation of positive changes within family dynamics. Within this setting, families acquire skills to enhance community safety, provide better supervision for the youth, nurture empathy in the youth, and instill hopeful values. As they exchange stories, families engage in the process of sharing and expressing emotions, fostering empathy for one another, and receiving practical feedback. Activities within these groups may encompass didactic instruction, video presentations, open discussions, and role modeling (Karam *et al.*, 2017).

Theories that explain the application of group therapy for individuals with mental illness include i) Group-as-a-whole theory, ii) Interpersonal theory, iii) Intrapsychic theory, and iv) General systems theory. According to the Group-as-a-whole theory (Bion, 1961), a group functions as a whole wherein each individual member in the group responds on behalf of and for all the members in the group. Group dynamics, a tacit characteristic of a group, plays an important role in the initiation of these responses. Interpersonal theory (Yalom, 1995) focuses on individuals in the group understanding themselves and others, leading to supportive interpersonal relationships. These supportive interpersonal relationships help in dealing with suppressed emotions.

According to Intrapsychic theory (Slavson, 1950), the group offers an opportunity for patients to regress to a state of internal conflict or developmental arrest, with a focus on unconscious processes. This theory uses the dyadic theory in groups. In General systems theory (Durkin, 1981), individuals are considered separate from their environment and the group itself. The subgroups formed during group therapy form the focus wherein members of subgroups are more equipped to deal with intrapsychic resistances and defenses because they are more aware of the similarities and distinctions among themselves.

CHARACTERISTICS OF GROUPS

Group Content and Process: In occupational therapy, groups comprise two key elements: content (what is done during group therapy) and process (how things are done in group therapy). Content pertains to what is shared and produced during group therapy, while process relates to the manner in which interactions unfold among group members, with the leader or therapist, the formation of subgroups, and the overall environment cultivated during the session. This includes emotional expressions, communication dynamics among members, and the therapeutic relationship established between the therapist and group participants. While both content and process are important and necessary components of group therapy, the emphasis may vary depending on the type of therapeutic group. Content may take precedence in groups focused on activities and tasks, while process gains prominence in functional and social groups.

Group dynamics: Group dynamics, as defined by Finlay in 2002, encompasses the various forces, social structures, behaviors, relationships, and processes that unfold within a group context. It has emerged as a significant facilitator, offering participants vital support in the pursuit of personal growth and goal attainment. Key factors contributing to this include the establishment of a strong sense of belonging and connection within the closed group structure, as well as the presence of peer support, both of which play pivotal roles in this dynamic.

Group cohesiveness: Group cohesion refers to the collective feeling of unity and mutual understanding among members within a group setting. This cohesion serves as a powerful motivator, encouraging clients to actively participate in group therapy sessions. It provides a supportive environment for group members to experiment with new skills, knowledge, and attitudes in a safer environment. The feedback received during these sessions facilitates valuable learning opportunities from one another. Consistent sessions centered around shared objectives are crucial in cultivating a strong sense of cohesiveness among group members. The therapeutic factors that are in-built into groups are effective only when there is group cohesiveness.

Group Culture (Norms): These are directives established by the group leader for the members during group therapy sessions. They encompass various aspects such as session schedules, venue, expected behaviors during sessions, the significance of mutual respect, confidentiality, and the establishment of specific goals for the group that need to be achieved. Additionally, rules pertaining to acceptable and unacceptable behaviors are outlined for group members. These group norms serve as a framework that aids both the therapist and clients in maintaining focus on the overarching group objectives, minimizing potential distractions. It is worth noting that group norms may adapt and develop over time as the group progresses and matures.

Group Goals: Group goals serve as targets that need to be achieved through the group sessions. They provide a clear direction for the group process, enabling members to focus their efforts effectively. Additionally, these goals foster a shared sense of identity among group members.

Group Roles: Within a group setting, members assume different roles, such as individual roles, task roles, or group maintenance roles. Task roles involve actions taken by group members to accomplish the specific task or activity at hand during the group session. Examples of task roles include initiators, coordinators, evaluators, and so forth. Group maintenance roles pertain to the dynamics and relationships among group members. Examples of such roles encompass encouragers, compromisers, followers, *etc*. These roles may be assigned by the group leader or voluntarily taken on by the group members themselves.

Group Leadership: In group therapy sessions, the therapist assumes the role of a leader. In this capacity, the therapist wields influence over the client's skills, knowledge, and attitudes by using himself/herself therapeutically through the effective use of activities and occupations, facilitating communication, setting boundaries, and conveying empathy during the sessions. This therapeutic leadership involves the use of different styles, such as directive, facilitative, or advisory, depending on the specific situation, the client's condition, and the group's objectives. When employing a directive style, the leader takes charge by selecting activities and providing clear instructions for the group session. In a facilitative approach, the leader empowers group members to make decisions while offering guidance and support. Whereas, in an advisory style, the leader allows group members to work independently but remains available for assistance when needed. These leadership styles are employed to demonstrate care and offer support to group members. They also contribute to knowledge enhancement as the leader imparts information, recommendations, and opinions. Moreover, group members acquire valuable skills, such as effective time management and emotional regulation, which are essential for collaborative work with others.

STAGES OF GROUP DEVELOPMENT

According to Tuckman (1965), there are four stages of group development.

1. Forming – The group is in its formative phase. Members may be uncertain about their roles and the overall purpose or function of the group.
2. Storming –At this point, group members may not be entirely receptive to one another or to each other's viewpoints. This can lead to conflicts and disagreements within the group.
3. Norming – In this stage, group members begin to find common ground and realize that achieving the group's goals is contingent on their ability to collaborate and accept one another.
4. Performing – In the performing stage, the group is focused on the collective objective. Members work together cohesively and explore various strategies to accomplish the set goals.

Gazda (1989) proposed stages of group development as follows:

1. Exploratory stage –This phase is leader-centered, where the leader communicates the group norms and goals. Group members use this time to acquaint themselves with one another.
2. Transition stage – During this phase, a sense of insecurity may emerge, leading to conflicts, defensiveness, and resistance among group members.
3. Action stage –In this stage, the group shifts its focus towards accomplishing the assigned task. Cohesiveness starts to develop, and group members begin to accept one another.
4. Termination stage – This marks the conclusion of the group's journey. It involves closure, saying goodbye, and moving forward from the group experience.

TYPES OF GROUPS

Based on the purpose of group interventions, groups are classified as follows:

Functional Groups: Functional groups aim to promote adaptation and enhance health through collective action and engagement in meaningful occupations. There are four types of actions integral to functional groups (Scaffa, 2019, p.

1381): (a) Purposeful Action: These are essential actions that benefit both individuals and the group as a whole; (b) Self-Initiated Action: This involves taking the initiative, whether through verbal or nonverbal means, to engage in activities; (c) Spontaneous Action: Actions that occur promptly in response to an opportunity; (d) Group-Centered Action: Behaviors of group members are interconnected and collaborative. In functional groups, the emphasis is placed not solely on the end result but on the process that transpires while creating the final product. When using functional groups in therapy, it is imperative for the therapist to ensure that the chosen occupations hold personal meaning for the client and align with their preferences, age, and performance level. This ensures that the activities are not only therapeutic but also relevant and engaging for the individual.

Bouzas, Celeiro, and Failde (2021) conducted a preliminary randomized controlled trial employing an aquatic-based occupational therapy group program for individuals with severe mental illness (SMI). The sessions commenced with a 30-minute activation of Activities of Daily Living (ADL) skills, followed by a 6-minute light warm-up, 20 minutes of group activities, 4 minutes of group feedback, and concluding with a 20-minute post-intervention activation of ADL skills. Prior to entering the aquatic environment, participants were required to perform fundamental ADLs and Instrumental Activities of Daily Living (IADLs), including tasks such as community mobility to access the swimming pool, donning appropriate swimwear, packing a bag filled with necessary items, toileting, showering, and personal hygiene. Familiarizing individuals with this routine at the outset facilitated their engagement and awareness throughout the process. The group dynamic encouraged mutual accountability and responsibility, fostering the establishment of a structured routine. Once in the water, participants engaged in low-intensity aerobic exercises, group games, and tasks designed to promote enjoyment and a positive experience. Pre-discussing activities with the group allowed for autonomy and consensus-building. Following the trial, the group exhibited notable improvements in the domains of impairment, symptoms, and social problems within the HoNOS subscale, as well as enhanced physical functioning, general health, vitality, social functioning, and mental health according to the SF-36 and the Activity and Social Relations scale.

Participation in the aquatic program led to a perceived reduction in self-assessed frequencies of nervousness, sadness, and need for encouragement. Additionally, individuals reported improvements in social activities, including seeking company, frequency of social contact, showing consideration, caring for others, and the need for support in social relations. The group environment facilitated the development of supportive relationships, promoting relaxation and confidence-building. The training in ADLs and IADLs within the community setting fostered greater independence. Engaging in recreational groups encouraged a focus on positive and gratifying stimuli, leading to increased patient engagement and, subsequently, enhancements in self-esteem and self-confidence. This, in turn, facilitated improved interpersonal functioning through the acquisition of social skills. The recreational context infused a sense of amusement and joy, nurturing team spirit without the pressure of competition and providing opportunities for meaningful social interaction. The aquatic medium further brought individuals closer, fostering the establishment of partnerships and the development of positive, inclusive relationships and friendships.

Task Groups: Task groups provide an opportunity for active engagement in meaningful activities within natural settings. They create a collaborative working environment that facilitates the seamless integration of thoughts, emotions, and behaviors. Task groups also offer a platform to enhance problem-solving abilities and skills. In these groups, members must collaborate effectively, communicate efficiently, rely on one another, and make collective decisions, thereby mirroring the demands of real-life situations. Task groups are particularly beneficial when the objective is to enhance performance in areas such as speed, precision, clarity, interest, motivation, planning, and organizational skills of performance. Therapists leverage activity analysis and synthesis skills to select suitable activities within task groups, ensuring they align with the therapeutic goals and individual needs of the participants.

In a study (Anderson *et al.*, 2022) on group therapy for adolescents with ADHD, the objectives were to educate about ADHD and provide psychological strategies for managing ADHD symptoms and related challenges. This intervention, structured in 12 weekly 90-minute sessions with a break, typically accommodated six participants per group. Sessions were scheduled after school hours, with transport assistance as needed and food provided upon arrival. The program utilized diverse teaching methods, including visual aids, modeling, group activities, and role-play. Handouts were given for reference and personal notes. Between sessions, a research assistant made follow-up calls to address homework and remind participants of the next meeting. The term 'coach' was used to denote this role. Sessions followed a consistent structure, covering agenda, past highlights, homework review, activities, psychoeducation, skills training, exercises, and homework preparation. Assignments were tailored to each session's focus and participant's needs. Cognitive behavioral techniques were emphasized, with structure, agenda, feedback, rewards, and active engagement. The group setting offered peer support and a secure space for skill practice, potentially reducing stigma and normalizing experiences for adolescents with ADHD. This was crucial given their potential feelings of social isolation and misunderstanding.

Activity Groups: Activity groups share a similar objective with task groups, aiming to engage group members in meaningful activities. However, activity groups are specifically designed to enhance communication skills, emotional regulation, and self-concept development among participants. These groups often incorporate a range of expressive arts, crafts, music, dance, role-playing activities, and other engaging pursuits to facilitate these therapeutic goals. Through such activities, members have an opportunity to express themselves, build relationships, and gain a deeper understanding of their own emotions and self-perceptions.

Ching-Teng *et al.* (2020) conducted a study examining the impact of group reminiscence therapy on depression levels and the perceived sense of meaning in life among veterans with dementia. The therapy involved a series of eight activities, encompassing greetings, childhood memories, reflections on school and military experiences, recounting wartime events, savoring traditional Chinese delicacies, celebrating Chinese New Year, expressing personal wishes, and bidding farewells. The resulting works and photographs from these activities were compiled into commemorative boards, which participants could proudly display in their bedrooms, serving as poignant mementos to evoke memories and enhance nostalgia. This comprehensive process enabled veterans with dementia to reflect on their aspirations and regrets in life, providing them with a platform to openly share their emotions, ultimately granting them a sense of tranquility. By revisiting and connecting with past experiences alongside their peers, they were able to re-immerse themselves in those moments, garner support, and alleviate negative emotions, including feelings of depression and loneliness.

Based on their nature, therapeutic groups can be as follows:

Client-centered Groups: In client-centered groups, the client possesses a clear understanding of what he/she wants out of therapy. The therapist respects the client's and caregiver's preferences and choices concerning the course of therapy. Creating an environment conducive to engaging in occupations that align with the client's chosen focus is a key priority for the therapist. This approach ensures that the therapy remains centered around the client's needs, goals, and aspirations.

The primary objective of a group compassion-focused therapy for adolescent girls (Bratt *et al.*, 2020) was to acquaint participants with one another and establish a safe and nurturing group environment. It was deliberately structured so that group leaders remained unaware of the specific psychiatric diagnoses or reasons for seeking group participation. Instead, participants were encouraged to articulate their challenges, aspirations, and concerns in their own words, allowing for a more organic exchange.

A central focal point of this session involved delving into the motivational underpinnings of emotions. They explored how the brain functions within the framework of the three circles model governing affect regulation: threat, drive, and soothing/safeness. Participants were introduced to the concept of their compassionate self and were equipped with tools to nurture and develop this intrinsic aspect of their being. Simultaneously, there was an ongoing exploration of understanding the role of self-critique within themselves. Integral to Compassion Focused Therapy (CFT), participants engaged in mindfulness and compassion-based exercises, which included practices such as soothing breathing techniques and the creation of a safe mental space. One particularly effective technique employed was chair-work, wherein participants occupied different chairs representing various emotions or facets of themselves. This facilitated a dialog between the compassionate self and other emotional aspects of the individual.

Furthermore, the adolescent girls were encouraged to involve their parents in completing homework assignments. This collaborative approach aimed to provide a holistic and supportive framework for their ongoing therapeutic journey. One of the outcomes of the group intervention was that the participants experienced a sense of clarity and relief. They felt connected as their apprehensions lessened when it became evident that fellow group members were ordinary girls of the same age. Trusting others proved difficult, with concerns about confidentiality outside the group. Some took longer to feel completely secure, while one girl struggled to fully integrate due to unfamiliarity and difficulty expressing herself. Nevertheless, she expressed a strong desire for the connectedness she observed in others. Initiating discussions about problems was initially daunting, as they were accustomed to concealing their feelings. However, as the therapy leaders fostered a safe and normalized environment, sharing became a relief and a more natural experience. The realization that many people experience distress, not just those in the group, provided a sense of security and calm. Engaging in discussions about difficult matters in the group generated a sense of being heard, seen, understood, and validated. For some, this was an entirely new experience.

Leaving the group after sessions often brought about feelings of energy and contentment. Feeling connected and not alone emerged as a paramount benefit for many. Recognizing shared experiences was a source of comfort. Some felt that others gained more from the group, while others expressed that it was the first time they truly felt understood. Hearing about others' experiences facilitated empathy and self-understanding.

The participants also learned the skill of asserting oneself by participating in group therapy. There was a transformative shift in self-perception. Rather than self-criticism for mental health struggles, it became acceptable to express emotions openly. This newfound acceptance led to positive changes in school, friendships, and at home. Seeking help became more natural, with the realization that support was available if needed. This shift in mindset brought about a growing sense of courage, enabling the setting and communication of boundaries when feeling mistreated. There was a newfound sense of participation and belonging, replacing feelings of isolation. However, this newfound strength had mixed consequences, as one girl felt a sense of loneliness.

For some, attendance at school improved significantly. One girl expressed a newfound enjoyment for school, even on days she struggled to attend. Improved communication with parents was a notable outcome. Parents who participated in the parental group demonstrated a better understanding of their daughters' situations. This led to a more supportive and less intrusive approach, creating an environment where self-acceptance flourished.

A bereavement group study (Mulligan & Karel, 2018) aimed at accepting the loss's reality and navigating life without the loved one, developing new roles and relationships. The group aimed to assist the bereaved individuals in harmonizing their acceptance of a spectrum of emotions associated with the loss while also allowing for breaks to engage in enjoyable activities. The sessions centered on setting group expectations and establishing ground rules while affording members the opportunity to introduce themselves and briefly discuss their reasons for joining. Participants were assured that they wouldn't be compelled to share their experiences but were encouraged to engage in group discussions to the extent they felt comfortable. Notably, in almost all cases, the veterans actively participated. Special attention was given to normalizing the diverse experiences associated with grief, dispelling misconceptions about the "correct way" to grieve, and underscoring the fluidity of grief-related emotions, thoughts, and behaviors over time. The sessions also focused on coping strategies, inviting group members to reflect on approaches that bring them comfort in their grief (*e.g.*, spending time with supportive others) as well as strategies that may provide temporary relief but ultimately exacerbate their feelings (*e.g.*, drinking, isolating). These sessions typically involved discussions around loss and restoration-oriented tasks as a framework for future group activities, as well as the importance of taking breaks to engage in enjoyable and valued activities. There were also group sessions on reflecting on past life successes and challenges from a lifespan developmental perspective, aiming to identify coping strategies, discussions of the positive and negative aspects of group members' relationships with their loved ones, with the hope of helping members consolidate positive memories and foster a balanced view of these relationships, enduring qualities, memories, and values of the deceased that have lived on. Group members were encouraged to engage in personalized activities to honor their loved ones' memories, such as continuing one of their traditions or volunteering for a cause they cared about. The goal was for members to reflect on both what is lost when someone dies and what things may endure. There were also group discussions about remaining significant relationships, identifying social and personal goals, and reflecting on successes and challenges with role changes and new responsibilities. Additionally, group members discussed any changes they noticed throughout the course of the group. Group treatment for bereavement was incredibly beneficial. It created a sense of belonging and shared experience, reducing the isolation that grieving individuals often feel. By interacting with others who have gone through similar experiences, participants gained valuable insights and support. Furthermore, the exchange of coping strategies within the group provided practical tools for healing and personal growth.

Developmental Groups: Mosey's developmental groups, as revised by Donohue (2010), illustrate a shift from leader-dependent to member-driven dynamics. These groups are not tied to specific age groups but rather emphasize the development of group skills in individuals. Donohue's model outlines five distinct stages of social participation: (a) Parallel Participation: Individuals work alongside others, acknowledging their presence, but engage in minimal to no interactions; (b) Associative Participation: Participants collaborate on tasks with a primary focus on the activity, with limited verbal or non-verbal exchanges; (c) Basic Cooperative Participation: Members work collectively on a project, engaging in interactions beyond the task itself, demonstrating cooperation and mutual respect; (d) Supportive Cooperative Participation: Emotional expressions become integrated with mutual cooperation and satisfaction in this stage; (e) Mature Participation: Members prioritize the process of task completion, addressing each other's emotional needs, while placing less emphasis on the final quality of the work itself.

Within a group of individuals with the same disorder, a Group Cognitive Behavioral Therapy (CBT) approach fostered a profound sense of belonging, acceptance, empathy, and mutual concern, effectively eradicating feelings of inferiority and stigma. This environment encourages the experience of sharing and altruism while simultaneously imparting valuable coping mechanisms. (Tong *et al.*, 2020)

Trans Diagnostic Groups: Trans diagnostic groups, wherein individuals have different comorbidities, help clients move away from emphasizing exclusively their symptoms. Participants begin to recognize how individuals with diverse symptoms all strive for the common goal of engaging in meaningful occupations. This collective understanding facilitates the identification of more effective coping strategies. As clients share their experiences and provide support for one another, group cohesion strengthens. A stable and positive group atmosphere encourages active participation and the development of a robust support network. A transdiagnostic approach also plays a vital role in integrating individuals with mental health disorders into mainstream society. It enables their interactions with individuals with physical ailments, thus creating awareness through psychoeducation, engendering different perspectives, reducing stigma, and diminishing the separateness between somatic and mental illness as they understand different hindrances towards ultimately participating in their valued occupations.

The LGBQ Wellbeing Group (Hambrook *et al.*, 2022) was created to support service users who identified as lesbian, gay, bisexual, queer, or as having other sexual-minority orientations and who were grappling with symptoms of depression, anxiety, and/or stress. The group was conceived as a step 2 'low-intensity' IAPT intervention, with the primary goal of imparting Cognitive Behavioral Therapy (CBT) skills and tools to assist patients in effectively managing low mood, anxiety, and stress. Simultaneously, it addressed the unique challenges associated with 'minority stress' factors, which research has highlighted as significantly affecting the mental well-being of sexual minority populations. These factors encompass internalized stigma, experiences of discrimination, feelings of loneliness, identity concealment, heightened sensitivity to rejection, and more. The LGBQ affirmative group encompassed a series of eight weekly 90-minute sessions. These sessions were designed to introduce participants to Cognitive Behavioral Therapy (CBT) techniques, delve into the mental health considerations specific to the sexual minority community, and address key areas such as overcoming avoidance behaviors, challenging negative thought patterns, and reevaluating self-perceptions. Additionally, the program explored vital aspects such as forging meaningful connections, effectively managing challenging emotions, cultivating confidence, resilience, and a sense of pride, as well as implementing strategies for relapse prevention. Remarkably, by the conclusion of the intervention, notable decreases were observed in both depressive and anxiety symptoms, alongside improvements in overall functional well-being.

Group members expressed a strong sense of normalization and validation through hearing others within the community share similar life experiences. They viewed the group as a distinctive and secure space that provided them with the opportunity to openly discuss the impact of minority stress on their lives. This environment fostered a profound sense of belonging and understanding among participants, contributing significantly to their overall well-being and mental health.

BENEFITS OF THERAPEUTIC GROUPS

Battling stigma: The therapy group serves as a crucial psychosocial intervention, effectively countering stigma through open discussion. Within this supportive environment, individuals with diverse experiences find common ground, receiving both therapeutic and educational support. This comprehensive approach complements the broader work in mental health groups within primary care settings. Through the collective exchange of experiences and the nurturing of a convivial atmosphere, the group endeavors to diminish societal stigma. This, in turn, cultivates a climate of increased tolerance and acceptance for all forms of individuality. Engaging with individuals experiencing psychological distress in the community serves as a powerful catalyst for expanding perspectives and dismantling entrenched stigmas. This multifaceted approach contributes significantly to personal growth and societal progress in understanding and supporting mental health.

Opportunity to learn from others: Group meetings provide invaluable opportunities for learning and instigating profound life changes. This is attributed to the therapeutic dynamic, where the exchange of ideas and emotions leads to a personal reevaluation of suffering within the context of shared existence. The group process facilitates a unique interchange of experiences and subjective shifts that surpass what can be accomplished in individualized care. These distinct features of group therapy directly correlate with the feelings of well-being, relief, and motivation expressed by participants. These positive emotions were exclusively experienced in the company of fellow group members, emphasizing the unparalleled value of collective support in the therapeutic journey.

Relational Technologies: In any healthcare approach, the interplay between professionals hinges on relational technologies, encompassing receptive assistance, bonding, communication, and trust – all indispensable tools in mental healthcare. Receptive assistance has a pivotal nature. Every interaction between a professional and a user relies on technological processes within the domain of relational technologies. Without receptive assistance, establishing bonds, fostering accountability, and consequently, problem-solving in health promotion would be untenable. It empowers clients to confront difficulties and seek professional assistance for their health conditions. Notably, receptive assistance can be administered by any healthcare worker, significantly enhancing the team's problem-solving capabilities, especially for users in need of psychosocial support. These relational technologies form the bedrock for the group's cohesion and progress and serve as a catalyst, encouraging users to accept invitations to participate, while communication, dialogue, and the exchange of experiences fortify the bonds of trust. Users feel a sense of confidence and comfort, enabling them to openly address their anguish and suffering, ultimately promoting mental health wellness and prevention.

The power of dialogue: Dialogue emerges as the guiding force in the group process. It serves as the linchpin for users to establish inclusive relationships with open channels of communication, allowing them to freely express their emotions once hidden beneath their symptoms. This newfound dialogue empowers users, leading to an increase in autonomy. Effective care hinges on the construction of a dialogical relationship between user-user and user-professional. This dynamic facilitates a deeper understanding of the unique realities and needs of each individual, ultimately elevating the standard of mental health care to a more comprehensive level. There is a need to recognize the imperative of a dialogical relationship in enhancing mental health practices in primary care and understand that this construction thrives when workers and users coexist in a group (Brunozi *et al.*, 2019).

CONDUCTING GROUPS

Cole's Seven Steps (Cole, 2012) of Conducting Groups

1. Step 1 - Introduction: Warm-up activity, set the mood, explain the purpose and introductory educational concepts, and outline the session
2. Step 2 – Activity: Selection of an activity based on activity analysis and activity synthesis, timing available, therapeutic goals, available skills of the clients, therapist`s knowledge and skills, and gradability of the activity
3. Step 3 – Sharing: Materials are removed and the product is shared, member contribution is acknowledged. Discussion-based activities do not require this step
4. Step 4 – Processing: Thoughts, feelings, difficulties, non-verbal aspects, *etc.*, faced during the activity are discussed
5. Step 5 - Generalizing: Mentally reviewing the group`s responses in the activity and summing them up with a few general principles
6. Step 6 – Application: Helping clients to apply the principles in day-to-day life
7. Step 7 – Summary: Reviewing the goals, content, and process so the group conducted

Coles Stages of Group Development: An example using Anger Management Group

Strategies for Improving Participation in Group Therapy

Participants' needs: The needs, preferences, and characteristics of the participants are to be considered. Groups need to be structured in a non-sequential and noncumulative way, thus including individuals who might miss sessions due to other appointments/ medical concerns.

Creating the group: Including individuals with similar health profiles would lead to improved engagement and better group dynamics. Individuals with differing functioning statuses might have certain reservations. Although differing functioning levels can help combat stigma and increase empathy, it could also evoke pre-existing negative stereotypes.

Onboarding for the group: Advertising in common areas in a safe and non-threatening manner to onboard more individuals in the group therapy program. For example, brochures for groups dealing with depression can be addressed in a non-stigmatized way by using words like "mood", "sadness", and "worry" which are generally deemed more acceptable. We need to take into account attitudes and stigma within the care providers and care recipients.

Selecting an activity: Selecting an activity that is universal and enjoyable, for example, listening to music will foster active engagement.

Minimizing conflict of schedules: A barrier towards group therapy is other appointments at a competing time. This could lead to perceptions of group therapy as being secondary. Scheduling appointments, if possible, must be made in a collaborative manner, thus increasing participation. This, however, requires changes at the grassroots level, such as attitudes, culture, and perception of importance.

Developing Group Protocols

A group protocol sets the overall goal of the group and the specific objectives of each session. Developing a group protocol involves the following processes:

1. Identifying the need for conducting a group intervention
2. Choosing the specific theory to use during the group intervention
3. Determining the type of group to be used for the clients based on available evidence
4. Setting goals as per the needs of the clients
5. Choosing appropriate activities or occupations to be used during group intervention
6. Setting logistics involved (time, resources, space, size, cost)
7. Setting the outcome criteria

Following is an example of a group protocol for clients with problems in social interaction:

1. By identifying the need to improve social interaction in a group of clients, a decision is made to conduct a group session.
2. Theoretical frameworks such as cognitive behavioral therapy are chosen in consideration of teaching social skills to the clients participating in the group therapy session.
3. We choose a task oriented group so as to facilitate group interaction while doing the task in a group.
4. Specific goals are set such as the client will be able to initiate a conversation without any prompts by the end of the session.
5. Activities like collage-making and montage creation are chosen based on the interests of the clients.
6. Logistical arrangements are made such as allocating 20-30 minutes duration for task performance in the clinical area and ensuring necessary supplies are available for the collage/montage activity.
7. Outcomes are defined, such as the goal is met if the client is able to initiate a conversation with other group members without any prompts.

Challenges, Barriers, and Issues in Conducting Groups

Despite benefits such as low costs, ease of providing services, and addressing an increased number of individuals with mental illnesses, group therapy has always been difficult to implement. The following are a few of them:

Timely attendance: Clients are not aware of the existence of a group session, likely due to their functional impairments. Some require assistance to perform their self-care and daily chores. Cognitive impairments also affect attending sessions. Within the group, the group leaders are required to tend to those with physical or cognitive impairments that lead to delays at the start of the session. Inadequate advertising leads to reduced awareness of sessions, timings, other appointments, and lack of time to prepare for the session.

Content irrelevance: This could lead to increased stigma, with clients believing they do not require therapy, and regarding it as an inefficient use of time.

Negative group dynamics: Differences within group members with differing functional capacities often lead to suboptimal group interactions. High-functioning individuals deem certain impairments as inappropriate behaviors. With inefficient group engagement stemming from conflicts, power struggles, and the formation of cliques, individuals may not experience a sense of security in the environment, thus leading to refusal to participate in the present group as well as future attendance.

Negative experiences: Group interventions involve clients with different communication styles, preferences for touch, diversity, trust, orientation levels, *etc.*, which are beneficial in learning skills and attitudes. However, the inability to cope with the expected amount of interpersonal skills may lead to many negative experiences as well. If not managed well, these may lead to the inefficacy of group interventions.

Client privacy: Maintaining the privacy of the client's information and the boundaries of social relationships is an issue in group interventions. Client information is received not only by the therapist but also by the other group members.

Transference and countertransference: Issues related to transference and countertransference may occur in group interventions. This may lead to disruption of client goal achievement and hence should be handled well by the therapist. Therapy may get biased due to transference or countertransference-related issues.

Documentation: Since group interventions involve multiple clients, document-ation can be challenging, and so is the payment for the services.

Therapists employ a range of effective strategies, including collaboration, empathizing, and encouragement, to address negative experiences that clients may encounter during group therapy. They emphasize the critical importance of maintaining confidentiality for all information shared during sessions. Social relationships outside the clinical setting should be avoided to provide interventions to clients that are ethically sound. To navigate issues related to transference and countertransference, therapists may adopt strategies like regular self-reflection on their own behavior or seek guidance from supervisors and colleagues for further insight and support. Additionally, therapists actively engage in the group therapy process, ensuring consistent interaction with clients in each session to appropriately address matters related to payment for services provided. This proactive involvement ensures that financial concerns are handled with transparency and sensitivity.

Group *vs.* Individual Therapy

Although group therapy holds significant benefits, it is essential to complement it with individual therapy. A study by Arntz *et al.*, (2022) focusing on schema therapy for individuals with borderline personality disorder demonstrated that the combination of individual and group therapy yielded superior outcomes compared to group therapy alone. This is attributed to the fact that individual therapy effectively addresses fundamental emotional needs that may not have been adequately met during childhood. In individual sessions, individuals have the opportunity to delve into topics at a deeper level, and the insights gained can then be leveraged to enrich the group dynamic.

Evidence for the Efficacy of Group Therapy

Group exposure therapy for adolescent anxiety disorder (Bertelsen *et al.*, 2022): The RISK-treatment protocol encompassed conventional CBT-based interventions tailored for children and adolescents grappling with anxiety. Additionally, it incorporated a significant emphasis on self-directed exposure exercises, with the involvement of therapists, family members, and peers. Parental participation and collaboration with school personnel were integral components of the treatment approach. A distinctive feature of the RISK treatment emerged during sessions 5, 6, 9, and 10, where an extended duration of four hours was dedicated to conducting exposure exercises in settings external to the clinical environment, such as at school or in public spaces like shopping centers and buses. During these sessions, adolescents were partnered with parents who were not their own, along with a group therapist. Clinicians oversaw smaller groups, typically comprising 1-3 adolescents along with their accompanying parents, as they ventured beyond the clinic premises. This innovative approach of mixing families provided a conducive environment for adolescents and parents to implement the techniques acquired in earlier sessions, free from the influence of existing family dynamics. The primary aim was to optimize the time spent by adolescents in actively engaging with exposure exercises, while simultaneously bolstering parents' confidence in their ability to support this process.

This study found that the adoption of a transdiagnostic group format holds significant advantages, particularly in routine-care settings where there may be constraints in patient flow and available resources, making it impractical to provide disorder-specific treatments for all forms of anxiety disorders. This format not only facilitates access to exposure therapy from qualified therapists for multiple adolescents simultaneously but also allows for extended session durations. This is a crucial implication, as time limitations and limited therapist availability have historically been primary impediments to the implementation of exposure interventions in routine care settings.

Group intervention program for individuals with Severe Mental Illness in jail (Leidenfrost *et al.*, 2017): The group intervention and its specific modules were meticulously designed to address the unique needs of seriously mentally ill individuals within a jail setting. These priorities encompass the seamless provision of mental health care and the imperative objective of reducing recidivism. Comprising a total of eight modules, each segment delves into distinct content areas. These modules are systematically administered on a weekly basis over the course of eight weeks.

Adhering to the recommendations outlined by Morgan *et al.* (2012), the groups are conducted in an open format, affording inmates the flexibility to initiate their participation at any juncture during the eight-week module rotation. This approach ensures accessibility and inclusivity. Furthermore, the groups are offered continuously, circling back to the initial module once all modules have been completed. The sequential order of module topics is as follows: discharge planning and release preparation (weeks one and five), safety planning (week two), courtroom behaviour (week three), treatment compliance (week four), mental health and substance use (week six), anger management and conflict resolution (week seven), and communication skills (week eight).

The study showed that 9 out of 10 participants reported the groups to be somewhat useful to extremely useful, and 58% found it extremely useful. The study also found associations between higher levels of motivation and recall of group topics. It also improved cognitive ability, psychiatric improvement, and increased motivation in the jail inmates.

Group intervention "Accept Voices" for management of auditory hallucinations (Langlois *et al.*, 2020): The group sessions adhered to a structured program known as "Accept Voices©". This program was specifically crafted for the management of Auditory Hallucinations (AHs) in patients contending with chronic psychotic disorders. It is rooted in a psycho-educational and cognitive-behavioral approach falling under the umbrella of 3rd wave therapeutic modalities. Each session, spanning approximately one to one and a half hours, was meticulously organized to address and alleviate AHs, following this structured breakdown:

The sessions centered on the exchange of representations and the phenomenological description of the participants' auditory experiences. It involved imparting knowledge about AHs, including relevant epidemiological data. Additionally, individual formulations of explanations for AHs were developed for each patient. Then, the focus was shifted to explanatory models, specifically delving into the stress vulnerability model and internal discourse. Mindfulness exercises were introduced alongside the sharing of coping strategies tailored to managing auditory experiences. The following sessions provided psychoeducation on the phenomenon of inner conflict with regard to thoughts and voices, which included grounding in the present moment and employing metaphors to highlight the futility of resistance. Additionally, participants learned a technique to regulate emotions, namely ventral breathing.

Anchoring techniques focusing on sensations and emotions, as well as defusion strategies, were initiated in the group. The practice of 3rd wave techniques was reinforced, and participants acquired new coping mechanisms tailored to voice management. Dedicated sessions were conducted to provide psychoeducation about antipsychotic treatments and their impact on AHs. Additionally, participants explored the influence of lifestyle choices on their auditory experiences. Finally, the sessions revolved around fortifying the participants' self-help networks and social support systems, all aimed at effectively addressing auditory experiences. The session also delved into the cultivation and exploration of individual values, empowering participants in their journey toward improved well-being.

This structured program was designed to holistically address the unique challenges posed by auditory hallucinations within the context of chronic psychotic disorders, employing a comprehensive and evidence-based approach. The findings indicate that the group intervention led to a notable reduction in the intensity of AHs among the participants. Additionally, the intervention yielded positive effects on depression and anxiety, with significant reductions observed after the intervention.

These favorable outcomes can be understood through several lenses. Firstly, the group setting and peer interactions may have alleviated the participants' sense of isolation (Mazmanian *et al*., 2015) and reduced the dramatization of their voices (Kingdon & Turkington, 2011; Romme & Escher, 2000). This potentially led to an increase in peer support (Leclerc & Lecomte, 2012; Lecomte *et al*., 2003) through shared experiences in understanding auditory phenomena (Penn *et al*., 2009; Romme & Escher, 2000; Wykes *et al*., 1999; Wykes *et al*., 2005). This, in turn, could have significantly diminished their feelings of helplessness in dealing with their voices and the associated distress, as indicated by the high depression scores at baseline. Additionally, the improvements observed in the voice competency scale suggest that participants felt better equipped to cope with their AHs as a result of the intervention.

Moreover, in addition to the reduction in the intensity of AHs, the group intervention also led to improvements in scores related to the acceptance of voices, along with a significant reduction in beliefs of malevolence associated with voices. This suggests that the acceptance process may necessitate some time for participants, especially for those who initially had lower average acceptance scores.

CONCLUSION

Occupational therapists often work with clients who have diverse diagnoses and can benefit from group sessions. The group itself serves as a therapeutic modality.

By organizing groups in a structured way, we can establish a sense of safety and trust among clients, reducing their fears and feelings of isolation. Encouraging clients to openly share in a non-judgmental and safe environment boosts their self-esteem. When individuals with similar conditions work together, group dynamics come into play, leading to the emergence of group cohesiveness. This helps them reevaluate biases and combat stigma.

The content and process of the group are essential components of therapeutic groups. The group leader sets norms and goals for the group to achieve. Throughout the process, each member takes on a specific role that enables the group to complete assigned tasks. The therapist plays a crucial role and adopts a directive, facilitative, or advisory leadership style. This contributes to knowledge enhancement and helps members acquire skills to collaborate effectively with others.

The type of group is defined by the purpose of the group intervention. A functional group promotes health through occupations as a means, while a task group provides an opportunity to engage in meaningful occupations, making occupation the end goal. Activity groups use meaningful activities to develop specific skills. Other types of groups, such as client-centered groups, developmental groups, and transdiagnostic groups, each contribute in their own way to involving clients in the therapy process and achieving a meaningful outcome.

By following a systematic approach as outlined by Cole, occupational therapy practitioners can enhance their ability to facilitate group sessions effectively. Various challenges may arise in implementing group therapy, but practitioners must establish goals, develop a group protocol, and employ strategies to enhance participation in therapy.

CONFLICT OF INTEREST

As authors of this chapter on group therapy in occupational therapy for mental health, we wish to transparently disclose any potential conflicts of interest:

FINANCIAL INTERESTS

Nil

PROFESSIONAL AFFILIATIONS

To address these potential conflicts, we have diligently ensured that the information provided is evidence-based, unbiased, and aligned with the best practices in the field of occupational therapy for mental health. Any references to specific products or services are based on factual information and do not imply endorsement.

Furthermore, this chapter underwent a rigorous peer review process to uphold its accuracy and credibility.

REFERENCES

Aboulafia-Brakha, T., Suchecki, D., Gouveia-Paulino, F., Nitrini, R., Ptak, R. (2014). Cognitive–behavioural group therapy improves a psychophysiological marker of stress in caregivers of patients with Alzheimer's disease. *Aging Ment. Health, 18*(6), 801-808.
[http://dx.doi.org/10.1080/13607863.2014.880406] [PMID: 24499394]

American Occupational Therapy Association. (2020). *Occupational therapy practice framework: Domain et process.*

Andersen, A.C., Sund, A.M., Thomsen, P.H., Lydersen, S., Young, S., Nøvik, T.S. (2022). Cognitive behavioural group therapy for adolescents with ADHD: a study of satisfaction and feasibility. *Nord. J. Psychiatry, 76*(4), 280-286.
[http://dx.doi.org/10.1080/08039488.2021.1965212] [PMID: 34410203]

Arntz, A., Jacob, G.A., Lee, C.W., Brand-de Wilde, O.M., Fassbinder, E., Harper, R.P., Lavender, A., Lockwood, G., Malogiannis, I.A., Ruths, F.A., Schweiger, U., Shaw, I.A., Zarbock, G., Farrell, J.M. (2022). Effectiveness of Predominantly Group Schema Therapy and Combined Individual and Group Schema Therapy for Borderline Personality Disorder. *JAMA Psychiatry, 79*(4), 287-299.
[http://dx.doi.org/10.1001/jamapsychiatry.2022.0010] [PMID: 35234828]

Bertelsen, T.B., Wergeland, G.J., Nordgreen, T., Himle, J.A., Håland, Å.T. (2022). Benchmarked effectiveness of family and school involvement in group exposure therapy for adolescent anxiety disorder. *Psychiatry Res., 313*, 114632.
[http://dx.doi.org/10.1016/j.psychres.2022.114632] [PMID: 35597139]

Bratt, A., Gralberg, I.M., Svensson, I., Rusner, M. (2020). Gaining the courage to see and accept oneself: Group-based compassion-focussed therapy as experienced by adolescent girls. *Clin. Child Psychol. Psychiatry, 25*(4), 909-921.
[http://dx.doi.org/10.1177/1359104520931583] [PMID: 32508169]

Brunozi, N.A., Souza, S.S., Sampaio, C.R., Oliveira Maier, S.R., Silva, L.C.V.G., Sudré, G.A. (2019). Therapeutic group in mental health: intervention in the family health strategy. *Rev. Gaúcha Enferm., 40*, e20190008.
[http://dx.doi.org/10.1590/1983-1447.2019.20190008] [PMID: 31664325]

Cole, M.B., Tufano, R. (2008). *Applied Theories in Occupational Therapy: A practical approach..* NJ, USA: SLACK Incorporated.

Ching-Teng, Y., Ya-Ping, Y., Chia-Ju, L., Hsiu-Yueh, L. (2020). Effect of group reminiscence therapy on depression and perceived meaning of life of veterans diagnosed with dementia at veteran homes. *Soc. Work Health Care, 59*(2), 75-90.
[http://dx.doi.org/10.1080/00981389.2019.1710320] [PMID: 31944912]

Hambrook, D.G., Aries, D., Benjamin, L., Rimes, K.A. (2022). Group intervention for sexual minority adults with common mental health problems: preliminary evaluation. *Behav. Cogn. Psychother., 50*(6), 575-589.
[http://dx.doi.org/10.1017/S1352465822000297] [PMID: 35950334]

Lapid, M.I., Atherton, P.J., Kung, S., Clark, M.M., Sloan, J.A., Whitford, K.J., Hubbard, J.M., Gentry, M.T., Miller, J.J., Rummans, T.A. (2022). A feasibility study of virtual group therapy to improve quality of life of cancer caregivers. *J. Psychosoc. Oncol., 40*(6), 854-867.
[http://dx.doi.org/10.1080/07347332.2021.2000550] [PMID: 34842060]

Langlois, T., Sanchez-Rodriguez, R., Bourcier, A., Lamy, P., Callahan, S., Lecomte, T. (2020). Impact of the

group intervention Accept Voices© for the management of auditory hallucinations. *Psychiatry Res., 291,* 113159.
[http://dx.doi.org/10.1016/j.psychres.2020.113159] [PMID: 32540685]

Leidenfrost, C.M., Schoelerman, R.M., Maher, M., Antonius, D. (2017). The development and efficacy of a group intervention program for individuals with serious mental illness in jail. *Int. J. Law Psychiatry, 54,* 98-106.
[http://dx.doi.org/10.1016/j.ijlp.2017.06.004] [PMID: 28655427]

Mulligan, E.A., Karel, M.J. (2018). Development of a Bereavement Group in a Geriatric Mental Health Clinic for Veterans. *Clin. Gerontol., 41*(5), 445-457.
[http://dx.doi.org/10.1080/07317115.2017.1409303] [PMID: 29279038]

Scaffa, M.E. (2019). *Willard and Spackman's Occupational Therapy.* Wolters Kluwer.

Sousa, J.M., Vale, R.R.M., Pinho, E.S., Almeida, D.R., Nunes, F.C., Farinha, M.G., Esperidião, E. (2020). Effectiveness of therapeutic groups in psychosocial care: analysis in the light of yalom's therapeutic factors. *Rev. Bras. Enferm., 73* (Suppl. 1), e20200410.
[http://dx.doi.org/10.1590/0034-7167-2020-0410] [PMID: 33295438]

Tong, P., Bu, P., Yang, Y., Dong, L., Sun, T., Shi, Y. (2020). Group cognitive behavioural therapy can reduce stigma and improve treatment compliance in major depressive disorder patients. *Early Interv. Psychiatry, 14*(2), 172-178.
[http://dx.doi.org/10.1111/eip.12841] [PMID: 31264787]

CHAPTER 13

Sensory Approaches, Attachment Theory, and Self-Regulation

Pamela Meredith[1,*]

[1] *Discipline of Occupational Therapy, University of the Sunshine Coast, Sunshine Coast, Queensland, Australia*

Abstract: Everyone experiences the world in unique ways based on their individual neurological systems, which have developed over time in an intricate and complex interplay between our genetic endowment, our sensory systems, and our past experiences of the world and the people in it. Convincing evidence has shown that people with mental illness and trauma histories have differences in their sensory processing patterns and also that they are more likely to be insecurely attached. In recognition of this, occupational therapists have shown a rapid increase in interest in the implementation of sensory approaches in mental health over the last 20 years. The relevance of attachment theory and the interrelationship between sensory and attachment systems have more recently been recognised in occupational therapy, with the recognition that these two systems develop at the same time within the same environmental conditions. In this chapter, an overview is provided of our sensory system, our attachment system, the interplay between these two systems, and the relevance of these systems in the fields of mental illness, trauma, and substance use. Understanding the sensory and attachment systems and the interrelationships between these can inform person-centred and trauma-informed occupational therapy for people with mental illness, ultimately improving occupational performance for clients with mental health conditions.

Keywords: Anxiety, Attachment theory, Co-regulation, Dysregulation, Individual, Intentional relationship, Mental health, Schizophrenia, Self-regulation, Sensory approaches, Sensory patterns, Stress, Substance use, Therapeutic relationship, Trauma.

INTRODUCTION

We each experience the world in unique ways based on our individual neurological systems, which have been developed over time in an intricate and complex interplay between our genetic endowment, our sensory systems, and our

---

[*] **Corresponding author Pamela Meredith:** Discipline of Occupational Therapy, University of the Sunshine Coast, Sunshine Coast, Queensland, Australia; E-mail: pmeredith@usc.edu.au

Tawanda Machingura (Ed.)

past experiences of the world and the people in it. In this chapter, an overview is provided of our sensory system, our attachment system, and the relevance of these systems in the fields of mental illness, trauma, and substance use. Understanding the sensory and attachment systems and the interrelationships between environmental and historical factors can inform person-centred and trauma-informed occupational therapy practice for people with mental illness. To begin, we need to understand the concepts of self-regulation and its related concepts.

Self-regulation, Co-regulation, and Dysregulation

Occupational therapy literature highlights the need for a person to be in the "just right state" to successfully achieve their functional goals. To learn at university, for example, we need to be both calm and alert at the same time. We can all relate to not being in quite the right frame of mind to engage in the activity in front of us. If I stay up too late studying last minute for a big exam at 8.00 am the next day, I may feel sluggish upon waking in the morning and look for something stimulating, like a quick run or a strong cup of coffee, to help me face the day. If, on the other hand, I have been celebrating with a friend after having aced the exam and come home happy and excited, I may find a warm shower or a warm glass of milk will calm me enough to sleep. Throughout our lives, we learn various behaviours to elevate our moods (alert us) and others' that can be more relaxing (or calming). We also learn when to use each of these strategies appropriately. This skill is known as our ability to self-regulate.

Self-regulationis the ability to maintain our level of arousal on a dimension from deep sleep through calmness to alertness, which permits us to engage in the occupations and activities we desire within the constraints of our environment. If I need to attend a lecture but I am agitated and not able to sit still, or if I am tired and dozing off, then I am not adequately regulated for that activity. Many people can recognise when they are insufficiently regulated and adeptly modify their behaviour to better support satisfactory functioning. There are several reasons, however, that people may not be able to do so. Infants and very young children will not yet have developed the skills to self-regulate, requiring the support of the caring adults in their lives to do so using co-regulation (*e.g.*, swaddling, feeding, rocking). We continue to need co-regulation throughout life as we draw on the support of others. For various reasons, some people may not have learned the skills to adequately self-regulate even though they are older, or the distress experienced may exceed their capacity to cope (*e.g.*, loss of a loved one or experience of a mental illness). Without the capacity to self- or co-regulate at any moment, we have the experience of being dysregulated (*i.e.*, an ongoing state of distress). In this chapter, sensory processing and attachment theories are considered, separately and together, to explain this challenge, with consideration to how this insight can inform occupational therapy and support more adaptive responses.

Our Senses

As human beings, we experience the world through our senses. Most people are aware of the five main senses: sight (vision), smell (olfactory), taste (gustatory), touch, and hearing (auditory). These senses are sometimes collectively referred to as "exteroception" because the stimuli for the sensations originate outside the body (*i.e.*, externally). Less commonly known senses are deep pressure and joint position (proprioception), motion (vestibular), pain (nociception), and other inner body sensory systems (interoception), such as when our bladder or bowel signals that we need to use the bathroom, when our stomach indicates we are hungry or full, and even our emotional experiences. We need these sensory stimuli to function adaptively and safely in our world. While we might presume everyday sensory experiences to be non-noxious, even non-noxious stimuli can become problematic, either by their presence or their absence. For example, consider the impact of a ticking clock or dripping tap when you are trying to get to sleep. Also, consider the experience of a lack of sensory stimuli (sensory deprivation), like being in a secure white hospital room.

It is important to distinguish between a stimulus itself (*e.g.*, a sharp pin), the signal arriving at our specialised peripheral nervous system receptors (a pinprick), the message that is received in the brain (a pin has pricked me, and it hurts), and the interpretation our brain makes of that message to instruct our body regarding how to respond. The brain's ultimate interpretation is nuanced for each person based on our unique past experiences and neurological systems. In the case of the pinprick, the interpretation and related body responses will vary for individuals who work in the clothing industry (who regularly encounter the sharp end of pins) compared to someone who was recently stuck by a discarded heroin needle left in the sand. The brain's ultimate interpretation might also be affected by the individual's neurological state. For example, a person with a trauma history or diagnosed with anxiety is more likely to have an activated neurological state and may experience a more extreme physical withdrawal reaction and/or emotional response to the pinprick.

In her seminal work, Winnie Dunn (Dunn, 1997; Dunn & Brown, 1997) recognised that one's sensory pattern is comprised of two dimensions. First, the neurological threshold (*i.e.*, the level of the sensation needed to trigger recognition by the body), which can be described as high or low. Second, our response to the stimuli, which might be more active (to avoid, minimise, or maximise the stimuli; also known as "counteract") or passive (little or no response; also known as "accordance"). Dunn (1997) detailed a Model of Sensory Processing based on the intersections of these two dimensions. People can be high or low on each dimension, delineating four categories, as detailed in Table **1**.

Table 1. Summary of elements of the Model of Sensory Processing (drawn from Dunn 1997 and Dunn and Brown 1997).

Sensory pattern	Dimensions	Characterised by	Example: Snow skiing
Sensory seeking	• High neurological threshold • Active response	• Finding pleasure in sensory-rich environments. • Engaging in behaviours high in sensory stimulation.	Will embrace this activity, enjoying the chill in the air, the movement, and the people on the slopes. Aware of others in the environment and will ski attentively and safely.
Sensory avoiding	• Low neurological threshold • Active response	• Trouble managing incoming stimuli • Adopting behaviours that limit exposure to sensory stimuli.	Will view this activity cautiously. Will likely avoid it altogether, participate at the edges of the ski slopes, or watch from the coffee shop.
Low registration	• High neurological threshold • Passive response	• Tendency to disregard sensation • Slow response to sensation.	Will usually engage in this activity without objection. May not notice the temperature, so may not dress appropriately. May also not be aware of others in the environment; may ski in front of others or engage in risky behaviour without awareness.
Sensory sensitivity	• Low neurological threshold • Passive response	• Trouble managing incoming stimuli • Discomfort with sensation • Distractibility	Will view this activity cautiously. May have a go, especially if others encourage this, but likely to experience heightened anxiety and caution in doing so. Likely to be hypervigilant to others in the environment and be secretly keen to end the session.

According to Dunn's Model of Sensory Processing, sensory processing patterns are stable trait-like characteristics; however, sensory processing can also be viewed as having a more state-like aspect. That is, as well as being impacted by our genetic or temperamental characteristics (traits), our inclination to detect and respond to stimuli is also based on recent life experiences, moods, mental state, substance use, weather, and other environmental phenomena (*i.e.*, states). The pinprick, mentioned earlier, provides a good example. If the person had not had the distressing experience with a sharp, possibly dangerous, needle, they might have had little reaction to the pinprick at all, depending on their trait sensory processing patterns described in Table **1**. Our nervous systems become custom-designed over time to survive in the world into which we are born. We have a lot of information entering our nervous system, and our nervous system is tasked with determining which information should be acted upon and which can be ignored. To use a different example, if I notice an ant crawling on my arm, how should I respond? How should my response differ if the ant is a sugar ant or a fire ant? How do I learn/know the difference? How might my response differ compared to a friend who has a different sensory pattern (trait) or different recent experiences (a different sensory state)? Personally, I tend to quickly notice things crawling on me, while a friend, who is high on low registration, swears she never notices such things as ants. Both perceptions have advantages; I am less likely to be bitten, which is great if the ant is venomous, while she is less likely to be distracted from her tasks. Of course, both also have obvious disadvantages! Even my low-registration friend will begin to notice ants for a time after experiencing a particularly painful bite.

Our temperament, diagnoses/neurological conditions, life experiences, and bodily changes such as pregnancy also affect sensitivity due to hormonal changes (*e.g.*, Geurdes, 2022). During pregnancy, food preferences may change, smells become more pronounced, and sensitivity to touch may increase. In a previous work role near a veterinary practice, dogs were routinely caged, awaiting intervention. While it was always a challenge to see so many dogs caged, when a colleague became pregnant, she found the smell intolerable and could no longer walk that way to her office.

For people with a mental illness, there is substantial evidence that the interpretation of sensory stimuli is altered compared to people without mental illness. In a comprehensive literature review of animal and human studies (Bailliard *et al.*, 2017) and in their other papers, Bailliard and colleagues (2015, 2023) demonstrated that adults with mental illness have atypical sensory processing patterns. There is also evidence that people with substance use disorders, often comorbid with mental illness, report altered sensory patterns compared to the norm (*e.g.*, Kelly *et al.*, 2021; Meredith *et al.*, 2020). People heavily using alcohol and other substances have described great differences in their sensory experiences compared to their experiences post-detoxification. For example, in his autobiography, A Million Little Pieces, James Frey recalled his early experiences in the medical unit of his substance use treatment facility:

I make my way through the Halls. Though the Sky is dark with night and weather, the Halls are still light, the overhead lamps are light, the walls are light, the carpet is light, the hanging pictures are light, the signs on the doors are light. I am uncomfortable in the light. I don't want to walk the Halls. The Halls are too light, and the light makes me uncomfortable. (Frey, 2003, pp. 88-89)

Close to discharge, however, he noted, "I walked to breakfast the Halls are bright I don't care about the halls anymore. They are what they are I can't change them." (Frey, 2003, p.454)

Previous experiences of trauma are also often comorbid with mental illness and substance use, as convincingly demonstrated in the Adverse Childhood Experiences (ACE) studies in America (Felliti *et al.*, 1998; Herzog & Schmahl, 2018). Trauma has also been associated with atypical sensory systems (Champagne, 2011; Jeon & Bae, 2022). This association appears bidirectional, with people who have experienced trauma being more likely to report extreme patterns of sensory processing (Harricharan *et al.*, 2021), while those high in sensory responsiveness are at risk of developing trauma symptoms in response to stressful experiences (Charney *et al.*, 2023).

As shown in the example in Table **1**, sensory differences can impact individual functioning, affecting the extent of engagement in meaningful occupations and life roles for all people. For people with mental illness, trauma histories, and/or substance use issues, sensory differences are typically more extreme, leading to challenges with self-regulation, social interactions, and adaptive functioning. This can be particularly exacerbated when hospitalised, where people have less control over their environment (lighting, noise, privacy) and less access to the occupations they typically use to self-regulate. It may no longer be possible to go for a run, have a cigarette, go for a drive, get away from other people, watch a movie, or many of the other myriad activities people may have previously used to self-regulate. Paradoxically, without awareness of sensory factors, inpatient settings designed to support mental health can *intensify* distress. Supporting an individual to gain insight into individual differences in sensory experience is a fabulous place to commence therapy, supporting strategies that can be used in various environments. Modifying hospitals and other environments using a sensory lens and supporting staff to understand how sensory experiences underpin behaviors, are equally important.

Relationships

When asked about their childhoods, people with mental illnesses often reveal a history of challenging and even traumatic interpersonal experiences. People may share stories of having spent a childhood in fear due to familial aggression or violence, of having experienced loss and great sadness, and of viewing the world of their childhood as unpredictable and unsafe. These experiences have often continued into adulthood, manifesting in romantic relationships and friendships. Perhaps just as likely, people will recall their childhood as "nothing out of the ordinary", and it is not until asked specific questions that a clearer picture might emerge about the challenges they experienced. Jane, for example, said that her childhood was "great" and "just like everyone else", but further questioning revealed that her mother had left the family when she was 4 years old and that she and her siblings had then spent several years living between her overwhelmed father and a helpful neighbour, with no knowledge of what had happened to her mother. She had never discussed this event, the challenging experiences it exposed her to, or the changes that occurred for her in the longer term as a result.

An underlying premise of attachment theory is that having caregivers during infancy and childhood who are consistent, responsive, attuned, and caring contributes to a feeling of safety. With this "felt safety", we can engage in the world, making the most of opportunities to learn and grow. When distressed "by pain, fatigue, an anything frightening…" (Bowlby, 1980/1998, p. 3), we have a safe place to return and be soothed or co-regulated. Within these relationships, we develop a sense of ourselves as being lovable and of others as being trustworthy and reliable. Without this experience, we are typically in a state of either arousal and emotional dysregulation (hyperactivation) or shutdown (deactivation), which makes learning more challenging or even impossible.

Approximately 50 years after the inception of attachment theory, Schore and Schore (2008) coined the term "modern attachment theory", suggesting that the theory has emerged, over time, to become a theory of affect regulation. It is within the relationships of our childhoods that we experience co-regulation, labelled by Schore and Schore (2008, p. 11) as "interactive psychobiological regulation." Ideally, children experience comfort and support from trusted others in their environment who might name and help them manage their distressing feelings with a soothing voice and a hug. It is also within these relationships that skills are developed to self-regulate, and an expectation arises that others will be available to guide and support us if needed. Those without such consistently supportive experiences will still develop strategies to cope with their environment. Sometimes, those strategies are helpful and adaptive and support them to function adequately in their world and even to become successful. For example, Samuel learned early in life that he could not rely on others to be there for him and that he could trust only himself. He generally avoided getting close to anyone and, instead, focused his emotional energy on working hard at school, getting good grades, and earning some money. While he went on to have a good career, it was hard for him to enjoy positive social relationships or to benefit from support. This became particularly problematic when he developed a painful back condition and could no longer work for the long hours he was used to. He felt his emotions were getting "out of control", and he did not know where to turn. He also felt he could not trust the advice or support of professionals or allow others to care for him. As experienced by Samuel, strategies that may be extremely helpful in the short term (and even in the longer term) may still have undesirable consequences over time.

Much has been written about the relevance of attachment theory in the fields of health and mental health. Patterns originating in childhood have been linked with the capacity to self-regulate and manage stress, seek support, and choose appropriate health behaviours. In contrast, less secure attachment patterns have been linked with risk factors for illness and injury (*e.g.*, smoking, risky sexual behaviours), ultimately leading to a greater risk of challenging health outcomes (Maunder & Hunter, 2001; Meredith, 2013; Meredith *et al.*, 2008; Meredith & Strong, 2019). Just as for sensory processing, people with more insecure patterns of attachment (*i.e.*, less favourable relational histories) are more likely to report personality pathology (*e.g.*, Goodwin, 2003; MacDonald *et al.*, 2013), mental illness (Goodwin, 2003; Vowels *et al.*, 2023), substance use (Flores, 2011; Reis *et al.*, 2012), and trauma history (Erozkan, 2016; Goodwin, 2003).

Meredith (2009) summarised how attachment theory informs occupational therapy clinical reasoning by supporting our understanding of: (a) individual health behaviours, emotions, and cognitions; (b) vulnerability to developing mental and physical health conditions; (c) individual needs and preferences; (d) distinctive subgroups of individuals who might respond to similarly tailored approaches; and (e) likely responses to different approaches. In a systematic review, Pearse and colleagues (2020) revealed associations between attachment and functioning for people with serious mental illness (SMI), highlighting "…the importance of considering attachment in relation to functional outcome when working with people with SMI" (p. 545).

Relationships and Our Senses

Evidence of links between attachment and sensory patterns has now emerged (for review, see Kerley *et al.*, 2022), with more extreme sensory perceptions consistently associated with attachment insecurity. Both sensory and attachment systems co-develop during similar key developmental periods, dependent on individual neurological and genetic factors interacting with the foetus/ infants' social and physical environments. Co-regulatory behaviours are also both sensory and relational – soothing rhythmic sounds, prosodic voice, rocking, swaddling, feeding, hugs, attuned facial expressions, and supportive actions. Over time, even thinking of a loved one (known as secure base priming) or handling a transitional object (*i.e.*, a tangible reminder of them, *e.g.*, a wedding ring) can elicit a calming response.

The possible direction of the association between attachment and sensory patterns is not easy to determine and is likely bidirectional (see Whitcomb, 2012). If a child has a caregiver who is not adequately attuned and not able to effectively support co-regulation when needed, the child's attachment system is not soothed, distress continues, the neurological system is activated, and sensory differences grow. On the other hand, a child with a condition predisposing to sensory processing differences (*e.g.*, cerebral palsy, autism spectrum disorder, attention deficit hyperactivity disorder) might not receive these efforts to soothe or coregulate in the expected way. They may be overwhelmed by efforts to soothe, increasing their levels of distress. They also may not be able to provide clear cues to their needs; thus, their needs may not be adequately met, resulting in the same heightening of the attachment system, distress/dysregulation, and ongoing sensory differences.

FOR OCCUPATIONAL THERAPY

Gaining an understanding of sensory and attachment systems and incorporating this understanding into our interventions may support occupational engagement of people with mental illness, trauma, and substance use. With this understanding, we can better explain behaviours and develop strategies with each person to improve their self-regulation, participation, and achievement of meaningful goals and roles. There are a range of interventions and a growing evidence base derived from sensory and attachment theories that an occupational therapist might consider when working in mental health settings. Several of these aspects are considered in more detail in this section.

Sensory-based Approaches

The use of sensory-based approaches in acute (inpatient) and community mental health services has grown exponentially for two main reasons. The first is the recognition that people with mental illness and trauma backgrounds are more likely to have atypical sensory processing patterns that impact their self-regulation and functioning. The second follows the work of Huckshorn (2004) and others regarding the need to reduce the use of seclusion and restraint in mental health services. Sensory-based approaches, described below, can be used to improve co- and self-regulation regardless of one's individual sensory processing pattern. They provide an avenue to de-escalate agitation, prevent aggression, and diminish the need for seclusion and restraint, including physical, environmental, mechanical, and chemical restraints. Champagne and Stromberg (2004) highlighted the person-centred, trauma-informed, and empowering nature of sensory-related approaches, with the potential to address individual needs, improve self-organisation, and strengthen the therapeutic relationship.

Sensory-based approaches in mental health include conducting sensory assessments to support improved self-awareness of sensory preferences, providing resources for people to learn about and address their sensory needs (*e.g.*, sensory rooms, carts, or kits), encouraging environmental modifications to support sensory needs (*e.g.*, allowing the person to control the light switch/put something over a bright light, painting one wall in blackboard paint for chalk drawing), developing "sensory diets" (Wilbarger & Wilbarger, 1991), and engaging in specific sensory programs (*e.g.*, Moore, 2008). These approaches can be conducted individually or in groups, and people can also engage in them independently. The sensory elements of animals are also now being recognised, with emerging evidence that dogs can be engaged in stressful settings, such as dental offices, to decrease anxiety (Cruz-Fierro *et al.*, 2019). Some of these approaches are considered further below.

Sensory assessments: Tools to assess for sensory patterns and preferences vary from standardised measures (such as the range of Sensory Profile measures by Dunn and colleagues) to tools, checklists, and even trial and error. Most measures involve self-reporting, although measures for younger people may include parent or teacher reports. Many services now use personal safety plans as a routine part of practice. A personal safety plan, also known as a safety tool, is typically conducted in an inpatient mental health unit. It involves talking with a person about their patterns of behaviour, emotional and behavioural triggers, what they find calming and alerting, and how they prefer to be supported when becoming distressed. A range of tools are freely available online, and many hospitals have developed their own versions. Lee and colleagues (2010) evaluated the use of a purpose-designed "safety tool", a brief sensory and risk assessment tool leading to early intervention for escalations of mood and behaviour. They reported high clinician acceptance of the tool and decreased rates of seclusion.

Resources to learn about and address sensory needs: One such resource, sensory rooms, takes many different forms, with three different types recognised: sensory modulation rooms (or comfort rooms); sensory integration rooms; and Snoezelen rooms or multisensory environments (Champagne, 2007, 2008). Sensory integration and Snoezelen (high-tech) rooms are beyond the scope of this chapter. Comfort rooms often contain resources such as controlled lighting, cooling, heating, a rocking chair or linear slide chair, a bean bag, art supplies, tactile resources (*e.g.*, lotions, soft fabrics, talc, a brush), auditory resources (*e.g.*, audiobooks, music, musical instruments), olfactory resources (*e.g.*, perfume, aromatherapy oils, scented teas), posters or paintings, crunchy food, thickened drinks, etc. Weighted animals are popular in inpatient units, along with other weighted modalities such as weighted vests, lap bags, blankets, and shoulder wraps. Fig. (**1**) shows a space in an adolescent inpatient unit. It exemplifies the importance of texture, shade/light, and colour, particularly capitalising on the beneficial influences of green and blue spaces.

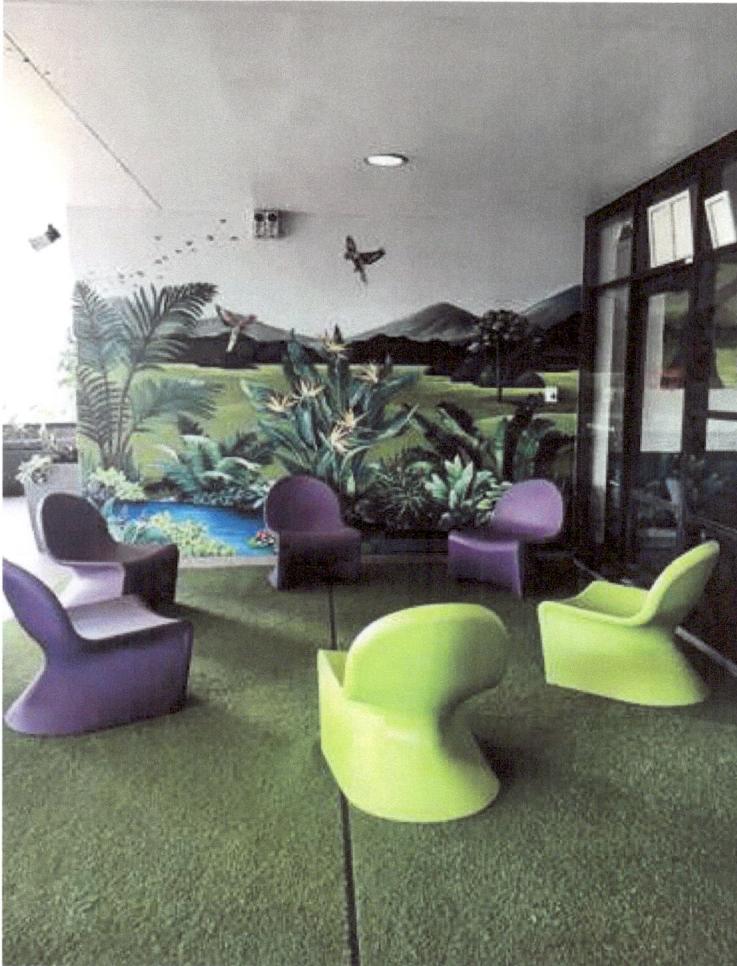

Fig. (1). An example of a space at an inpatient mental health facility designed with sensory features in mind.

Sensory kits are co-created collections of items that are personalised to the individual's preferences. There may be different themes or foci of different kits for use at different times. For example, a person might have kits dedicated to grounding, sobriety, and self-soothing, depending on their needs. Fig. (**2**) shows one example of a sensory kit, which includes fidget toys, sweets, warm drinks, fluffy textured cloth, stress ball, and putty. Such contents are stored in a portable bag or box, which can be carried by the person wherever they go. Sensory items can also be stored in a drawer or trolley in a hospital ward, permitting people to access them as needed to self-soothe (Fig. **3**).

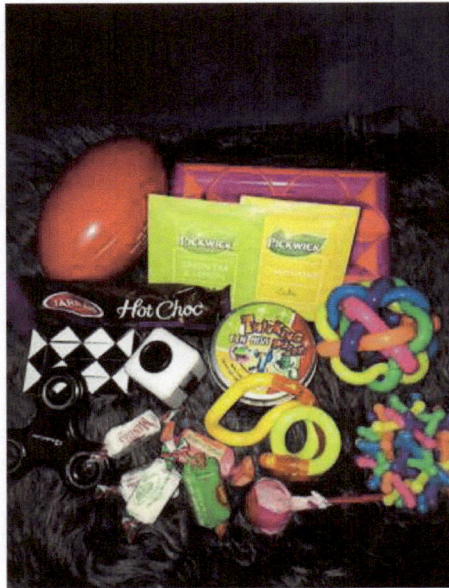

Fig. (2). A sensory kit.

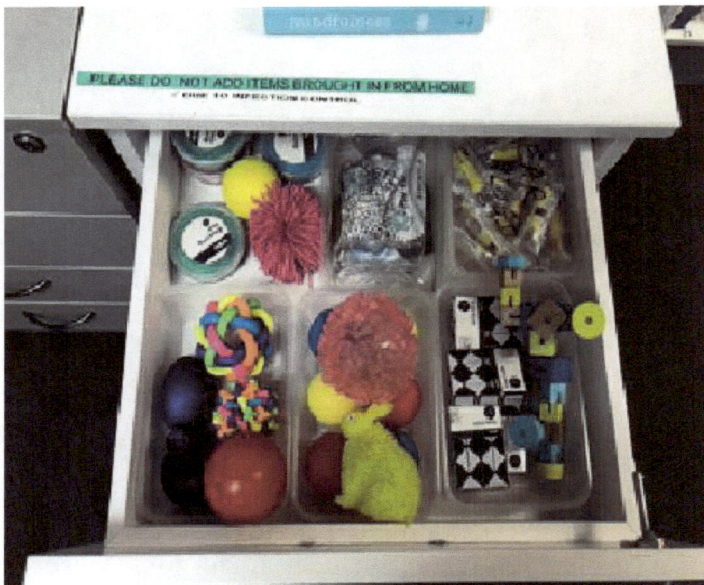

Fig. (3). Sensory items stored in a hospital drawer.

Considerable modifications have been made in practice internationally to support the delivery of a range of sensory-based programs and approaches, and growing empirical evidence suggests that these changes have resulted in improved clinical outcomes and the desired reduction in seclusion and restraint. For example, in America, Champagne and Sayer (2003) reported that, of 96 sensory room sessions, 47 mental health consumers indicated that they had derived a positive outcome in 89% of sessions. Chalmers *et al.* (2012) reported on the outcomes of implementing a sensory program, including a sensory room, a sensory group, and a personal safety plan, within an acute care setting. Preliminary findings suggested that both consumer and clinician ratings of distress were significantly reduced from entering to exiting the sensory room. Findings of the group program suggested similarly significant improvements in arousal levels.

When implementing sensory-based approaches in mental health settings, Champagne and Sayer (2003) noted the need for training of direct care staff, the development of policies and procedures, and the involvement of both staff and consumers in setting up environmental changes. Other researchers have observed challenges to the implementation of the approaches and made recommendations for future practice (Chalmers *et al.*, 2012; Lee *et al.*, 2010; Wright *et al.*, 2022, 2023a and b).

Attachment-informed Approaches

While there are interventions specifically designed to help people develop attachment security, this is not a focus for occupational therapists. Unlike sensory approaches, it is not a typical goal of occupational therapy to help people understand or change their attachment patterns. Instead, having a sound understanding of the theory helps us to guide our understanding of behaviour and supports our clinical reasoning and development of a positive therapeutic relationship (Goodwin, 2003; Meredith, 2009). When our attachment system is activated by pain, fear, or distress, we are motivated to seek our attachment figures to obtain support. If our history has taught us that others are not safe or trustworthy, or if we do not have trustworthy people in our lives, it can be difficult to obtain comfort from others. This extends to the willingness to trust a therapist. Recognising that a person might be reluctant to engage with us or, alternatively, may want to engage with staff excessively due to their relational history helps us to manage such behaviour without judgement. Safety and trust in therapy are enhanced by being clear about the boundaries of therapy, including confidentiality, exceptions to confidentiality, and the length of time any therapy session might take. Much has been written about the relevance of attachment theory to the therapeutic relationship, including the attachment patterns of both therapist and client. Better understanding individual differences in the person's and our own attachment patterns will inform the intentional relationship (Taylor, 2020).

Occupational therapists need to encourage the trust of their clients to establish strong therapeutic alliances. Guidance is provided in a tutorial paper by Clarke and colleagues (2018), who defined the construct of epistemic trust as the ability, developed in relationships with our earliest caregivers, to accept information and assistance from others. As summarised by Clark *et al.* (2018), the trustworthiness of a relationship is marked by four specific behaviours: mirroring, responsiveness, cueing, and language that describes emotions, wishes, and beliefs. These behaviours can be intentionally utilised in therapeutic situations. In terms of *mirroring*, we can hold "mirrors" to clients during our interactions to assist them in understanding their thoughts, feelings, and behaviours, as well as the thoughts, feelings, and behaviours of those around them. We might name feelings they express while returning facial expressions consistent with those feelings (*e.g.*, stating "Oh, that sounds frightening!" with a concerned, fearful expression). We demonstrate *responsiveness* by being in tune with the person, curious about their experiences, and empathic. *Cueing* includes the use of eye contact, tone of voice, increasing the use of gestures and pointing, and the use of one's name. Some of these strategies are also recognised as minimal encouragers. The use of *language* that describes the person's emotions, wishes, and beliefs is also part of establishing trust. This was mentioned briefly earlier in relation to mirroring. Taken together, these responses communicate to the person that they are seen and that their needs are important to the therapist.

Consider an example of engaging in collaborative goal setting as part of building trust. Therapists who are attuned to the person will develop truly shared goals and take care to explain why each aspect of a program was selected for that individual. The importance of collaboration and cooperative goal-setting in fostering trust between clients and clinicians has been well-described in the literature.

While relevant to the therapeutic relationship, it is also important to provide a physically and psychologically safe therapeutic space. For example, where possible, we might check with each person about where they feel most comfortable meeting and who they are comfortable with attending meetings. Some people prefer to meet in their own homes, a local coffee shop, or park. If inpatient, there may be some rooms that are more acceptable as meeting spaces; for example, some people indicate a preference to meet with their occupational therapist in the sensory room.

Neurosequential Model of Therapeutics

Bruce Perry's (2009) Neurosequential Model of Therapeutics is an interesting approach that brings together both sensory and attachment precepts. According to this approach, "We must regulate people, before we can possibly persuade them with a cognitive argument or compel them with an emotional affect" (Brous, 2014, n.p.). Perry (2009) emphasised the six "R's" of treatment when working with people who have experienced trauma:

1. Relational (interpersonally safe)
2. Relevant (developmentally matched to the individual)
3. Repetitive (use of repeated or patterned activities increases a sense of safety)
4. Rewarding (pleasurable)
5. Rhythmic (rhythm that is resonant with neural patterns is regulating, *e.g.*, tapping, drumming, clapping, dancing)
6. Respectful (of the individual, the family, and the culture)

In this approach, developmentally tailored therapy is informed by neuroscience and sensory understanding and "…is combined with rich relationships with trustworthy peers, teachers, and caregivers" (Perry & Hambrick, 2008, p. 38). Perry noted that interventions adhering to the 5 R's can literally change the brain.

CONCLUSION

People who have experienced trauma in the past and/or present and those with substance use and/or mental health concerns are more likely to experience both sensory and relational challenges that impact their engagement in occupations and their quality of life. It is important that occupational therapists understand these theories and the importance of taking sensory and attachment theories into consideration when working with people in this field. While a sound understanding of the theories will usefully guide daily practice, numerous interventions exist, including emerging and evidence-based approaches, to support therapists in providing optimum interventions.

Key Points

- An individual's sensory and attachment patterns develop at the same time within the same social and physical environment.
- Sensory- and attachment-based approaches are interrelated.
- Sensory and attachment theories are important to inform clinical reasoning and the therapeutic relationship when working with people with mental illness.
- Occupational therapists can use insights and approaches based on sensory and attachment theories to improve occupational performance for clients with mental health conditions.

REFERENCES

Bailliard, A.L. (2015). Habits of the sensory system and mental health: Understanding sensory dissonance. *Am. J. Occup. Ther., 69*(4), 6904250020p1-, 6904250020p8.
[http://dx.doi.org/10.5014/ajot.2015.014977] [PMID: 26114463]

Bailliard, A., Lee, B., Bennett, J. (2023). Polysensoriality and aesthetics: The lived sensory experiences of adults with mental illness. *Can. J. Occup. Ther., 90*(1), 103-113.
[http://dx.doi.org/10.1177/00084174221145811] [PMID: 36632011]

Bailliard, A.L., Whigham, S.C. (2017). Centennial Topics—Linking neuroscience, function, and intervention: A scoping review of sensory processing and mental illness. *Am. J. Occup. Ther., 71*(5), 7105100040p1-, p18.
[http://dx.doi.org/10.5014/ajot.2017.024497] [PMID: 28809649]

Bowlby, J. (1969). *Attachment and loss: Volume 1 Attachment* (Vol. 1). New York: Basic Books.

Bowlby, J. (1980/1998). *Attachment and Loss: Loss, Sadness and Depression.* (Vol. 3). New York: Basic Books.

Brous, K. Perry: Rhythm Regulates the Brain. Available from: https://attachment-disorderhealing.com/developmental-trauma-3/. (2014).

Chalmers, A., Harrison, S., Mollison, K., Molloy, N., Gray, K. (2012). Establishing sensory-based approaches in mental health inpatient care: a multidisciplinary approach. *Australas. Psychiatry, 20*(1), 35-39.
[http://dx.doi.org/10.1177/1039856211430146] [PMID: 22357673]

Champagne, T. (2011). *Sensory Modulation & Environment: Essential Elements of Occupation.* (3rd ed.). Sydney: Pearson.

Champagne, T., Sayer, E. The effects of the use of the sensory room in psychiatry. Available from: https://www.ot-innovations.com/wp-content/uploads/2014/09/qi_study_sensory_room1.pdf. (2003).

Champagne, T., Stromberg, N. (2004). Sensory approaches in inpatient psychiatric settings: innovative alternatives to seclusion & restraint. *J. Psychosoc. Nurs. Ment. Health Serv., 42*(9), 34-44.
[http://dx.doi.org/10.3928/02793695-20040901-06] [PMID: 15493494]

Clarke, A., Meredith, P.J., Rose, T.A., Daubney, M. (2018). A role for epistemic trust in speech-language pathology: A tutorial paper. *J. Commun. Disord., 72*, 54-63.
[http://dx.doi.org/10.1016/j.jcomdis.2018.02.004] [PMID: 29471178]

Cruz-Fierro, N., Vanegas-Farfano, M., González-Ramírez, M.T. (2019). Dog-assisted therapy and dental anxiety: A pilot study. *Animals (Basel), 9*(8), 512.
[http://dx.doi.org/10.3390/ani9080512] [PMID: 31370328]

Dunn, W. (1997). The impact of sensory processing abilities on the daily lives of young children and their families: A conceptual model. *Infants Young Child., 9*(4), 23-35.
[http://dx.doi.org/10.1097/00001163-199704000-00005]

Dunn, W., Brown, C. (1997). Factor analysis on the Sensory Profile from a national sample of children without disabilities. *Am. J. Occup. Ther., 51*(7), 490-495.
[http://dx.doi.org/10.5014/ajot.51.7.490] [PMID: 9242854]

Erozkan, A. (2016). The link between types of attachment and childhood trauma. *Universal Journal of Educational Research, 4*(5), 1071-1079.
[http://dx.doi.org/10.13189/ujer.2016.040517]

Felitti, V.J., Anda, R.F., Nordenberg, D., Williamson, D.F., Spitz, A.M., Edwards, V., Koss, M.P., Marks, J.S. (1998). Relationship of childhood abuse and household dysfunction to many of the leading causes of death in adults. The Adverse Childhood Experiences (ACE) Study. *Am. J. Prev. Med., 14*(4), 245-258.
[http://dx.doi.org/10.1016/S0749-3797(98)00017-8] [PMID: 9635069]

Flores, P.J. (2011). *Addiction as an attachment disorder.*. Rowman & Littlefield Publishers.

Geurdes, J. (2022). Hormonal and sensory changes during pregnancy. *Maternal and Paediatric Nutrition,*

7(2), 1-2.

Goodwin, I. (2003). The relevance of attachment theory to the philosophy, organization, and practice of adult mental health care. *Clin. Psychol. Rev., 23*(1), 35-56.
[http://dx.doi.org/10.1016/S0272-7358(02)00145-9] [PMID: 12559993]

Harricharan, S., McKinnon, M.C., Lanius, R.A. (2021). How processing of sensory information from the internal and external worlds shape the perception and engagement with the world in the aftermath of trauma: Implications for PTSD. *Front. Neurosci., 15*, 625490.
[http://dx.doi.org/10.3389/fnins.2021.625490] [PMID: 33935627]

Herzog, J.I., Schmahl, C. (2018). Adverse childhood experiences and the consequences on neurobiological, psychosocial, and somatic conditions across the lifespan. *Front. Psychiatry, 9*, 420.
[http://dx.doi.org/10.3389/fpsyt.2018.00420] [PMID: 30233435]

Huckshorn, K.A. (2004). Seclusion & restraint: Where have we been? Where are we now? Where are we going? *J. Psychosoc. Nurs. Ment. Health Serv., 42*(9), 6-7.
[http://dx.doi.org/10.3928/02793695-20040901-01] [PMID: 15493490]

Jeon, M.S., Bae, E.B. (2022). Emotions and sensory processing in adolescents: The effect of childhood traumatic experiences. *J. Psychiatr. Res., 151*, 136-143.
[http://dx.doi.org/10.1016/j.jpsychires.2022.03.054] [PMID: 35477078]

Kelly, J., Meredith, P.J., Taylor, M., Morphett, A., Wilson, H. (2021). Substances and your senses: The sensory patterns of young people within an alcohol and drug treatment service. *Subst. Abus., 42*(4), 998-1006.
[http://dx.doi.org/10.1080/08897077.2021.1901177] [PMID: 33750274]

Kerley, L.J., Meredith, P.J., Harnett, P.H. (2023). The relationship between sensory processing and attachment patterns: A scoping review. *Can. J. Occup. Ther., 90*(1), 79-91.
[http://dx.doi.org/10.1177/00084174221102726] [PMID: 35611458]

Lee, S.J., Cox, A., Whitecross, F., Williams, P., Hollander, Y. (2010). Sensory assessment and therapy to help reduce seclusion use with service users needing psychiatric intensive care. *J. Psychiatr. Intensive Care, 6*(2), 83-90.
[http://dx.doi.org/10.1017/S1742646410000014]

Maunder, R.G., Hunter, J.J. (2001). Attachment and psychosomatic medicine: developmental contributions to stress and disease. *Psychosom. Med., 63*(4), 556-567.
[http://dx.doi.org/10.1097/00006842-200107000-00006] [PMID: 11485109]

MacDonald, K., Berlow, R., Thomas, M.L. (2013). Attachment, affective temperament, and personality disorders: A study of their relationships in psychiatric outpatients. *J. Affect. Disord., 151*(3), 932-941.
[http://dx.doi.org/10.1016/j.jad.2013.07.040] [PMID: 24054918]

Meredith, P. (2009). Introducing attachment theory to occupational therapy. *Aust. Occup. Ther. J., 56*(4), 285-292.
[http://dx.doi.org/10.1111/j.1440-1630.2009.00789.x] [PMID: 20854529]

Meredith, P.J. (2013). A review of the evidence regarding associations between attachment theory and experimentally induced pain. *Curr. Pain Headache Rep., 17*(4), 326.
[http://dx.doi.org/10.1007/s11916-013-0326-y] [PMID: 23456784]

Meredith, P.J., Kerley, L., Moyle, R. (2020). Substance use: Links with attachment, sensory sensitivity, distress, and health-related quality-of-life in young adults. *Subst. Use Misuse, 55*(11), 1817-1824.
[http://dx.doi.org/10.1080/10826084.2020.1766502] [PMID: 32441186]

Meredith, P.J., Strong, J. (2019). Attachment and chronic illness. *Curr. Opin. Psychol., 25*, 132-138.
[http://dx.doi.org/10.1016/j.copsyc.2018.04.018] [PMID: 29753973]

Meredith, P.J., Strong, J., Ownsworth, T. (2008).

Moore, K. (2008). *The Sensory Connection Self-Regulation Workbook.*. NH, US: The Sensory Connection

Program.

Pearse, E., Bucci, S., Raphael, J., Berry, K. (2020). The relationship between attachment and functioning for people with serious mental illness: a systematic review. *Nord. J. Psychiatry, 74*(8), 545-557. [http://dx.doi.org/10.1080/08039488.2020.1767687] [PMID: 32692588]

Perry, B.D. (2009). Examining child maltreatment through a neurodevelopmental lens: Clinical applications of the Neurosequential Model of Therapeutics. *J. Loss Trauma, 14*(4), 240-255. [http://dx.doi.org/10.1080/15325020903004350]

Perry, B.D., Hambrick, E.P. (2008). The Neurosequential Model of Therapeutics. *Reclaiming Child. Youth, 17*(3), 38-43.

Reis, S., Curtis, J., Reid, A. (2012). Attachment styles and alcohol problems in emerging adulthood: a pilot test of an integrative model. *Ment. Health Subst. Use, 5*(2), 115-131. [http://dx.doi.org/10.1080/17523281.2011.619503]

Schore, J.R., Schore, A.N. (2008). Modern attachment theory: The central role of affect Regulation in development and treatment. *Clin. Soc. Work J., 36*(1), 9-20. [http://dx.doi.org/10.1007/s10615-007-0111-7]

Taylor, R. (2020). *The Intentional Relationship: Occupational Therapy and Use of Self.* F. A. Davis.

Vowels, L.M., Vowels, M.J., Carnelley, K.B., Millings, A., Gibson-Miller, J. (2023). Toward a causal link between attachment styles and mental health during the COVID-19 pandemic. *Br. J. Clin. Psychol., 62*(3), 605-620. [http://dx.doi.org/10.1111/bjc.12428] [PMID: 37300241]

Whitcomb, D.A. (2012). Attachment, occupation, and identity: Considerations in Infancy. *J. Occup. Sci., 19*(3), 271-282. [http://dx.doi.org/10.1080/14427591.2011.634762]

Wilbarger, P., Wilbarger, J. (1991). *Sensory defensiveness in children ages 1 - 12: An intervention guide for parents and other caretakers..* Santa Barbara, CA: Avanti Educational Programs.

Wright, L., Meredith, P., Bennett, S. (2022). Sensory approaches in psychiatric units: Patterns and influences of use in one Australian health region. *Aust. Occup. Ther. J., 69*(5), 559-573. [http://dx.doi.org/10.1111/1440-1630.12813] [PMID: 35706333]

Wright, L., Bennett, S., Meredith, P., Doig, E. (2023). Planning for change: Co-designing implementation strategies to improve the use of sensory approaches in an acute psychiatric unit. *Issues Ment. Health Nurs., 44*(10), 960-973. a [http://dx.doi.org/10.1080/01612840.2023.2236712] [PMID: 37643312]

Wright, L., Bennett, S., Meredith, P. (2023). Using the Theoretical Domain Framework to understand what helps and hinders the use of different sensory approaches in Australian psychiatric units: A survey of mental health clinicians. *Aust. Occup. Ther. J., 70*(5), 599-616. b [http://dx.doi.org/10.1111/1440-1630.12889] [PMID: 37259982]

CHAPTER 14

Child and Youth Mental Health

Tawanda Machingura[1,*] and **Moffat Makomo**[2]

[1] Head of Discipline Occupational Therapy Program, University of Notre Dame Australia, Sydney, Australia

[2] Occupational Therapist, Manchester University NHS Foundation Trust, Manchester, England, United Kingdom

Abstract: Mental health affects a large number of children and young people worldwide. The role of child and youth mental health services is to provide timely assessment and interventions to improve the well-being and standard of life of children and youth with mental health conditions, foster child development, and ultimately save lives. This chapter explores the role of occupational therapists when providing services to children, families, and carers. The chapter summarises common models of practice used by occupational therapists and provides a synopsis of common conditions seen in child and youth mental health settings. The chapter then introduces common recovery-oriented interventions used when working with children and young people experiencing mental health problems and their carers and families.

Keywords: Occupational therapy, Models, Sensory, Multidisciplinary, Child and youth mental health, Multidisciplinary team, Mental health disorders, Anxiety, Depression, Bipolar, Sensory integration, Sensory modulation, Parents and family interventions.

INTRODUCTION

Worldwide, one in seven 10- to 19-year-olds experience a mental illness of some sort, and this accounts for 13% of the burden of disease for this age group (WHO, 2021). Globally, suicide is the fourth leading cause of death among 15–29-yea--olds (WHO, 2021). Mental health conditions in early life years can extend into adulthood and increase the risk of substance misuse, poverty, reduced life satisfaction, poor job satisfaction, and impaired relationships (Reardon *et al.*, 2017). Whilst early intervention is paramount to limiting the development of these issues, having the knowledge and awareness of finding the most effective services for the child can be difficult to navigate (MacDonald *et al.*, 2018). Given this responsibility largely falls on the parent or guardian, it is important that their

---

[*] **Corresponding author Tawanda Machingura:** Head of Discipline Occupational Therapy Program, University of Notre Dame Australia, Sydney, Australia; E-mail: tawanda.machingura@nd.edu.au

experiences within the health system are considered. Parental involvement in Child and Youth Mental Health Services (CYMHS) is essential (Brown, 2020). The parent's role is also to facilitate appointments and help implement treatments recommended by treating clinicians during sessions (Haine-Schlagel & Walsh, 2015).

Occupational therapists play a very important role in mental healthcare for children and youth. By working in a multidisciplinary team, they support the development of life skills and promote engagement in meaningful activities (American Occupational Therapy Association [AOTA], 2020). Recently, the impact of the COVID-19 pandemic on children and youth has further impacted this group. With the introduction of lockdowns, school closures, and social distancing, daily lives and daily routines were disturbed and limited (Loades *et al.*, 2020). It is also important to acknowledge the impact of traumatic events such as natural disasters, like fires, and domestic abuse on children and youth (Leed *et al.*, 2020).

Child Youth Mental Health Services (CYMHS) are usually public mental health services, although private child and youth mental health services also exist, particularly in Western countries. The importance of CYMHS is to provide timely assessment and interventions to improve the well-being and quality of life of children with mental health conditions, foster child development, and ultimately save lives (Reardon *et al.*, 2017). Occupational therapists are often employed and work within child and youth mental health services. Occupational Therapy (OT) is a key component of mental health service delivery and provides support to consumers who have difficulties completing daily occupations (Nardella *et al.*, 2018).

Role of Occupational Therapy in CYMHS

Occupational Therapy (OT) is a key component of mental health service delivery and provides support to consumers who have difficulties completing daily occupations (Nardella *et al.*, 2018). Occupational therapists utilise client-centred approaches to make improvements to health and well-being by using targeted interventions that increase functionality. Transition to adulthood is an important role for OTs in CYMHS, as they aim to equip the youth with the necessary skills to attain independent living and successfully integrate into adult life (Bazyk, 2017). Emotional regulation is another focus area addressed by OTs, who use different therapeutic techniques, including sensory integration, to improve coping mechanisms and promote self-regulation among young individuals (Schaaf & Mailloux, 2015). OT strategies may include providing enabling environments and other environmental modifications, behavioral interventions, and psychoeducation focusing on addressing the functional impairments associated with the psychiatric disorders (AOTA, 2014).

Other OT roles and interventions in CYMHS include:

- Clinic Interventions,
- Home interventions,
- School-based interventions, and
- Community-based programs.

Models of Practice

In occupational therapy, models and frames of reference are used to guide practice. This helps the occupational therapist to be theory-informed when identifying challenges and difficulties and formulating the interventions and strategies. In occupational therapy, there are a variety of well-established models and frames of reference that are commonly used when working with children and youth with mental health problems. In this chapter, we briefly overview the common models as another specific section of this book is dedicated to discussing models in more detail.

Model of Human Occupation (MOHO)

This is one of the most utilised models in mental health occupational therapy. In this model, the focus is on how human occupation is chosen and how and when it is done (patterned and performed) in context (Kielhofner, 2008). When used with children, the occupational therapist is interested in the individual's motivation to do, their habits, roles, routines, and performance abilities within their environment (Kiefhofner, 2008). The occupational therapist focuses on how the child's condition and difficulties impact their motivation, routines, and performance.

Person Environment Occupation Model (PEO)

This model's focus is on the fit between the person, environment, and occupation (Law *et al.*, 1996). The occupational therapist will assess the transactions and fit between the child's abilities and capacities (person), their occupations *e.g.*, play, and their environment. The occupational therapist would then work with the child and their significant others, including caregivers, to increase the fit. This includes considering environmental factors such as family dynamics and fiscal environment and how they impact performance and function.

Sensory Integration Model

The Sensory Integration framework was developed by A. Jean Ayres. It looks at how the child's brain takes in information and makes sense of it to produce a favourable response. Challenges with integrating sensory information can impact the child's learning, daily activities, participation, and behaviour. An example when this framework can be used is creating an enabling sensory environment for a child with sensory processing difficulties associated with a mental illness or autism spectrum disorder.

Trauma-informed Care

This approach acknowledges the impact of trauma and affects growth and mental development. It aims to create environments that promote healing and resilience (SAMHA 2014). This approach is useful when working with children and youth, particularly those who have gone through adverse childhood experiences and other types of traumas. Strategies that focus on trust empowerment and building resilience are used. As an example, an occupational therapist may use sensory-based interventions to help a child feel more grounded and safer within their body, thus reducing the symptoms of trauma.

Multidisciplinary Approach

The importance of CYMHS is to provide timely assessment and interventions to improve the well-being and quality of life of children with mental health conditions, foster child development, and ultimately save lives (Reardon *et al.*, 2017). Mental health conditions in early life years can extend into adulthood and increase the risk of substance misuse, poverty, reduced life satisfaction, poor job satisfaction, and impaired relationships (Reardon *et al.*, 2017). Whilst early intervention is paramount to limiting the development of these issues, having the knowledge and awareness of finding the most effective services for the child can be difficult to navigate (MacDonald *et al.*, 2018). Given this responsibility largely falls on the parent or guardian, it is important that their experiences within the health system are considered. Parental involvement in Child and Youth Mental Health Services (CYMHS) is essential (Brown, 2020). The parent`s role is also to facilitate appointments and help implement treatments recommended by treating clinicians during sessions (Haine-Schlagel & Walsh, 2015).

CYMHS are commonly staffed by a range of health professionals who work collaboratively to determine and facilitate the most appropriate treatment plan for the children. Health professionals who work in mental health, particularly with children, focus on developing a positive alliance with families and include them in the treatment process (Brown, 2020). The lived experience provides a unique and valuable input to the design and delivery of health programs (Schlichthorst *et al.*, 2020). A multidisciplinary team in CYMHS usually consists of professionals from different fields who work together to provide care to children and adolescents with mental health concerns. The team may include:

- Child and Adolescent Psychiatrists
- Clinical Psychologists
- Psychiatric Nurses
- Social Workers
- Occupational Therapists
- Speech and Language Therapists
- Educational Psychologists
- Family Therapists
- Art Therapists
- Music Therapists
- Experiential counsellor

This multidisciplinary team works together to assess, diagnose, and come up with personalized treatment plans to address the unique needs of children and adolescents within the services. Those who work in child and youth mental health services complete comprehensive assessments by talking to the child or young person as well as collaborating with teachers and parents and observing the activities of the children in the natural environment (Arbesman *et al.*, 2013).

Conditions that Impact Occupational Performance

Mental health conditions can affect children and youth in their ability to participate in activities of daily living, take part in social interactions, and engage in study or schoolwork. Mental health conditions have unique, different signs and symptoms, and they also affect the child's occupational performance. The following are some of the conditions or mental health-related problems that an occupational therapist is likely to encounter in child and youth mental health services (Table **1**):

In this chapter, we briefly overview the common conditions as another specific section of this book is dedicated to discussing conditions in more detail. It is worth noting that most mental health conditions in early life years can extend into adulthood and, therefore, increase the risk of other challenges such as substance abuse, poverty, reduced life satisfaction, poor job satisfaction, and impaired relationships (Reardon *et al.*, 2017).

Table 1. Common conditions needing OT Intervention in CYMHS

Condition	Types
Anxiety Disorders	• Generalized anxiety disorder (GAD), • Social anxiety disorder, • Specific phobias. • Obsessive-Compulsive Disorder (OCD):
Depression	• Major depressive disorder • Persistent depressive disorder
Attention Deficit Hyperactivity Disorder (ADHD)	• Combined Type • Inattentive type • Hyperactive and impulsive type
Autism Spectrum Disorder (ASD)	• Level 1 • Level 2 • Level 3
Behavioural Disorders	• Oppositional defiant disorder (ODD) • Conduct disorder
Eating Disorders	• Anorexia nervosa • Bulimia nervosa • Binge-eating disorder • Avoidant restrictive food intake disorder
Trauma and Stressor-Related Disorders	• Post-Traumatic Stress Disorder (PTSD
Psychotic Disorders:	• Schizophrenia spectrum disorders • Bipolar Disorder • Other psychotic illnesses
Others	• Suicidal Ideation • Substance Use Disorders • Personality Disorders

Anxiety Disorders

This is among the most common mental health conditions in children and youth. Anxiety can affect a child's ability to participate in schooling, social interaction, and hobbies. This can result in masking and being compliant at school. In this scenario, the child might be so anxious within the school context that they comply; however, when they return home, they have emotional regulation difficulties that are not seen at school.

Depressive Disorders

The child will present with low motivation and energy to engage in social activities, play, and school activities. This can lead to poor school outcomes, challenges with social participation isolation, and reduced participation in meaningful activities.

Attention Deficit Hyperactive Disorder (ADHD)

The child may struggle with focusing, attention, concentration, following instructions, and memory. The child may present as not organised and may have difficulties with completing tasks. This often results in challenges with organisational skills, executive functioning skills, behavioural challenges, and learning. At home, the child or young person may have difficulties with performing activities of daily living and can haveunsatisfying daily routines.

Autism Spectrum Disorder (ASD)

Although not a mental illness, ASD affects the child's ability to socially interact, communicate appropriately and effectively, andengage in play. Sensory processing difficulties may also lead to poor performance in activities of daily living and being overwhelmed in social settings. An enabling environment and routines are often required by this group of children to reduce the impact of unpredictability.

Suicidal Ideations and Self-harm

Suicidal ideation and self-harm can result in strained relationships for the child with their family and other social connections. The occupational therapist may need to enable the child or young person's access to acute intensive care to ensure their safety and support for recovery. The occupational therapist may also work with the individual to identify triggers and support networks as well as coping strategies. Another key role the occupational therapist may take is risk assessment. This includes considering the environment, support systems, and coping mechanisms developed in the individual's safety plan to reduce risks and promote resilience (Quinlan *et al.*, 2021). Essential elements identified for suicide prevention at a state level by the US Suicide Prevention Resource Centre are shown in Fig. (**1**) below:

Gaming Disorder

This disorder is often seen when children develop impaired control and give increased priority to gaming to the extent that it takes precedence over activities of daily living. The occupational therapist would assess the impact of gaming on schooling, ADLs, and social relationships.

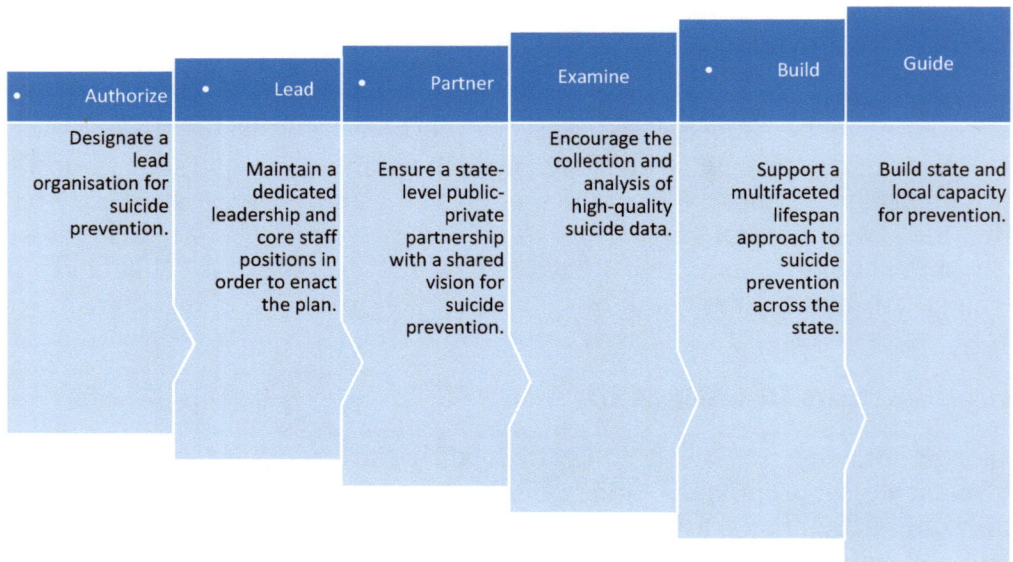

Fig. (1). Recommendations for suicide prevention programs.

Problems Related to the use of Social Media and Technology

Technology and social media have positive impacts on social connection and provide educational and recreational opportunities; however, overuse of these can have negative implications on the child's mental health. Addictions to technology and cyberbullying can have negative consequences.

Interventions and Recovery Strategies

Children and youth occupational therapists tailor interventions to address the unique presentations. For instance, they may use play strategies aimed at promoting engagement, developing skills, enhancing well-being, improving social communication and emotional regulation, and providing transactional support within their environmental settings. The occupational therapist would work collaboratively with the child or youth and their families to identify meaningful goals and objectives regarding their activities of daily living, social participation, and functional skills. Using activity analysis, the occupational therapist would create goals that are specific, measurable, achievable, relevant, and time-bound (AOTA, 2020). The occupational therapist will also use purposeful and meaningful activities that target those specific therapeutic goals. Interventions include a range of activities such as sensory activities, play, creative arts, experiential counselling, social skills training, and life skills development activities (Parham & Fazio, 2008). Below are some of these specific interventions:

Sensory Integration Therapy and Sensory Modulation

This is mainly used for children who have heightened sensitivity to sensory input or who have sensory registration difficulties. Children who also present with sensory modulation difficulties may require the use of sensory interventions such as a sensory diet to provide the sensory input that they might be seeking, as well as to calm and organise their central nervous system. Activities may include sensory circuits, deep pressure, movement breaks, and equipment such as noise-cancellation headphones.

Social Skills Training (SST)

SST can be done with individuals or groups. The focus is on educating and teaching the child or youth the necessary skills for successful social interaction and participation. The occupational therapist would use activities such as role-playing, modelling, and social stories to assist the child and youth in learning socially appropriate behaviours, communication skills, and problem-solving skills.

School-based Interventions

The occupational therapist works closely with educators within the school environment. This includes working with the teachers, administrators, teachers' assistants, school counsellors, and the school special education needs coordinators. The occupational therapist creates supportive, enabling environments. Enabling environments are developed by providing accommodations, adaptations, modifications, direct therapies, and opportunities for emotional regulation. When the occupational therapist promotes inclusion and participation, the children and youth are bound to thrive within the school setting (Case-Smith & Holland 2009).

Telehealth and Digital Interventions

Post the COVID-19 pandemic, the use of telehealth and other digital technologies in occupational therapy practice increasingly became important in children and youth mental health services and occupational therapy services in general. Occupational therapists use video conferencing, telephone calls, mobile apps, and virtual reality platforms to deliver services remotely to children, youth, and their families and to provide continuing care (Campden & Silva, 2021).

Impact of Parental Mental Illness on Children

Parental involvement in CYMHS can be part of the treatment process through family therapy, communication with home programs, and finding out the family relational context to provide other clinicians with relevant information (Brown, 2020). The parent's role is also to facilitate appointments and help implement home programs recommended by treating clinicians during sessions (Haine-Schlagel & Walsh, 2015). Health professionals who work in mental health, particularly with children, want a positive alliance with families, so it is important to have them involved in the treatment process (Brown, 2020). The clinician is employed to work with the child, and parental influence can become overwhelming, impacting the clinician and child relationship (Brown, 2020). Likewise, children with parents who experience a mental illness may be more vulnerable to developing mental health issues and conditions themselves. Accessing and providing support for children will help promote their own mental health and well-being and assist in preventing mental health issues in the future. Talking to children about their understanding of living with a parent who is experiencing mental illness may help to validate and shield the young person. Family work in mental health practice requires the practitioner to develop an understanding of many factors that influence people's reactions to major life events. This includes the common sense of loss when relatives realise that the illness is going to affect the hopes they had for the person's (and their) future and the social and economic consequences of having an ill family member. Some other factors are shown in Fig. (**2**).

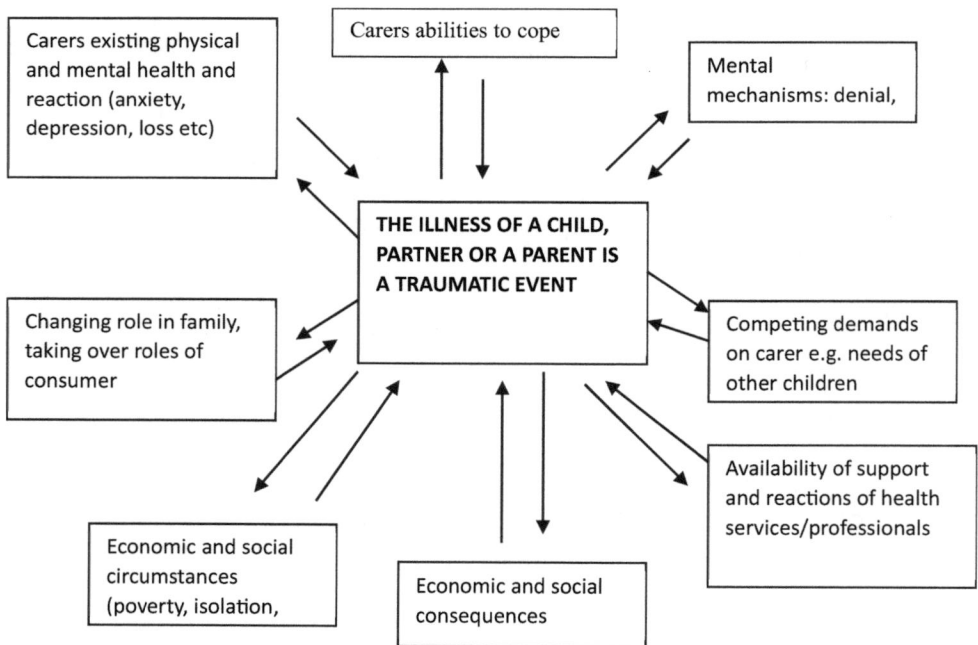

Fig. (2). Factors influencing people's reactions to major life events.

Discovering that a family member has a mental illness can bring great stress to a family. Family members may experience a whole range of emotions, including confusion, grief, and a sense of loss. Australian surveys have found that between 29% to 35% of clients in the mental health sector are female parents of dependent children under the age of 18 years. In the 2002 National Survey of Mental Health & Wellbeing, it was indicated that 15% of boys and 14.4% of girls between the ages of 4 to 12 had some type of mental health problem.

Clear information about mental illness for all family members can assist them in coming to terms with what is happening. It can help them understand their current situation and then prepare for the future.

Effects of Parental Mental Illness on Child Wellbeing

Bipolar Disorder

There may be a disruption to the continuity of care, which results in the child becoming fearful and distressed, especially after encountering manic behavioural disturbances. The greatest risk to children is through a manic relapse during post-partum pregnancy within the first 90 days, which places the child at a greater risk of emotional and physical neglect.

Depression

Some long-term effects include social and occupational difficulties. According to Beardslee *et al.*, by the age of 20, children with parents who have depression have a 40% chance of having an episode of major depression.

Schizophrenia

The child will be more vulnerable to developmental delays and emotional problems. Studies have shown that the child-rearing environment is characterised by less play, fewer learning experiences, and less emotional and verbal involvement.

Personality Disorder

Behaviours associated with personality disorder include domestic violence, substance misuse, and social impairment, which leads to difficulties meeting the child's needs, emotional well-being, and physical safety. Children are at risk of disruption and discontinuities of early child-parent involvement.

Substance Misuse

The impact of parental drug and alcohol problems can include psychological difficulties (poor self-esteem, anxiety, withdrawal, hyperactivity), physical illnesses, social and interpersonal problems, academic problems, and behaviour problems. These are due to the potentially large effects on family functioning that can occur, such as serious disruptions in schooling, work, or social functioning.

Children's Experience

A systematic review of qualitative studies identified four themes to describe children's experiences of living with a parent with mental illness (Yamamoto & Keogh, 2018). The summary of Yamamoto and Keogh's (2018) findings were as follows:

- Children's understanding of parental mental illness- Children want to know what is happening to their parents, but only a few are told.
- Children's relationship with parents- Children's connections with their parents are broken, and yet children want to spend time with their parents.
- Coping strategies- Children need to develop positive coping strategies, and this can be difficult.
- Social connections of children – Children experience social connection problems because of their parents.

In view of the above factors, it can be concluded that to a large extent, children with parents with a mental illness experience:

- Self-isolation due to stigma,
- Educational disruption, tardiness, and nonattendance, leading to underperformance, and
- Display loyalty towards parents through guilt and fear (Yamamoto & Keogh, 2018).

How to Work with Families and Carers

The first thing is to understand how family members react to illness. Fig. (**2**) presents an explanation of family reactions in the form of a diagrammatic representation or model. Explanatory models are often understood as simply personal explanations of the illness one has, its course, and what is causing it (Mathews *et al*., 2019). The lived experience provides a unique and valuable input to the design and delivery of health programs (Sunkel & Sartor, 2022).

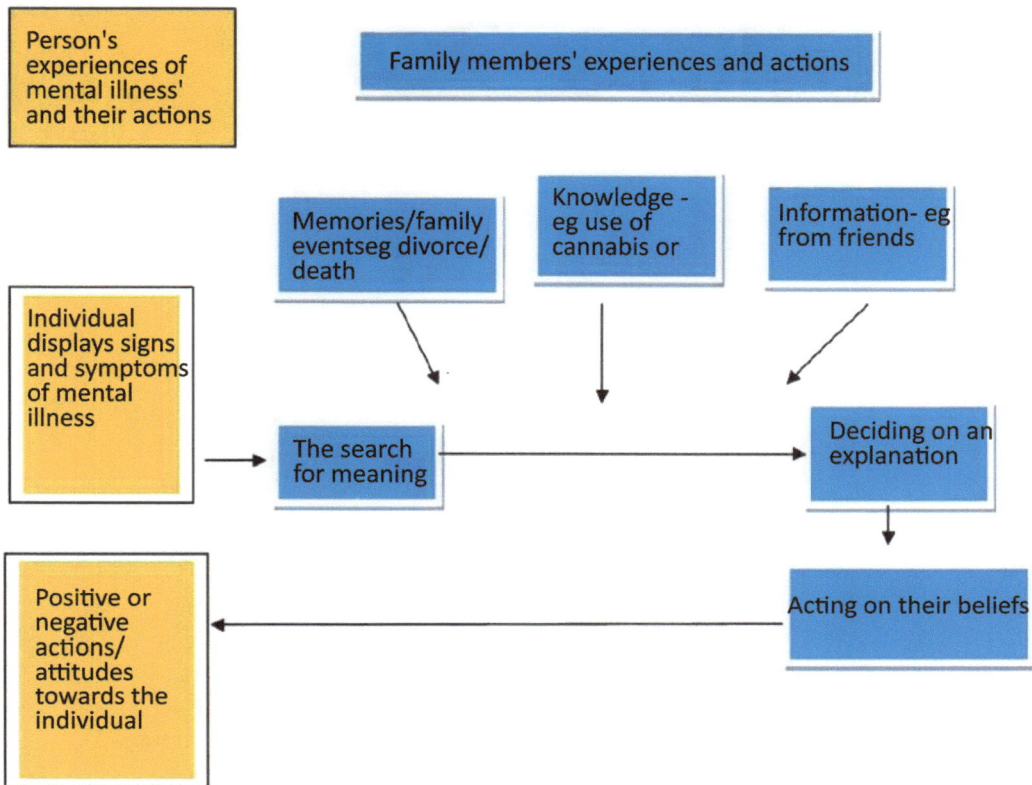

Fig. (3). An explanatory model of family members' reactions to mental illness.

The importance of the family members' beliefs about the consumer's behaviour can be seen in the following example using the A-B-C process (Activating event-Belief- Consequence) in Fig. (**4**) below:

Once unhelpful beliefs like these have been identified, relatives and carers can be helped to change them using structured work, often starting with information and education. When beliefs change, the consequences (feelings and behaviour) will change.

Interventions Tailored to Supporting Families

Families and carers should be recognised, respected, and supported as partners in providing care to the consumer. Some practical ways of ensuring family and carer involvement are below Fig. (**3**).

Activating event	Beliefs	Consequences
Son stays in bed, neglects hygiene and appearance, and does not tidy the room.	*"He could do it if he wanted, he can control it, he's being lazy, he needs a good push to get better"* OR *"He cannot do anything, I've let him down, I have to be there to help and do it for him"*	Feeling: Irritated, frustrated, angry Behaviour: Critical comments, nagging OR Feeling: Guilty, hopeless, sad Behaviour: Self-sacrificing, overcompensating.

Fig. (4). Example using the A-B-C process.

- Families and carers should be fully involved in aspects of the consumer's care when/wherever possible.
- Families and carers should be engaged as early as possible in the episode of treatment and care.

Also, provide children with the opportunity to talk about their experiences.

- Introduce yourself, tell them who you are and what your job is.
- Tell them what is going to happen next.
- Give children as much information as possible.
- Talk to children and listen to them.
- Ask children what they know and what they think- they live with their parents; they know how they are behaving- so ask them.
- Keep them informed.

The process provides information, promotes understanding, and facilitates harmonious relationships within families. Waid & Kelly (2020) state that early assessment and care planning should also include discussion and planning for service provider and community-level factors that could impact sustained engagement with mental health services. They also made suggestions for interventions as listed below:

- Find out what they know already and respect their own explanatory model. Practitioners must be wary of within-family variability, such as different perspectives between parents and children about the nature and extent of the presenting problems and motivations to engage with services.
- Recognition of the consumer/client as a parent. Take time to empower families by providing clear and accurate information about the range of available services to the client's needs and preferences.
- Acknowledgement of the presence of children and their individuality.
- Engaging and forming a relationship with the parent/carer and child- a collaborative process (talking, not telling). Take time to explore and validate the client's feelings of skepticism and ambivalence about mental health services and treatment.
- Explore the parent's concerns about issues of confidentiality and discuss the benefits to children of receiving accurate and age-appropriate information.
- Promote children's access to age-appropriate information about the parent's mental illness while maintaining the right of the consumer to confidentiality.
- Provide opportunities for children to have their questions answered about their own risk of developing a mental illness and any concerns they may have about this on their future lifestyle.
- Ensure that young people who have major caregiving responsibilities for their parents have access to relevant information about their parent's treatment and involvement in their parent's discharge planning if they are admitted.
- Advocate for and provide services to assist children to remain well by having access to services that increase resilience, such as:
  - Having a contact person in the event of a crisis regarding their parent.
  - Knowing someone to talk with; opportunities to meet adults with whom they can develop supportive links.
  - Participation in activities where they can meet other children (peer support).
  - Provide opportunities for the children to develop coping skills and age-appropriate problem-solving capacities.

Using a checklist when working with families and carers may be helpful. The Table **2** below presents an example of such a checklist.

FAMILY AND CARERS ASSESSMENT CHECKLIST TABLE 2

Name(s) of family members involved/ relationships	
Assessed by_____ **date**_____ **Assessed**	
1	**Genogram.** Who is in the family, and who does the consumer live with and see regularly?
2	**Family timeline.** Growing up and early life experiences, the onset of problems, and since then, family events that may have affected the consumer, *i.e.*, bereavement, divorce, *etc.*
3	**Diagnosis/problem.** What have you been told? Do you know the diagnosis? What do you think it is?
4	**Aetiology.** What do you think is the cause of 'X's problems? Biological illness/upbringing/ inherited? The main cause (what is the family/carer explanatory model for the problem?)
5	**Course/prognosis.** Might the problem occur, what could make it worse/ bring it back? What if the person stops taking their medication?
6	**Main problem areas for the consumer** – What are they? Are they 'X's natural self or illness? Can X help/ control them? Ask for examples (the 'family Questionnaire (FQ) can be used to assess the following sections.)
	Does X have problems with negative symptoms?
	Does X have problems with 'difficult' behaviour?
	Does X have problems with relationships?
	Does X have problems with mood or mood changes (anxiety, depression, high moods, and irritability)?
	Does X have problems with psychotic or illness symptoms?
7	**MAIN PROBLEMS – FOR RELATIVE/CARER**
	Do you have someone to contact from services about concerns or advice?
	Would you like more information about … (the illness)?
	Would you like to learn how to monitor illness signs to get help early if needed?
	Have there been changes in your well-being since X became unwell? How has it affected you?
	Have there been changes in your relationship with X since s/he became unwell?
	Have there been changes in the relationship between X and… (other family members) since X became ill?
	Have you had to change your work pattern in the last year due to Xs illness?
	Have you had more responsibilities at home in the last year due to Xs illness?
	Have you reduced your social activities or seeing friends because of 'X's illness?
8	**What helps?** Is there anything you can do to help? Anything you should not do? (are there signs that the relative/carer uses criticism or over-involvement to help the consumer)
9	**Medication** – Does the relative/carer know if any is prescribed? What for? Name? How often is it taken? Taken for how long? Who will stop them? Side effects?
10	**What help would you like from our service?** For 'X'? For yourself? For the family together?

Name(s) of family members involved/ relationships
Assessed by_____ date_____ Assessed

11	Case formulation What is the problem? What precipitated the problem? What is perpetuating the problem? What are the predisposing factors and the protective factors?

Self-Care Strategies for Family Members

There are ways to incorporate self-care into daily routines. Clearing space in life for self-care often means shifting priorities or tasks to make that space. It is important for family members to try various self-care activities and find the ones that work best for them. Here are some practical suggestions for family members:

- Take one thing at a time.
- Solve little problems.
- Be realistic.
- Be flexible.
- Adopt a positive attitude.
- Avoid over-scheduling.
- Learn to relax.
- Treat your body well. Adopt a healthy lifestyle. ♦ Eat healthy food. ♦ Exercise. ♦ See your doctors regularly. ♦ Get enough sleep as often as you can. ♦ Take time off when you are sick.
- Watch what you are thinking.
- Share your feelings.
- Talk about stress with friends and family.
- Talking to a doctor, spiritual advisor, or other professional might also help.
- Learn to ask for help.
- Be aware of your limitations.
- Personalize your work and home environment.
- Take time for self-reflection.
- Say "no."
- Limit your exposure to media (*e.g.*, news stories, movies) that deals with sad, violent, or tragic themes.

SUMMARY

Mental health problems in children and young people can extend into childhood, so providing timely assessments and interventions to improve the outcomes and prognosis for children and young people is very important. CYMHS are commonly staffed by a range of health professionals that work collaboratively to determine and facilitate the most appropriate treatment plan for the children. Health professionals who work in mental health, particularly with children, must focus on developing a positive alliance with families and include them in the treatment process. OTs utilise client-centred therapy to make improvements to health and well-being by using targeted interventions that increase functionality. Occupational therapists work in multidisciplinary teams and play a key role in completing comprehensive mental health assessments of children and youth, which improves the understanding of the roles of the child or youth and the provision of appropriate interventions by collaborating with other health professionals, teachers, and parents and observing activities of the individual in their context.

REFERENCES

Arbesman, M., Bazyk, S., Nochajski, S.M. (2013). Systematic review of occupational therapy and mental health promotion, prevention, and intervention for children and youth. *Am. J. Occup. Ther., 67*(6), e120-e130.
[http://dx.doi.org/10.5014/ajot.2013.008359] [PMID: 24195907]

Brown, J. (2020). Engaging with Parents in Child and Adolescent Mental Health Services. *Aust. N. Z. J. Fam. Ther., 41*(2), 145-160.
[http://dx.doi.org/10.1002/anzf.1409]

Camden, C., Silva, M. (2021). Pediatric Teleheath: Opportunities Created by the COVID-19 and Suggestions to Sustain Its Use to Support Families of Children with Disabilities. *Phys. Occup. Ther. Pediatr., 41*(1), 1-17.
[http://dx.doi.org/10.1080/01942638.2020.1825032] [PMID: 33023352]

Haine-Schlagel, R., Walsh, N.E. (2015). A review of parent participation engagement in child and family mental health treatment. *Clin. Child Fam. Psychol. Rev., 18*(2), 133-150.
[http://dx.doi.org/10.1007/s10567-015-0182-x] [PMID: 25726421]

Healthdirect. (2021). Mental Health and Wellbeing. Available from: https://www.healthdirect. gov.au/mental-health-and-wellbeing.

Mathews, M., Bhola, P., Herbert, H., Chaturvedi, S.K. (2019). Explanatory models of mental illness among family caregivers of persons in psychiatric rehabilitation services: A pilot study. *Int. J. Soc. Psychiatry, 65*(7-8), 589-602.
[http://dx.doi.org/10.1177/0020764019866228] [PMID: 31385555]

MacDonald, K., Fainman-Adelman, N., Anderson, K.K., Iyer, S.N. (2018). Pathways to mental health services for young people: a systematic review. *Soc. Psychiatry Psychiatr. Epidemiol., 53*(10), 1005-1038.
[http://dx.doi.org/10.1007/s00127-018-1578-y] [PMID: 30136192]

Nardella, M. S., Carson, N. E., Colucci, C. N., Corsilles-Sy, C., Hissong, A. N., Simmons, D., Taff, S. D., Amin-Arsala, T., DeAngelis, T., Fitzcharles, D., Grajo, L. C., Higgins, S., Gray, J. M., Stoll, M., Harvison, N. (2018). Importance of collaborative occupational therapist-occupational therapy assistant intraprofessional education in occupational therapy curricula. *The American journal of occupational therapy, 72(Supplement_2)*.
[http://dx.doi.org/10.5014/ajot.2018.72S207]

Preventing suicide among men in the middle years: Recommendations for Suicide Prevention Programs.

Queensland Government, (2021). Children's Health Queensland Hospital and Health Service. Available from: https://www.childrens.health.qld.gov.au/service-mental-health-community-clinics/.

Quinlan, K., Nickerson, K., Ebin, J., Humphries-Wadsworth, T., Stout, E., Frankini, E. (2021). Supporting a

public health approach to suicide prevention: Recommendations for state infrastructure. *Suicide Life Threat. Behav., 51*(2), 352-357.
[http://dx.doi.org/10.1111/sltb.12711] [PMID: 33876497]

Reardon, T., Harvey, K., Baranowska, M., O'Brien, D., Smith, L., Creswell, C. (2017). What do parents perceive are the barriers and facilitators to accessing psychological treatment for mental health problems in children and adolescents? A systematic review of qualitative and quantitative studies. *Eur. Child Adolesc. Psychiatry, 26*(6), 623-647.
[http://dx.doi.org/10.1007/s00787-016-0930-6] [PMID: 28054223]

Sunkel, C., Sartor, C. (2022). Perspectives: involving persons with lived experience of mental health conditions in service delivery, development and leadership. *BJPsych Bull., 46*(3), 160-164.
[http://dx.doi.org/10.1192/bjb.2021.51] [PMID: 33977895]

Waid, J., Kelly, M. (2020). Supporting family engagement with child and adolescent mental health services: A scoping review. *Health Soc. Care Community, 28*(5), 1333-1342.
[http://dx.doi.org/10.1111/hsc.12947] [PMID: 31951087]

World Health Organisation, (2021). Mental health of adolescents. Available from: https://www.who.int/news-room/fact-sheets/detail/adolescent-mental-health.

Yamamoto, R., Keogh, B. (2018). Children's experiences of living with a parent with mental illness: A systematic review of qualitative studies using thematic analysis. *J. Psychiatr. Ment. Health Nurs., 25*(2), 131-141.
[http://dx.doi.org/10.1111/jpm.12415] [PMID: 28776896]

Young, E., Green, L., Goldfarb, R., Hollamby, K., Milligan, K. (2020). Caring for children with mental health or developmental and behavioural disorders: Perspectives of family health teams on roles and barriers to care. *Can. Fam. Physician, 66*(10), 750-757.
[PMID: 33077456]

CHAPTER 15

COVID-19, Mental Health, and Occupational Therapy

Tawanda Machingura[1,*]

[1] *Head of Discipline Occupational Therapy Program, University of Notre Dame Australia, Sydney, Australia*

Abstract: The COVID-19 pandemic has significantly impacted global health, prompting widespread public health measures that inadvertently disrupted occupational engagement and mental health. This chapter highlights the specific challenges presented by COVID-19 with a focus on mental health. This chapter focuses on mental health, a key strategy in responding to the pandemic, as identified by the World Health Organisation (WHO). Key mental health-related impacts of the COVID-19 pandemic on the world's population included occupational disruption, increased mental health issues, and a marked impact on vulnerable populations such as children and those with pre-existing mental conditions. Telehealth emerged as a crucial adaptation in occupational therapy, facilitating continuity of care. However, disparities in access to these services persist, necessitating further attention to health equity. Lessons learned are ongoing and point to the use of virtual/ teletherapy technologies, the need for integrated health services, and ongoing support for mental health care in future pandemics.

Keywords: COVID-19, Health service delivery, Mental health, Occupational engagement, Occupational therapy, Pandemic preparedness, Psychological distress, Social isolation, Telehealth, Vulnerable populations.

INTRODUCTION

Many pandemics and epidemics have been known to have occurred throughout human history. In the last century, the world has seen the Spanish flu (1918-1920), the Asiatic flu (1956-1957), the severe acute respiratory syndrome (SARS, 2002-2003), the "Swine" flu (2009), the Ebola (2013-2014) and many others. Psychological distress in the population has been reported in all previous pandemics and epidemics (Talevi *et al.*, 2020). Despite this historical context, the world was seemingly surprised and unprepared when the COVID-19 pandemic

[*] **Corresponding author Tawanda Machingura:** Head of Discipline Occupational Therapy Program, University of Notre Dame Australia, Sydney, Australia; E-mail: tawanda.machingura@nd.edu.au

started. The purpose of this chapter is to assist the reader in understanding the impact of the measures taken and the lessons learned from the experience.

COVID-19

The World Health Organization declared that the widespread severe acute respiratory syndrome coronavirus 2 (SARS-CoV-2), which soon became known as the coronavirus disease 2019 (COVID-19), was a global pandemic in March 2020. Many public health measures were implemented, such as 'lockdowns' and 'social distancing', and other infection control measures to contain the COVID-19 pandemic. Inadvertently, these measures also had unintended consequences, disrupting occupational engagement to many people across the world (Culleton, 2022) as well as forcing people to adapt to new ways of living (Maynard, 202). The impact of COVID-19 on mental and neurological health and substance use services (MNS) has now been evaluated, and leading causes of disruptions are identified in below (WHO, 2020).

Table 1. Leading causes of disruptions in MNS-related intervention/services

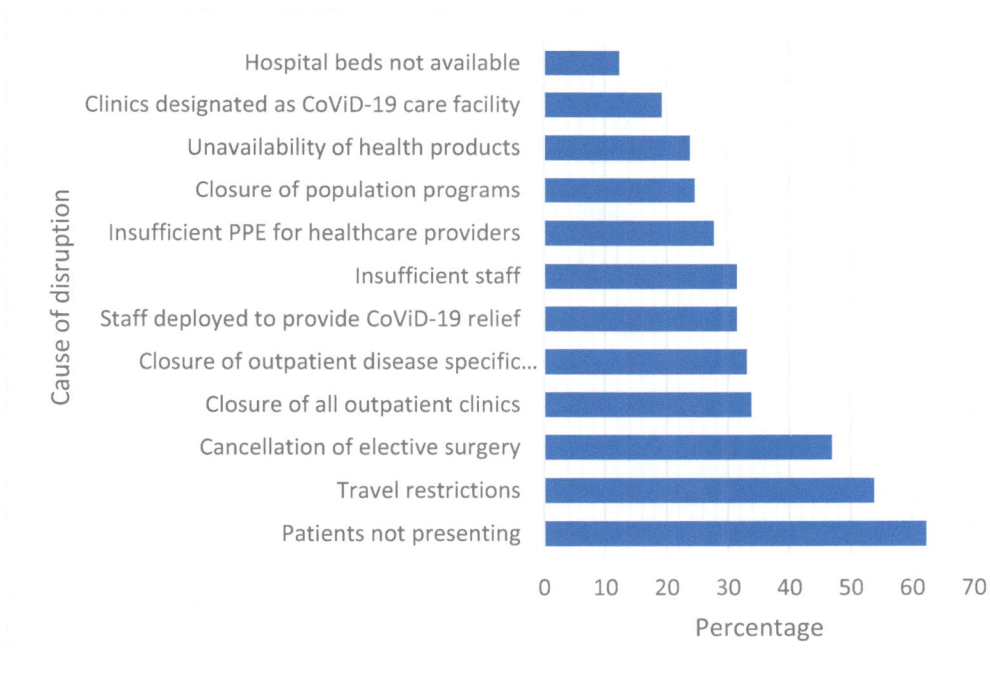

*Data sourced from WHO 2020, under the Creative Commons Attribution-licence-NC-SA 3.0 IGO; https://creativecommons.org/licenses/by-nc-sa/3.0/igo).

The occupational balance and mental health of the population, especially those who already had a previous history of mental illness, were affected negatively (WJHO, 2021). There were also negative effects on people's physical health, including pulmonary, cardiac, and muscular problems and neurological manifestations that directly affect mobility (Grabowski *et al.*, 2020) and the performance of activities of daily living (Grabowski *et al.*, 2020; Sánchez-Guarnido *et al.*, 2021).

Measuring the Impact of COVID-19

According to Moreno *et al* (2020), p.819, the following indicators should be continuously assessed during and after the pandemic and compared with corresponding indicators before the pandemic to establish pandemic-related changes in local and national delivery systems for mental health:

- The proportion of all mental health services provided in inpatient, emergency, institutional (*e.g.*, prisons), outpatient, community, and home-based settings
- Rates of face-to-face, video, and telephone contact with different types of mental health providers
- Rates of prescription and use of psychiatric medication
- Access to, and use of, different mental health services both by people with pre-existing mental health disorders and those with new incident cases of mental illness, and the sociodemographic characteristics of these users
- Quality of care of different mental health services (including acceptability and satisfaction with health-care providers), with a focus on user expectations and satisfaction and on functional, vocational, and clinical outcomes (including families' or carers' views)
- Disparities in mental healthcare, with socioeconomic, race, and ethnicity data linked to quality measures
- Integration of mental health services with general health services, social welfare, and other institutions (*e.g.*, schools, prisons) and community associations
- Governmental and non-governmental financial support for mental health and social care services and for research focusing on the monitoring and improvement of mental health services" p. 819.

During the COVID-19 pandemic, these measures were not reported. In this chapter, the author will not be reporting on the outcomes as the purpose is to alert the reader to future practice rather than dwell on history. The reader is encouraged to reflect on these outcome measures in their own country and context.

What were the Effects of COVID-19?

Occupational Disruption

The lockdown measures implemented by many governments across the world slowed down the spread of the COVID-19 virus but impacted people's engagement in occupations and caused major changes in people's behavioural patterns There was an interruption of people's daily routines and occupations; people had to modify their habits and adopt new and/or previously unperformed roles. During the pandemic, it became impossible to carry out the usual habits and rituals that formed part of the individual's occupational identity before the pandemic (Muñoz-Valverde *et al.*, 2020). These measures resulted in reduced access to everyday community resources necessary for everyday life, for example, assess to shops, leisure facilities, cultural supports and facilities, and social and economic hubs and facilities (Culleton, 2022). As a result, high unemployment rates resulting from the implementation of lockdowns were reported in some countries, such as Brazil (Ricci *et al.*, 2020). The impact on students came in the form of the suspension of face-to-face classes (Gomez, 2020).

Increased Alcohol Consumption and Other Social Problems

The were negative impacts associated with lockdown measures during the COVID-19 pandemic. Many preventable lifestyle risks for both premature death and disease burden were amplified (Guignard *et al.*, 2021). Many studies reported that there was an increased alcohol consumption in the general population in many countries (Guignard *et al.*, 2021; Pannoi *et al.*, 2024). The lockdowns also led to social isolation, loss of income, loneliness, inactivity, limited access to basic services, increased access to and use of food, tobacco, alcohol, online gambling, and decreased family and social support, especially in older and vulnerable people (Guignard *et al.*, 2021; Moreno *et al.*, 2020).

Increased Mental Health Problems

There were adverse mental health effects in previously healthy people, and these effects were more marked in people with pre-existing mental health disorders (Moreno *et al.*, 2020). Problems such as stress, anger, and an increase in risky behaviours, for example, online gambling, were reported in the general population (Moreno *et al.*, 2020). An increase in alcohol consumption and domestic violence because of alcohol consumption were also reported (Moreno *et al.*, 2020). People with COVID-19 or those recovering from it were found to have higher rates of post-traumatic stress disorder, particularly after severe coronavirus infections (Moreno *et al.*, 2020). Individuals with pre-existing mental health conditions had a higher risk of infection with SARS-CoV-2 (Moreno *et al.*, 2020).

Impact on Children and Young People

A higher-than-expected prevalence of late talkers (below the 10th percentile) was reported among females and children born during the first wave of the pandemic (Giesbrecht, 2024). Young children were at increased risk of acute stress disorders, anxiety, adjustment disorders, and grief (Moreno *et al.*, 2020).

Impact on Health Service Delivery

During the pandemic, access to other types of healthcare was restricted as a key method for controlling the spread of COVID-19. However, this measure limited treatment to other life-threatening conditions, leading to delays in accessing treatment for those with other conditions, sometimes with serious consequences, including loss of life for those affected (Moreno *et al.*, 2020). Furthermore, the focus during this time was on physical health, which meant that the mental health of populations was largely ignored.

The positive impact to come out of the COVID-19 pandemic was the increased use of telehealth. Prior to the pandemic, telehealth was rarely used by health services around the world; however, it rapidly became a commonly used tool during the pandemic (Mann *et al*, 2020).

What Lessons were Learned?

- The main educational focus during the pandemic was on physical health (Moreno *et al.*, 2020). Health services have since been promoting changes to facilitate access to mental health services, including the widespread use of telehealth and virtual meetings for medication management, nursing, case management, vocational interventions, and peer support (Moreno *et al.*, 2020).
- The facilitation of diverse and flexible access to mental healthcare is particularly important and can have longer-term advantages and help reduce disparities in healthcare.
- Mental health professionals should also advise regulators to develop, implement, and assess strategies for dealing with the pandemic and its aftermath (Moreno *et al.*, 2020).
- World Federation of Occupational Therapists (WFOT) issued a statement stating that occupational therapists' role would be to work with people "…to develop strategies to facilitate continued access to their occupations. These will include, but will not be limited to, individual, family, community, social and environmental adaptation, mental health, assistive technology, and telehealth" (WFOT, 2020, p. 1).
- Evidence-based clinical practice guidelines recommend offering occupational therapy to people with severe mental disorders (SMDs) during both the acute

phase and the recovery phase [Galletly *et al.*, 2020)], as this has proven useful in improving social functioning and reducing the number of readmissions (Mann *et al.*, 2020).
- There is a need to consider the special needs of children and young people in disaster preparation and response, and this includes pandemics such as COVID-19 (Giesbrecht, 2024).

Changes to Occupational Therapy Mental Health Practice Due to COVID-19

In occupational therapy practice, there was a change from face-to-face interventions to online interventions (Sánchez-Guarnido *et al.*, 2021). Telehealth use has increased in occupational therapy practice and, more generally, in mental health (Sánchez-Guarnido *et al.*, 2021). Video conferencing was particularly reported to have high levels of satisfaction on the part of the users who receive it (Aleman, 2018; Sánchez-Guarnido *et al.*, 2021), and it was found to aid relapse prevention in different mental disorders (Hennemann *et al.*, 2018). Telehealth, such as video conferencing, also led to improvements in treatment adherence, social functioning, and quality of life, even in some cases, similar to those observed in face-to-face intervention (Backhaus *et al.*, 2012).

Ongoing Challenges to Practice

The use of digital technology-based therapy is also known to be lower for people with psychosis than for the general population (Culleton, 2022; Robotham *et al.*, 2021). This implies that there is potential for an exacerbation of inequalities in access to healthcare (Moreno *et al.*, 2020).

Reflect
<ul><li>Do you prefer to receive health services using digital technologies rather than face-to-face?</li><li>In your context, do or will all your clients have access to the digital technologies they need?</li><li>In your context, is there a possibility of exacerbating inequalities in accessing healthcare?</li><li>What can you do in your context to mitigate these risks?</li></ul>

CONCLUSION

The COVID-19 pandemic affected the physical as well as the mental health of the world's population. Both physical and mental health effects are still ongoing for many people around the world. People with pre-existing mental illnesses, children, and young people, as well as healthcare workers, were found to be particularly vulnerable, and more needs to be done to protect them in the current and future pandemics. More research is needed to ensure better preparedness for future pandemics and epidemics.

Chapter Summary

This chapter examines the effects of the COVID-19 pandemic on mental health and occupational engagement. The pandemic's onset led to drastic public health measures, including lockdowns and social distancing, which severely disrupted daily routines and occupational identities. The chapter discussed the surge in mental health issues, particularly among individuals with pre-existing conditions, and highlighted increased alcohol consumption and social isolation as significant concerns.

Children and young people faced unique challenges, with reports of heightened anxiety and developmental delays. Access to healthcare, especially for non-COVID-19-related conditions, was restricted, leading to serious health consequences. The transition to telehealth in occupational therapy emerged as a vital response, offering new means of support despite presenting challenges in access for marginalised groups. The chapter concludes with recommendations for future pandemic preparedness, emphasising the importance of addressing mental health needs and ensuring equitable access to care.

REFERENCES

Aleman, A., Enriquez-Geppert, S., Knegtering, H., Dlabac-de Lange, J.J. (2018). Moderate effects of noninvasive brain stimulation of the frontal cortex for improving negative symptoms in schizophrenia: Meta-analysis of controlled trials. *Neurosci. Biobehav. Rev., 89*, 111-118.
[http://dx.doi.org/10.1016/j.neubiorev.2018.02.009] [PMID: 29471017]

Backhaus, A., Agha, Z., Maglione, M.L., Repp, A., Ross, B., Zuest, D., Rice-Thorp, N.M., Lohr, J., Thorp, S.R. (2012). Videoconferencing psychotherapy: A systematic review. *Psychol. Serv., 9*(2), 111-131.https://psycnet.apa.org/buy/2012-14616-001
[http://dx.doi.org/10.1037/a0027924] [PMID: 22662727]

Culleton, B. (2022). Exploring the professional experiences of mental health occupational therapists during a period of COVID-19. *Irish Journal of Occupational Therapy, 50*(1), 3-9.
[http://dx.doi.org/10.1108/IJOT-04-2021-0012]

Galletly, C., Castle, D., Dark, F., Humberstone, V., Jablensky, A., Killackey, E., Kulkarni, J., McGorry, P., Nielssen, O., Tran, N. (2016). Royal Australian and New Zealand College of Psychiatrists clinical practice guidelines for the management of schizophrenia and related disorders. *Aust. N. Z. J. Psychiatry, 50*(5), 410-472.
[http://dx.doi.org/10.1177/0004867416641195] [PMID: 27106681]

Giesbrecht, G.F., van de Wouw, M., Watts, D., Perdue, M.V., Graham, S., Lai, B.P.Y., Tomfohr-Madsen, L., Lebel, C. (2024). Language learning in the context of a global pandemic: proximal and distal factors matter. *Pediatr. Res.,* 1-11.
[http://dx.doi.org/10.1038/s41390-024-03583-9] [PMID: 39294240]

Gomez, I.N.B. (2023). Reflections on the role of occupational therapy programmes on the mental health of stakeholders' transition to e-learning during the COVID-19 pandemic. *World Federation of Occupational Therapists Bulletin, 79*(1), 4-8.
[http://dx.doi.org/10.1080/14473828.2020.1836791]

Grabowski, D.C., Joynt Maddox, K.E. (2020). Postacute care preparedness for COVID-19: thinking ahead. *JAMA, 323*(20), 2007-2008.
[http://dx.doi.org/10.1001/jama.2020.4686] [PMID: 32211831]

Guignard, R., Andler, R., Quatremère, G., Pasquereau, A., du Roscoät, E., Arwidson, P., Berlin, I., Nguyen-Thanh, V. (2021). Changes in smoking and alcohol consumption during COVID-19-related lockdown: a cross-sectional study in France. *Eur. J. Public Health, 31*(5), 1076-1083. https://academic.oup.com/eurpub/article/31/5/1076/6214519
[http://dx.doi.org/10.1093/eurpub/ckab054] [PMID: 33826721]

Hennemann, S., Farnsteiner, S., Sander, L. (2018). Internet- and mobile-based aftercare and relapse prevention in mental disorders: A systematic review and recommendations for future research. *Internet Interv., 14*, 1-17.
[http://dx.doi.org/10.1016/j.invent.2018.09.001] [PMID: 30510909]

Mann, D.M., Chen, J., Chunara, R., Testa, P.A., Nov, O. (2020). COVID-19 transforms health care through telemedicine: Evidence from the field. *J. Am. Med. Inform. Assoc., 27*(7), 1132-1135.
[http://dx.doi.org/10.1093/jamia/ocaa072] [PMID: 32324855]

Moreno, C., Wykes, T., Galderisi, S., Nordentoft, M., Crossley, N., Jones, N., Cannon, M., Correll, C.U., Byrne, L., Carr, S., Chen, E.Y.H., Gorwood, P., Johnson, S., Kärkkäinen, H., Krystal, J.H., Lee, J., Lieberman, J., López-Jaramillo, C., Männikkö, M., Phillips, M.R., Uchida, H., Vieta, E., Vita, A., Arango, C. (2020). How mental health care should change as a consequence of the COVID-19 pandemic. *Lancet Psychiatry, 7*(9), 813-824.
[http://dx.doi.org/10.1016/S2215-0366(20)30307-2] [PMID: 32682460]

Muñoz-Valverde, V., Zujeros, S.M. Guía clínica de intervención de terapia ocupacional en pacientes con Covid-19. Recensión. *Revista Terapia Ocupacional Galicia, 17*(2), 225-228.Available from: https://www.revistatog.es/ojs/index.php/tog/article/view/92. (2020).

Pannoi, T., Sottiyotin, T., Waleewong, O., Adulyarat, N. (2024). Perceived social measures and drinking behavior during the COVID-19 pandemic in Thailand. *J. Public Health Policy, 45*(4), 700-713.
[http://dx.doi.org/10.1057/s41271-024-00521-1] [PMID: 39294344]

Ricci, É.C., Dimov, T., da Silva Cassais, T., Dellbrügger, A.P. (2021). Occupational therapy in Brazil during the COVID-19 pandemic: peer support groups as mental health intervention strategy. *World Federation of Occupational Therapists Bulletin, 77*(1), 33-35.
[http://dx.doi.org/10.1080/14473828.2020.1840767]

Robotham, D., Satkunanathan, S., Doughty, L., Wykes, T. (2016). Do we still have a digital divide in mental health? A five-year survey follow-up. *J. Med. Internet Res., 18*(11), e309.
[http://dx.doi.org/10.2196/jmir.6511] [PMID: 27876684]

Sánchez-Guarnido, A.J., Domínguez-Macías, E., Garrido-Cervera, J.A., González-Casares, R., Marí-Boned, S., Represa-Martínez, Á., Herruzo, C. (2021). Occupational therapy in mental health *via* telehealth during the COVID-19 pandemic. *Int. J. Environ. Res. Public Health, 18*(13), 7138.
[http://dx.doi.org/10.3390/ijerph18137138] [PMID: 34281072]

Talevi, D., Socci, V., Carai, M., Carnaghi, G., Faleri, S., Trebbi, E., di Bernardo, A., Capelli, F., Pacitti, F. (2020). Mental health outcomes of the CoViD-19 pandemic. *Riv. Psichiatr., 55*(3), 137-144.
[http://dx.doi.org/10.1708/3382.33569] [PMID: 32489190]

World Health Organization. (2020). The impact of COVID-19 on mental, neurological and substance use services: results of a rapid assessment. Available from: https://apps.who.int/iris/handle/10665/335838.

Part 4
Recovery-Oriented Occupational Therapy Practice in Mental Health

CHAPTER 16

Social Determinants of Mental Health: A Critical Occupational Perspective

Clement Nhunzvi[1,*] and Roshan Galvaan[2]

[1] *Occupational Therapy Program, Bond University, Gold Coast, Australia*

[2] *Department of Occupational Therapy, University of Cape Town, Cape Town, South Africa*

Abstract: Living a healthy lifestyle is influenced by personal agency and societal structures, which contribute to a continuum of physical and mental health. The social determinants of mental health offer a perspective on how structural factors may influence a person's lifestyle. These determinants include the conditions in which people are born, live, grow up, and age, shaped by policy decisions and resource distribution within their communities and societies. These social, political, cultural, and economic conditions, along with spiritually problematic situations, may disrupt optimal mental health, increase the risk of mental disorders, and worsen outcomes among those affected. The concept of social inclusion holds great potential in the rights-based examination and redress of challenging social determinants of mental health. Further to this, the chapter proposes drawing on a critical occupational perspective as a paradigm shift from an individualistic medicalised view to a more collective and justice-oriented approach, challenging the taken-for-granted ways of participation and centering participation in meaningful occupations for all.

Keywords: Africa, Disability, HIV/AIDS, Mental health, Occupation, Occupational justice, Occupational perspective, Poverty, Social determinants, Social exclusion, Social inclusion.

INTRODUCTION

Maintaining mental and physical health is important for sustainable human development across the lifespan. Healthy lifestyles are integral, however, there are contextual factors to consider that may be facilitative or restrictive in nature. It has long been demonstrated that healthy lifestyles occur through an interaction between many factors, which could be viewed as including the broad categories of personal agency and societal structures. Some geopolitical situations are historically positioned for worse outcomes because of the social determinants of health dominant in these contexts.

* **Corresponding author Clement Nhunzvi:** Occupational Therapy Program, Bond University, Gold Coast, Australia; E-mail: clemynhu@gmail.com

Tawanda Machingura (Ed.)

There are ongoing contestations over how much personal agency compared to societal structures influences the achievement of healthy lifestyles (Cockerham, 2005). Nevertheless, it is evident that agency, which involves the capacity to utilise various causal abilities, and structure, which encompasses established laws and resources within society, both contribute to a continuum of physical and mental health (World Health Organization and Calouste Gulbenkian Foundation, 2014). However, healthy lifestyles are challenged in conditions of ill health and disability and are usually complicated by social inequalities that could lead to social exclusion (Ikkos, 2023). Mental health has been traditionally neglected, and there is a need to explore the complex factors and propose sustainable solutions. To this end, social determinants of mental health offer a perspective with which to understand how structural factors may influence a person's lifestyle, health, and well-being. This chapter begins with a description of the social determinants of mental health and then draws on a critical occupational perspective to discuss how mental illness and the associated exclusions may be addressed.

Mental health is influenced by the social determinants of health, which are social conditions that people experience throughout their lives, such as where they are born, live, grow up, and grow old. These conditions are shaped by policy decisions and the allocation of resources and opportunities in their communities and societies (Sen *et al*., 2007; Shim & Compton, 2020; Silva *et al*., 2016). This means that the environments where people live, and work have an impact on their mental health (Marmot, 2005). The idea of the social determinants of mental health has been widely adopted in the fields of population health, where there is a growing interest in how the social determinants of mental health interact with lifestyle-related diseases (Shim & Compton, 2020). These social, political, cultural, and economic factors, as well as spiritually challenging situations, can affect mental health negatively, increase the likelihood of mental disorders, and worsen the outcomes for those who are already affected (Lund *et al*., 2018a; Shim & Compton, 2020). There have been many efforts to better understand and address the social determinants of mental health, as shown by the increasing number of publications, commissions, reports, and task forces on this topic (Satcher & Shim, 2015; Sen *et al*., 2007; Shim & Compton, 2020; Silva *et al*., 2016). All are designed to promote good mental health in an inclusive and equitable society.

Good mental health is a function of equitable and supportive human and non-human environments. When environments are unsupportive, such as when health inequities prevail, then health disparities exist between population groups (Lund *et al*., 2018a; Shim & Compton, 2020) and poor mental health may occur. Since the social determinants of mental health shape access to and distribution of opportunities and resources for mentally healthy lifestyles, addressing the social determinants of mental health becomes a necessary priority. It is important to do this in a manner that challenges and changes the values and policies sustaining the normative influences of the social determinants of mental health. Even more, applying this position to the everyday lives and realities of those affected and or at risk of social exclusion can enhance the mental health outcomes of a population.

Addressing Social Determinants of Mental Health in Developing Settings

Mental health challenges in developing settings remain prevalent and complex, with multiple causal roots disproportionately affecting already marginalised population groups. When contemplating what lifestyle changes could promote good mental health in low-resource settings, the historical origins of the political, social, economic, cultural, and physical factors of the environment should be considered. This is necessary since prevalent social inequalities, many of which have colonial descendance, have been implicated in major risk factors for most mental disorders (Lund *et al.*, 2018a; World Health Organization & Louste Gulbenkian Foundation 2014) (Fig. **1**). Little has been done beyond blueprints to seek redress to these challenges in most developing countries. Generally, these conditions remain under-researched with scant attention to how they could be considered in the prevention of mental disorders across the lifespan. Understanding social determinants of mental health and other associated concepts as they apply to marginalised population groups is drawn from the first author's doctoral thesis which explored the experience of social inclusion among young adults dually afflicted with substance use disorders and Human Immunodeficiency Virus (HIV) in Zimbabwe, Africa (Nhunzvi, 2021).

There is a need to deliberately target social determinants such as poverty, lack of education, unemployment, conflicts, political and economic crises, and adverse life experiences which continue to drive the unfair distribution of opportunity for lifestyles that promote good mental health. Most of these social determinants are influenced by the geopolitical locations, especially the characteristics of people's immediate neighbourhoods (Silva *et al.*, 2016). For example, in the first author's doctoral study with young adults dually afflicted with substance use disorders and HIV in Zimbabwe, unsupportive environments, poverty, unemployment, and political and economic crises were some of the major determinants of mental health (Nhunzvi, 2021). Also major was the challenge of access to resources and opportunities for healthy lifestyles even when one was considering recovery. Below we share P Jay[1]'s situation, emphasising the presence of social determinants of mental health.

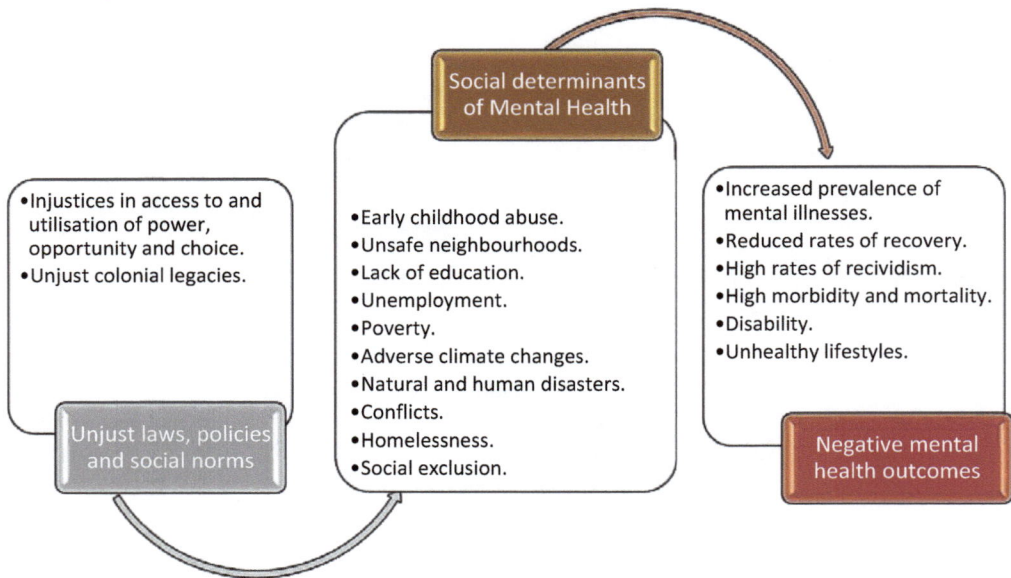

Fig. (1). Social determinants of mental health and their causes and consequences.

To address the outcomes of the social determinants of mental health in disadvantaged contexts, multisectoral and collaborative approaches that apply biopsychosocial models (models that look at the interconnection between biology, psychology, political and socio-environmental factors) are required (Frazier, 2020). These approaches should be guided by critical explorations of how to best respond and disrupt the pathways that lead to adverse mental health outcomes. Fig. (1) below depicts how the pathways between adverse mental health outcomes and Fig. (1) inequities and inequalities in opportunities are mediated through different types of social determinants of mental health (Compton & Shim, 2020). The seemingly predictable trajectory between adverse outcomes and inequitable and unjust opportunities could be disrupted to foster lifestyles that promote mental health.

P Jay

P Jay is a young adult residing in one of Harare's underdeveloped and poorly managed high-density suburbs. He is struggling with substance use disorder with the comorbidity of a poorly controlled HIV infection. In his narrative of seeking social inclusion and better mental health, several adverse social determinants of mental health are apparent, including the marginalised and crime infested neighbourhood, a function of the colonial past and a failing corrupt post-independence government. The quality of P Jay's neighbourhood and childhood have a tremendous effect on the course of his life. Access to decent shelter, food, basic education, productive engagements, and generally a conducive environment for growth remain a pipe dream for him and many in his community. P Jay is not battling mere substance use disorder and HIV, and he is not to blame for what he is going through. Stigma and discrimination against substance use disorders and HIV are prevalent in his community. Under-resourcing and non-implementation of policies and strategies is the order of the day. Worse, the hope for a mentally healthy lifestyle vanished too early for him and his siblings when they lost both parents to HIV/AIDS in a poverty-stricken context leaving them vulnerable and predisposed to injustices and exclusion.

Reflective Questions

• How can you use a critical occupational perspective to P Jay's situation?

• What are the social determinants of mental health that affect P Jay and his community, and how can you address them in your practice?

• How can you reduce stigma and discrimination against substance use disorder and HIV in P Jay's community, and promote social inclusion and good mental health?

• Identify key stakeholders in this situation and describe how you will collaborate them? Consider stakeholders such as other young adults in the community, policy makers, service providers, and community leaders, to advocate for the rights and needs of P Jay and his community?

Most adverse social determinants of mental health in most low-resource settings are a breeding ground for human rights violations, where those with mental disorders are disproportionately affected (Patel *et al.*, 2016). In these situations of human rights violations, quality of life is neglected and lifestyle diseases surge. Attending to these social determinants should therefore be treated as an urgent human rights issue (Patel *et al.*, 2016) if healthy lifestyles for all are to be achieved. In the example of P Jay, the starting point should be upholding his basic human rights, including access to food, shelter, healthcare, education, and all this in a supportive and nurturing neighbourhood. Poverty eradication should go beyond academic and political talk, into transforming human lives. Symptomatic relief and prescribed medication adherence alone are too superficial for complex challenges as shown in P Jay's situation, and hence the need for the critical approach we here propose.

Targeting Poverty and Stigma

Despite the deliberate efforts through the Sustainable Development Goals (SDGs) led by the United Nations, poverty and disability continue to complicate and negatively influence health outcomes (Hák *et al.*, 2016; Sachs, 2012). Poverty has remained a reality globally and even more in low-resource settings such as in some African countries, where some of the world's poorest economies are found (Reynolds, 2021). Lifestyle opportunities and choices possible in these conditions of lack render the promotion of mental health more difficult. There is empirical evidence associating poverty with common mental disorders in LMIC (Lund *et al.*, 2010). The relationship between poverty and mental health is bi-directional, for example, in South Africa poverty predicted worse depression, and depression contributed to a spiraling poverty cycle (Lund & Cois, 2018). Given that depression is one of the leading causes of disability (Friedrich, 2017; World Health Organisation (WHO), 2017), a concerted effort is needed to reduce its impacts through eradicating poverty. This will contribute to decreasing disability and the global disease burden mediated through depression. The poverty–disability cycle in Fig. (2) below should be broken for the betterment of mental health and healthy lifestyles for all.

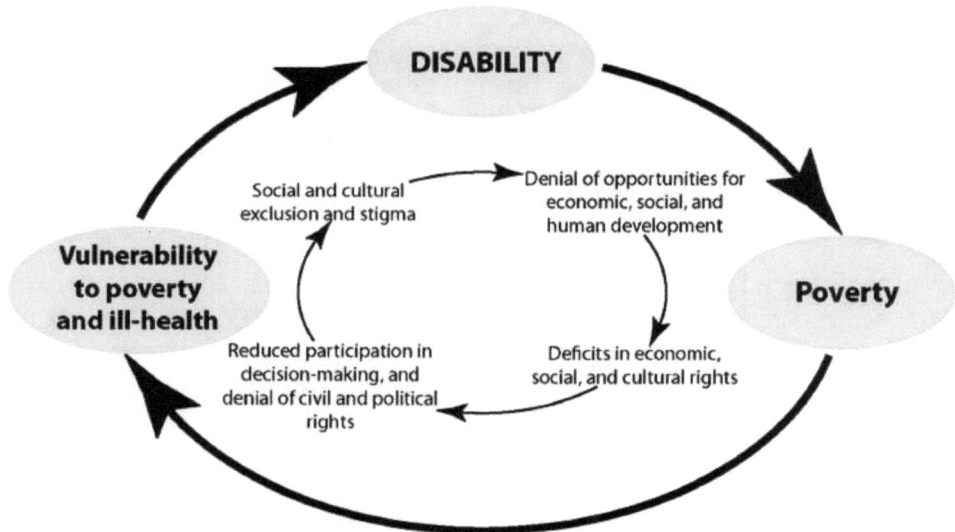

Fig. (2). The Poverty – Disability Cycle.

Note. Adapted from U.K. Department for International Development, 2000 (UK Department for International Development (DFID), 2000)

Stigma and discrimination against persons with mental illness are significant factors sustaining the disability–poverty cycle and consequently limiting the promotion of mental health and healthy lifestyles (Patel *et al.*, 2010; Ridley *et al.*, 2020). Stigma and discrimination occur in diverse ways. The power associated with different categories of social identities, such as race, ethnicity, citizenship status, sexual orientation, and occupational status intersects in different situations to produce different prejudices and privileges for different people. The way that this occurs should be explored in relation to the influences it may have on the social determinants of mental health (Alegría *et al.*, 2018). Stigma is a barrier to accessing health and social care services and thus may limit health-seeking behaviours that could promote healthy lifestyles and mental health. Shunned intersectional identities drawing from stigmatised and discriminated against conditions of substance use and HIV, made it very difficult for young adults such as P Jay, with a dual affliction of substance use disorders and HIV to access even those underdeveloped services (Nhunzvi, 2021).

To address social determinants of mental health, service providers, researchers, and advocates need to employ a revolutionary, human rights-based approach, entailing moving away from their traditional roles in biomedical approaches (Shim & Compton, 2020). In this chapter, we propose that a critical and exploratory research agenda to understand social inclusion holds promise to this effect since most disorders are associated and or made worse by social injustices and inequality. Strategic players in this case are urged to act further upstream to focus on mental health-promoting environments, environments that allow every citizen to flourish whilst leading a lifestyle they have reason to value (Shim & Compton, 2020).

Understanding the Value of Social Inclusion for Good Mental Health

A critical understanding and appreciation of social inclusion has the potential to prompt adaptive perspectives in comprehensively examining and challenging social determinants of mental health. The dominant social inclusion and mental health narrative has for long excluded the realities of those disenfranchised by disease and geopolitical forces in the Global South (Nhunzvi, 2021). With a particular focus on mental health, Allman (2013) argues for social inclusion as the needed doorway to greater social justice, equity, and collectivism in response to situations of injustice, oppression, and global crises including the growing burden of mental disorders (Allman, 2013). Social inclusion offers a way of focusing on population groups that are marginalized from mainstream society, including those with mental disorders (Nhunzvi, 2021) in order to understand the complex drivers of their non-health-promoting lifestyles. We propose investing in processes that enhance social justice and equality for all as a way of promoting social inclusion and mental health among the underclass and excluded groups. We take it that the lack of targeted focus on social fairness and equal opportunities, and poor mental health lifestyles will increase among the marginalised and disadvantaged. It also has to be acknowledged that, ignoring the social inclusion needs of some population groups will ultimately put the whole society at risk of social instability (The World Bank, 2013). Appreciating this perspective offers a foundation for advocating for global equity and self-determination of those marginalised, for a more meaningful, healthy life and a sense of belonging in society to occur. This would however call for critical perspectives to be applied. A critical occupational perspective, as way of exploring and seeking understanding of what surrounds everyday activities and occupations in society is presented next.

A Critical Occupational Perspective of Social Determinants of Mental Health and Social Inclusion

There is a paucity of literature on the critical occupational perspective of social determinants of mental health, including situations of social inclusion or exclusion. However, here we propose using the constructs of occupation and occupational choice as possibilities for understanding and applying this perspective even more in traditionally marginalised groups, inclusive of persons with mental illnesses.

Occupational therapy and occupational science primarily draw on the idea that occupation is fundamental to human life and that engagement in meaningful occupations is vital for sustainable human existence, health, and well-being (Nhunzvi, 2021; Wilcock, 2006; Yerxa, 2000). Meaningful occupations are foundational for mental health and a basic human right. Equitable access to and participation in such occupations have the potential to significantly transform the lives of those experiencing ill health or injuries (Christiansen & Townsend, 2009; Hammell & Iwama, 2012; Hammell, 2007; Kielhofner, 2009). In this area, social inclusion refers to the actions and results that tackle disparities hindering complete engagement in essential community roles, including educational, employment, and social activities. It is realized through active involvement in these roles and aligns seamlessly with the goals of occupational therapy in mental health settings. (Harrison & Sellers, 2008). In occupational therapy and occupational science, meaningful occupational participation and engagement can be considered to be fundamental human rights, and hence social determinants of mental health (Pereira *et al.*, 2020).

These everyday occupations encompass what people need to do, are expected to do, and want to do, and be in occupying their everyday lives (Harrison & Sellers, 2008). Adverse social determinants such as poverty leading to social exclusion, segregate people from those everyday occupations. These situations increase the risk for mental disorders and or worsen the outcomes in those already affected, hence should be a target for occupational therapy. Acting further upstream, at the level of social determinants, prioritising people's everyday doings, is what a critical occupational perspective advocates for. A critical occupational perspective calls for all mental health players to have a paradigm shift, moving away from a narrow-medicalised focus on symptomatic management. But rather to also address the underlying social determinants across the full continuum of mental health and well-being, even more with occupational rights in mind. The literature in occupational science and therapy suggests that social exclusion from active engagement in family and community life is often a consequence of the societal structures shaped by history, society, culture, and economy.(Barros *et al.*, 2011; Farias & Rudman, 2019; Kantartzis, 2018; Malfitano & Lopes, 2018; Malfitano *et al.*, 2014; Pereira, 2015; Pereira *et al.*, 2020); hence, the call for a departure from the individualist, reductionistic focus, and instead deliberate engagement with the macro factors influencing occupational access, opportunities, and participation (Frank & Muriithi, 2015; Laliberte Rudman, 2013; Malfitano *et al.*, 2021) and mental health and well-being.

Practice Example

Consider a case study of Mary, a 35-year-old woman with bipolar disorder who has been dismissed from work and is facing rejection among friends and relatives in a context with poor legislative frameworks to uphold the rights of persons with mental health challenges.

Using a critical occupational perspective, occupational therapists deliberately dare to challenge all the systems sustaining the injustices, from legislation to practice. The occupational therapist takes a collaborator explorative stance, whilst practicing professional advocacy. All key stakeholders are engaged to support Mary's participation in an equitable and just manner in her community, including policy makers, employers, and community leaders.

The ideal will be liberated participation in an occupation-centred and community-based occupational therapy program. The program should aim to promote social inclusion and recovery by facilitating access and participation in meaningful activities and social connections within Mary's community. The devised interventions should help Mary to develop a sense of belonging, identity, and purpose, and even more advocacy for her own rights.

This approach doesn't negate traditional occupational therapy goals but just focuses further upstream for sustainable and emancipatory work. Mary should still receive her client-centred occupational therapy to improve her condition management, self-esteem, coping skills, mood stability and more. Such a program demonstrates how the occupational perspective of social inclusion can enhance

Applying the critical occupational perspective would entail challenging the taken for granted ways of participation in society while pursuing social transformation and equitable justice to meaningful occupations (Barros *et al.*, 2011; Farias & Rudman, 2019; Kantartzis, 2018; Malfitano & Lopes, 2018; Malfitano *et al.*, 2014; Pereira, 2015; Pereira *et al.*, 2020; Whatley *et al.*, 2015). This in turn creates a fertile ground for the promotion of meaningful occupations and mental health for all. Fostering social inclusion and encouraging active engagement in meaningful activities form a compelling rationale for occupational therapists and researchers to address situations where adverse social factors negatively impact mental health. Their efforts should aim to cultivate lifestyles that promote positive mental well-being. This approach is flourishing among South American scholars and Brazil, in particular, through the genesis of social occupational therapy (Barros *et al.*, 2011; Jorge *et al.*, 2017; Malfitano, 2005; Malfitano & Lopes, 2018; Malfitano *et al.*, 2014; Muñoz, 2018; Pereira, 2015; Vinzón *et al.*, 2020). Their efforts promote and advocate for an occupational therapy service that is socially engaged and transformative, operating beyond the confinements of the healthcare system. This approach is aimed at investigating and tackling the underlying structures that contribute to social exclusion and injustice affecting individuals, groups, and communities(Barros *et al.*, 2011; Malfitano *et al.*, 2014).

"Healthy lifestyles which promote mental health should be commonly reflected in everyone's everyday occupations they have" resources and opportunities to access.

The critical occupational perspective emphasizes the need to examine the broader systemic and structural factors that impact an individual's ability to engage in meaningful occupations and maintain mental well-being. This approach highlights the issue of social exclusion, which manifests as a denial or deprivation of the fundamental rights to participate in occupations that promote health and personal fulfillment (Hammell, 2017; Hammell, 2020). To address this form of social exclusion, the individual or group of persons in this case mental health service users experiencing difficulties should be capacitated to participate in meaningful and socially inclusive occupations, while, at the same time, efforts to remove participation barriers should be directed at a societal level (Harrison & Sellers, 2008; Kantartzis, 2018). From the critical occupational perspective, addressing participation barriers entails working with the real context. The real context is understood as the locus for many sectors of life; it is the context within which occupations are realized, subject to the possibilities and limitations imposed by socioeconomic determinants (Malfitano, 2005). By moving occupational therapy away from solely addressing health conditions, this perspective encourages practices that empower individuals, dismantle societal barriers, and foster an inclusive environment where diverse abilities are embraced and accommodated. It recognizes the need to shift from a purely medical approach to one that addresses the complex interplay of individual, environmental, and societal factors influencing participation and well-being (Barros *et al.*, 2005). This perspective yielded transformative insights in the context of a dominant biomedical disease model and prevalent systemic and structural factors around the social inclusion of young adults with dual affliction of substance use disorders and HIV in Zimbabwe (Nhunzvi, 2021).

Collective occupations are another way of enabling the social inclusion of all. This has been proposed, though not yet well-researched. The importance of collective occupations in challenging injustice and promoting social inclusion among marginalised groups has started to garner attention (Kantartzis, 2018; Kantartzis & Molineux, 2017; Ramugondo & Kronenberg, 2015), something that can be extended to those with stigmatised comorbidities like the mental health service users. Kantartzis and Molineux posit that collective occupation is defined "by its unique construction through the numerous people engaged in it and the power that is thereby produced, as well as by its intention or purpose towards the social fabric" (Kantartzis & Molineux, 2017, p.173). Kantartzis suggests that communities can achieve social inclusion through collective occupations which serve as social transformational tools to address the unjust conditions of many people's lives in our societies today (Kantartzis, 2018). Occupations are inherently social activities that bring people together. This shared and communal aspect is clearly evident in collective occupations undertaken by groups. However, there is a risk that certain collective occupations, despite fostering togetherness, may inadvertently exclude or discriminate against individuals perceived as different or as outsiders(Ramugondo & Kronenberg, 2015; Rudman, 2015).

Critical perspectives in occupational science and occupational therapy emphasize the importance of occupational justice for promoting social inclusion. Occupational justice refers to a restorative approach aimed at achieving social justice and inclusion by identifying and addressing inequalities that prevent people from engaging in meaningful occupations. Proponents argue that for true occupational justice to exist, the ability to participate in occupations must be viewed as a fundamental human right, rather than merely an optional lifestyle choice. By treating occupation and participation as rights, occupational scientists seek to dismantle barriers and ensure equitable opportunities for all individuals to engage in purposeful activities that enhance their well-being and enable their full participation in society. (Christiansen & Townsend, 2004; Harrison & Sellers, 2008; Kantartzis, 2018). If occupational therapy and other mental health players take insights from this position, Christiansen and Townsend (2004) posit that it will be possible to pursue the principle of an occupationally just world, a world where everyone can participate equitably and fully (Christiansen & Townsend, 2004). While occupational justice is often viewed as an idealistic concept, it serves as a robust theoretical foundation that compels occupational therapists to actively promote social inclusion and advocate for lifestyles conducive to good mental health for everyone. Beyond mere aspirations, this principle provides a practical framework for occupational therapists to champion equitable access to meaningful occupations and activities that foster well-being across all segments of society. (Corbett & Howe, 2007).

A Lifestyle Approach to Mental Health and Social Inclusion

Within the provisions of the context, mental health and social inclusion can be enhanced through a lifestyle approach. Embedding inclusive and mental health-promoting activities in everyday routines and as habits for all concerned, can help overcome the barriers for specified population groups. A collective approach further aids the inclusivity goals, where all stakeholders are given an equal opportunity and resources to routine community engagements of meaning and value. A lifestyle change should be influenced by the desire for all to do and be for the common good.

A lifestyle approach to mental health emphasising social inclusion should support everyone to live fulfilling and meaningful lives in their communities. Everyone within the community should have equitable access to resources that help them to identify and pursue their personal and collective goals, interests, and values, and to develop healthy habits and routines that promote both individual and collective well-being.

In refection: Consider, Kuda, a 40-year-old man who was diagnosed with schizophrenia and is feeling socially isolated. He recounts his situation as being like many others he met at a local mental health hospital when they were admitted. Like his counterparts, Kuda is struggling with a drug use problem, has low self-esteem, and feelings of depression. John joined a Using Kuda as the index case, we reach out to others in his situation and consider even those as risks.

We then devise a community-based occupational lifestyle program that offers psychoeducational support, life coaching, behaviour change support, group activities, and peer support, embedded in the everyday activities of the community. In such a program, Kuda rediscovers himself, his passions, those sharing similar hobbies, engages in a collective, is trusted by the community and further opportunities become available, including enrolling for further skills development through local institutions. The lifestyle programs are embedded in communities, reignite hope, and help people like Kuda to find a sense of purpose and belonging in their life.

It remains elusive to guarantee good mental health in the dynamic world, but efforts can be made to continually improve the conditions of everyday life for everyone, despite naturalised differences which may exist. The actions for an inclusive and conducive environment for all should begin before birth (focusing on planned healthy pregnancies) and progress into the post-natal period and early childhood, older childhood and adolescence, young adulthood and working ages, and through to old age. Action throughout these life stages would provide opportunities and resources for both improving the population's mental health and for reducing the risk of those mental disorders that are associated with social inequalities and unhealthy lifestyles.

Key Points

- Injustice in laws, policies, social norms, and values should be addressed for mentally healthy lifestyles.
- Social determinants of mental should be targeted for population-level goals of mentally healthy lifestyles.
- A critical occupational perspective of social inclusion holds promises of situating and actioning the equity and justice-oriented interventions to promote good mental health for all.

REFERENCES

Allman, D. (2013). The Sociology of Social Inclusion. *SAGE Open,* *3*(1), 2158244012471957. [http://dx.doi.org/10.1177/2158244012471957]

Barros, D.D., Ghirardi, M.I.G., Lopes, R.E. (2005). Social occupational therapy: A socio-historical perspective. In: Kronenberg, F., Algado, S.S., Pollard, N., (Eds.), *Occupational therapy without borders: Learning from the spirit of survivors.* Elsevier Science/Churchill Livingstone.

Barros, D.D., Ghirardi, M.I.G., Lopes, R.E., Galheigo, S.M. (2011). Brazilian experiences in social occupational therapy. In: Kronenberg, F., Pollard, N., Sakellariou, D., (Eds.), *Occupational therapy without borders. Towards an ecology of occupation-based practices.* (Vol. Vol. 2, pp. 209-215). Edinburgh: Elsevier.

Christiansen, C., Townsend, E. (2004). The occupational nature of communities. *Introduction to occupation: The art and science of living,* 141-172.

Christiansen, C., Townsend, E.A. (2009). *Introduction to Occupation: The art of science and living.* Prentice Hall.

Cockerham, W.C. (2005). Health lifestyle theory and the convergence of agency and structure. *J. Health Soc. Behav., 46*(1), 51-67.
[http://dx.doi.org/10.1177/002214650504600105] [PMID: 15869120]

Corbett, P., Howe, H. (2007). Bridge building in mental health. *Occupational Therapy News, 15*(1), 24-25.

Farias, L., Rudman, D.L. (2019). Challenges in enacting occupation-based social transformative practices: A critical dialogical study. *Can. J. Occup. Ther., 86*(3), 243-252.
[http://dx.doi.org/10.1177/0008417419828798] [PMID: 30803264]

Frank, G., Muriithi, B.A.K. (2015). Theorising social transformation in occupational science: The American Civil Rights Movement and South African struggle against apartheid as 'Occupational Reconstructions'. *S. Afr. J. Occup. Ther., 45*(1), 11-19. http://www.scielo.org.za/scielo.php? script=sci_arttext&pid=S2310-38332015000100003&nrm=iso
[http://dx.doi.org/10.17159/2310-3833/2015/v45no1a3]

Frazier, L.D. (2020). The past, present, and future of the biopsychosocial model: A review of The Biopsychosocial Model of Health and Disease: New philosophical and scientific developments by Derek Bolton and Grant Gillett. *New Ideas Psychol., 57*, 100755.
[http://dx.doi.org/10.1016/j.newideapsych.2019.100755]

Friedrich, M.J. (2017). Depression Is the Leading Cause of Disability Around the World. *JAMA, 317*(15), 1517-1517.
[http://dx.doi.org/10.1001/jama.2017.3826] [PMID: 28418490]

Hák, T., Janoušková, S., Moldan, B. (2016). Sustainable Development Goals: A need for relevant indicators. *Ecol. Indic., 60*, 565-573.
[http://dx.doi.org/10.1016/j.ecolind.2015.08.003]

Hammell, K.R.W. (2017). Critical reflections on occupational justice: Toward a rights-based approach to occupational opportunities. *Can. J. Occup. Ther., 84*(1), 47-57.
[http://dx.doi.org/10.1177/0008417416654501] [PMID: 27402705]

Hammell, K.R.W., Iwama, M.K. (2012). Well-being and occupational rights: An imperative for critical occupational therapy. *Scand. J. Occup. Ther., 19*(5), 385-394.
[http://dx.doi.org/10.3109/11038128.2011.611821] [PMID: 21905983]

Hammell, K.W. (2008). Reflections on...well-being and occupational rights. *Can. J. Occup. Ther., 75*(1), 61-64.
[http://dx.doi.org/10.2182/cjot.07.007] [PMID: 18323370]

Hammell, K.W. (2020). Action on the social determinants of health: Advancing occupational equity and occupational rights. *Cadernos Brasileiros de Terapia Ocupacional, 28*(1), 387-400.
[http://dx.doi.org/10.4322/2526-8910.ctoARF2052]

Harrison, D., Sellers, A. (2008). Occupation for mental health and social inclusion. *Br. J. Occup. Ther., 71*(5), 216-219.
[http://dx.doi.org/10.1177/030802260807100509]

Ikkos, G. (2023). Social Inclusion and Mental Health: Understanding Poverty, Inequality and Social Exclusion By Jed Boardman, Helen Killaspy and Gillian Mezey 2nd edn. *The British Journal of Psychiatry* (Vol. 223, pp. 494-494). Cambridge University.(4)
[http://dx.doi.org/10.1192/bjp.2023.73]

Jorge, C., Debra, R.W., James, G.L., Emanuel, A. (2017). The role of the family in defining and managing disability of persons with schizophrenia in Chile: Meeting objective and subjective criteria of social inclusion. *International Journal of Sociology and Anthropology, 9*(12), 166-172.
[http://dx.doi.org/10.5897/IJSA2017.0742]

Kantartzis, S. (2018). Perspectives on occupation-based social inclusion: Collective occupation in the local, social world. *Japanese Journal of Occupational Science, 12*(1), 14-37.

Kantartzis, S., Molineux, M. (2017). Collective occupation in public spaces and the construction of the social fabric. *Can. J. Occup. Ther., 84*(3), 168-177.
[http://dx.doi.org/10.1177/0008417417701936] [PMID: 28569548]

Kielhofner, G. (2009). *Conceptual foundations of occupational therapy practice..* FA Davis.

Laliberte Rudman, D. (2013). Enacting the Critical Potential of Occupational Science: Problematizing the 'Individualizing of Occupation'. *J. Occup. Sci., 20*(4), 298-313.
[http://dx.doi.org/10.1080/14427591.2013.803434]

Malfitano, A.P.S. (2005). Intervention fields and centers in social occupational therapy. *Journal of Occupational Therapy. University of São Paulo, 16*(1), 1-8.
[http://dx.doi.org/10.11606/issn.2238-6149.v16i1p1-8]

Malfitano, A.P.S., Lopes, R.E. (2018). Social occupational therapy: Committing to social change. *N. Z. J. Occup. Ther., 65*(1), 20-26.
[http://dx.doi.org/10.3316/informit.779763971754213]

Malfitano, A.P.S., Lopes, R.E., Magalhães, L., Townsend, E.A. (2014). Social occupational therapy. *Can. J. Occup. Ther., 81*(5), 298-307.
[http://dx.doi.org/10.1177/0008417414536712] [PMID: 25702374]

Malfitano, A.P.S., Whiteford, G., Molineux, M. (2021). Transcending the individual: The promise and potential of collectivist approaches in occupational therapy. *Scand. J. Occup. Ther., 28*(3), 188-200.
[http://dx.doi.org/10.1080/11038128.2019.1693627] [PMID: 31774692]

Muñoz, C.G. (2018). Challenges in occupational justice and social inclusion: Selected experiences within Valdivia's civil society. *J. Occup. Sci., 25*(4), 486-496.
[http://dx.doi.org/10.1080/14427591.2018.1517404]

Nhunzvi, C. (2021). *A case study exploring an occupational perspective of social inclusion among young adults dually afflicted with substance use disorder and hiv/aids in zimbabwe.* [Doctoral, University of Cape Town]. South Africa.

Patel, V., Lund, C., Hatherill, S., Plagerson, S., Corrigall, J., Funk, M., Flisher, A. J. (2010). Mental disorders: equity and social determinants. *Equity, social determinants and public health programmes,* 115-134.

Pereira, R. (2015). *Enabling social transformation through occupation for citizens living with mental illness.*

Pereira, R.B., Whiteford, G., Hyett, N., Weekes, G., Di Tommaso, A., Naismith, J. (2020). Capabilities, Opportunities, Resources and Environments (CORE): Using the CORE approach for inclusive, occupation-centred practice. *Aust. Occup. Ther. J., 67*(2), 162-171.
[http://dx.doi.org/10.1111/1440-1630.12642] [PMID: 31957045]

Ramugondo, E.L., Kronenberg, F. (2015). Explaining Collective Occupations from a Human Relations Perspective: Bridging the Individual-Collective Dichotomy. *J. Occup. Sci., 22*(1), 3-16.
[http://dx.doi.org/10.1080/14427591.2013.781920]

Ridley, M., Rao, G., Schilbach, F., Patel, V. (2020). Poverty, depression, and anxiety: Causal evidence and mechanisms. *Science, 370*(6522), eaay0214.
[http://dx.doi.org/10.1126/science.aay0214] [PMID: 33303583]

Rudman, D.L. (2015). Situating occupation in social relations of power: Occupational possibilities, ageism and the retirement 'choice'. *S. Afr. J. Occup. Ther., 45,* 27-33.

Sachs, J.D. (2012). From millennium development goals to sustainable development goals. *Lancet, 379*(9832), 2206-2211.
[http://dx.doi.org/10.1016/S0140-6736(12)60685-0] [PMID: 22682467]

The World Bank. (2013). Inclusion Matters: The Foundation for Shared Prosperity. In. Washington, DC: World Bank. License: Creative Commons Attribution CC BY 3.0.

UK Department for International Development (DFID). (2000). *Disability, Poverty and Development..* London, UK.

Vinzón, V., Allegretti, M., Magalhães, L. (2020). An overview of occupational therapy community practices in Latin America. *Cad. Ter. Ocup. UFSCar,   28*(2), 600-620.https://doi.org/http://dx.doi.org/10.4322/2526-8910.ctoAR1891 [Um panorama das práticas comunitarias da terapia ocupacional na América Latina].

Whatley, E., Fortune, T., Williams, A.E. (2015). Enabling occupational participation and social inclusion for people recovering from mental ill□health through community gardening. *Aust. Occup. Ther. J.,   62*(6), 428-437.https://onlinelibrary.wiley.com/doi/abs/10.1111/1440-1630.12240 [http://dx.doi.org/10.1111/1440-1630.12240] [PMID: 26530278]

Wilcock, A.A. (2006). *An occupational perspective of health..* Slack Incorporated.

World Health Organisation (WHO). 2017 *Depression and other common mental disorders: global health estimates.* (p. 24). Geneva: World Health Organization.

World Health Organization and Calouste Gulbenkian Foundation. (2014). *Social determinants of mental health.*https://apps.who.int/iris/bitstream/handle/10665/112828/9789241506809_eng.pdf.

Yerxa, E.J. (2000). Occupational science: a renaissance of service to humankind through knowledge. *Occup. Ther. Int.,   7*(2), 87-98.https://doi.org/https://doi.org/10.1002/oti.109 [http://dx.doi.org/10.1002/oti.109]

CHAPTER 17

Models of Recovery-Oriented Practice & Recovery-Oriented Assessment and Intervention

Maya Hayden-Evans[1,*], Patricia Tran[1], Rachel Oliver[1], Sonya Girdler[1] and **Ben Milbourn[1]**

[1] *Faculty of Health Sciences, Curtin School of Allied Health, Curtin University, Perth, Australia*

Abstract: This chapter views recovery through multiple perspectives, focusing on the lens of personal recovery in the mental health context. The process of personal recovery may be as unique as the individuals experiencing it. However, some common themes are discussed, including the presence of connection, hope, optimism, identity, meaning, and empowerment. This chapter draws on the lived experience of mental health consumers to highlight the role of occupational therapists in recovery and breathe life into the theoretical concepts discussed throughout. Examples of how occupational therapists may use strengths-based and person-centred approaches to facilitate recovery and engage consumers in the occupational therapy process are provided. In addition, this chapter emphasises the importance of shared decision-making and describes the unique considerations when working with diverse populations including culturally and linguistically diverse individuals, individuals who identify as LGBTQIA+, and individuals who are neurodivergent.

Keywords: Mental health, Neurodivergent, Occupational therapists, Personal recovery, Recovery.

INTRODUCTION

In the context of mental health, the term 'recovery' has diverse implications and meanings. Recovery could mean the person is no longer experiencing the symptoms of a mental health condition, or it could mean these symptoms are no longer impacting their ability to engage in their usual life activities. For others, recovery might be about experiencing their challenges or symptoms differently (for example, using their experiences of their voices or suicidality as a way of tracking unnoticed fears or burnout), or simply finding new ways to do the things they used to enjoy, or trying new things altogether. Some may find faith as their source of recovery and others may feel that they have nothing to 'recover from'

---

* **Corresponding author Maya Hayden-Evans:** Faculty of Health Sciences, Curtin School of Allied Health, Curtin University, Perth, Australia; E-mail: ben.milbourn@curtin.edu.au

Tawanda Machingura (Ed.)

and therefore have no use for this term. Every individual will have their unique relationship with this word, and as occupational therapists, it is important to explore how the individual views recovery, and work within their preferred framework.

In this chapter, three dominant discourses around recovery are defined and discussed: clinical recovery, social recovery, and personal recovery. This chapter presents current models of recovery relevant to occupational therapy practice and provides examples of how occupational therapists can use a recovery-oriented approach to support clients experiencing distress and/or uncommon realities in their recovery journey. Occupational therapists play an important role in promoting the positive shift in attitudes and language within the mental health sector, moving away from entrenched 'illness' talk towards exploring 'valued roles.' In using a holistic, person-centred approach, occupational therapists can begin to contextualise a person's previous experience and meet them where they are, to walk with them to where they want to be.

This chapter blends theoretical concepts defined in the literature with real stories of recovery, told from the lived experience perspective. These rich narratives will provide readers with a deeper understanding of how their theoretical knowledge can be applied in practice to support people on their recovery journey. In addition, these stories highlight some examples of harmful or unhelpful interactions between clinicians and individuals with mental health lived experiences, from which students and clinicians can learn.

What is Recovery?

Recovery is a complex and multifaceted concept in that it can mean different things to different people, or the meaning may shift depending on where the person is in their recovery journey. Because of this, there is no single, universally accepted way to define the term 'recovery'. Instead, multiple complementary definitions of recovery have been proposed in the literature, reflecting different understandings of health and wellbeing, which can be broadly categorised under the following three domains.

Clinical Recovery

Clinical, sometimes referred to as symptomatic, recovery takes a medicalised approach to recovery with a focus on symptoms, or lack thereof. Unlike the other categories of recovery described in this chapter, clinical recovery does not consider the person's unique contextual factors, and can therefore limit one's ability to achieve 'recovery' by this definition.

"Clinical recovery refers to the absence of symptoms, either as a result of them being eradicated by treatment, or because the treatment is suppressing or controlling them. The essential concept of clinical recovery is that the recovery process occurs because of the effectiveness of the clinical treatment." (Coleman, 2011, p. 31)

The concept of clinical recovery refers mostly to reducing or eradicating symptoms of mental ill health through the use of psychological and/or pharmacological interventions (Pelletier *et al.*, 2020). Access to evidence-based interventions and the opportunity to continue accessing services long-term is essential for facilitating clinical recovery (Lloyd *et al.*, 2008). However, it is important to note that, even with ongoing access to treatments and services, total recovery from a clinical perspective may not be an achievable outcome for all individuals experiencing a mental health condition. Unlike recovery from a physical ailment such as a broken leg, the road to mental health recovery may be filled with peaks and troughs and individuals may encounter setbacks in their recovery as a result of adverse life events outside of their control. It is for this reason that other, less limiting definitions of recovery have been suggested.

Societal Recovery

"Social recovery ... views the recovery process as the person's ability (or lack of) to interact in a particular way within society." (Coleman, 2011, p. 53)

Societal, or social, recovery incorporates functioning and the person's ability to participate in such areas of their life as work/productivity, social interactions and relationships, and housing/independent living (Castelein *et al.*, 2021). Societal recovery is grounded in the premise that one does not have to be clinically recovered to begin taking control of their life and returning to community activities that were perhaps made difficult by the presence of mental health symptoms. This approach involves acknowledging the need for ongoing support to develop skills and capacity, while providing the person with opportunities to build or re-build their identity in terms of social roles (Tew *et al.*, 2012).

Personal Recovery

Personal recovery is a term created by lived experience and fought for by the consumer/ survivor/ex-patient (CSX) movement (Morrison, 2009). It was the lived experience response to the pathologizing and limiting (clinician-led) clinical recovery and social recovery. It is no small feat that lived experience has seen this term accepted and embedded within mental health services across the globe. Arguably the most important concept of recovery in the context of mental health, personal recovery refers to *"shifting emphasis from clinical symptom reduction toward reclaiming personal agency and creating meaning-filled lives despite the presence of distressing experiences"* (Sokol *et al.*, 2023, p. 842). This domain of recovery highlights the 'personal' nature of the process and goes beyond the reductive approach reflected in clinical recovery and the need to meet societal expectations to achieve societal or social recovery. Instead, personal recovery considers a multitude of factors with the potential to influence the recovery process, including identity, meaning, hope, empowerment, choice and control, support, relationships, and spirituality (Leamy *et al.*, 2011).

The following definition proposed by Anthony (1993) is widely used to describe the concept of personal recovery, although it is important to be mindful that each person may have their definition of what recovery means for them.

"Recovery is a deeply personal, unique process of changing one's attitudes, values, feelings, goals, skills, and/or roles. It is a way of living a satisfying, hopeful, and contributing life even within the limitations caused by illness. Recovery involves the development of new meaning and purpose in one's life as one grows beyond the catastrophic effects of mental illness." (Anthony, 1993, p. 15).

Unlike clinical recovery, which may be considered an outcome or endpoint, personal recovery is often perceived as a process. Pat Deegan, an expert in mental health recovery with lived experience, describes the process of recovery as "the urge, the wrestle, and the resurrection", one where the personal relationship with anguish and hope is transformed (Deegan, 1988, p. 15). The road to recovery is unlikely to follow a linear trajectory. The personal approach to recovery acknowledges that this is normal and a natural part of human life.

While recovery is considered personal and unique to each individual, Glover (2012) proposed a model of recovery that suggests it is the perpetual movement between, and self-righting within, different states (with the act of self-righting being the process of recovery).

Self-righting states:

1. Passive to active sense of self.
2. Hopelessness to hope.
3. Others in control to being in control of one's self.
4. Alienation to discovery.
5. Disconnectedness to connectedness.

These can be used to guide the conceptualisation of personal recovery, acknowledging that each process may look different for each person. For example, what sparks hope for one person may not necessarily do so for someone else.

Lived Experiences of Recovery

As demonstrated in the examples provided below, no two journeys of recovery will be the same. Recovery is influenced and affected by a multitude of unique contextual factors, which should be considered when entering into a therapeutic relationship with someone already on, or about to commence, their recovery journey. Social determinants, experiences of war, political and legal power over minorities, displacement, disempowerment, trauma, adverse childhood experiences, colonisation, and even service use influence how a person perceives and engages with their recovery.

Trish

I consider myself as a child of trauma. I grew up around alcoholism, housing, and food insecurity, family domestic violence, intergenerational trauma, and sexual predation. Due to the turbulent nature of my living arrangements, my autism, and ADHD went unrecognised. For most of my life, I have lived with the terrible belief that there was 'something wrong with me' and that I was not 'normal'. When I was eventually channelled into mental health services as a young adult due to repeated suicide attempts, this gave me a sense of belonging whilst also confirming my worst fears about myself – that there was something terribly different about me. In a quest for belonging and normalcy, I took the medication prescribed, attended the appointments, and worked hard to be a 'good patient' – even researching symptoms so I could correctly 'fit' the diagnosis. For me, masking was my life and patienthood was no different. Sadly, mental health services had not considered screening for autism and ADHD and I was caught in a system that failed to help me, failed to give me the tools to understand myself, and failed to create the conditions where I could find recovery. I was not sick. I was not broken. I did not need psychotropic medications. I was an undiagnosed autistic living with complex trauma in a neurotypical world, which continued to contribute to the ongoing trauma. I needed someone to work with me in this context, not sedate and further stigmatise me.

Personal recovery for me, therefore has been about self-discovery and unlearning false narratives. Discovering myself, my needs, and my autistic relationship with distress. It is not about sanitising the life of my fears and trigger points. My recovery has been about changing my relationship with distress and suicidality and seeing these experiences now as 'the canary in the mine' – telling me to attend to something that has fallen out of balance. It has now become the pathway to self-understanding, which helps me navigate my way through a neurotypical world that I still struggle to comprehend.

From a service perspective, what I needed from service providers was acceptance and respect, connection and curiosity. I needed them to put aside their textbooks about what my frequent presentations meant and explore with open minds and hearts – what unnoticed drivers were beneath such things. I needed them to see my autism and to inspire me with the hope that I could have a life of belonging and connection. This leads me to ask myself, "What is that invisible substance that transmutes recovery-oriented practice into inspiration?" Inspiration comes from the Latin word "inspirare" which means something akin to 'to breathe or blow life into' the darkness. How do service providers inspire me to believe that I am whole and capable – an equal member of society and someone who holds the respect of others? How do they project the image to me that I am 'normal' and not a stigmatised fringe dweller amongst the 'capable'?

I have experienced many voluntary and involuntary hospitalisations during my twenty-year service use. It was often reinforced to me (through the way I was treated and talked to), that I was an underserving system drainer who needed to be treated coldly so I got the message that I should not return. However, there was one occupational therapist (OT) who had been working on the ward throughout my hospital admissions and who interacted with me as if I were an equal and someone deserving of respect and connection. Whenever I was admitted to the ward, she would make it her priority to come and personally greet me. Often, I would be crumpled on the floor in deep distress at having failed yet another suicide attempt. She would come and sit with me on the floor and express how great it was to see me, despite how I must have looked and interacted with her. She would inquire about my children and share a bit about her progress . She showed me, through these brief interactions, that I was a person who could hold someone's respect regardless of the circumstances I found myself in. Over time, I came to believe (uncomfortably and confusedly at first), that I was worthy of this type of interaction and began to look forward to her greetings. Eventually, despite my distress, whenever she came up to greet me, I would rise from my crumpled position and stand and talk with her and momentarily forget that I was 'different' and 'undeserving'. I can see now that she had used the Rogerian approach on me. She knew that I had everything I needed within me and was already utilising these resources towards my personal recovery. She also recognised she could either hinder or hamper this access by the way she interacted with me. She kept unhelpful judgements and 'helping' outside of our relationship and provided me with the experience of having her respect and being seen as her equal, her peer. Not broken and not requiring sympathy.

That OT has not seen me for decades now and is quite unaware of how much I have achieved and my work within the mental health space but *I still remember her* and how she came into my darkness and breathed light into it through a relationship. She may not have noticed my autism and ADHD but she protected my identity and that kept me going, that kept me intact.

For me, recovery is ignited when the service provider sees the person as their equal and treats them with respect which extends beyond words.

In summary, the factors that helped in my recovery journey were:

- Having an OT who would take a few moments to 'sit with me' and interact with me as a person and not a patient;
- Having an OT who knew that they did not have to 'activate' my personal recovery for me – that connection was enough;
- Having an OT who gives me the same respect they would accord a colleague or friend; and
- Having an OT who respects my autonomy and personal agency (this was observable in their language use and non-verbal interactions).

Factors that did not help were:

- Service providers felt the need to send me a 'strong message' around how 'unacceptable' my frequent presentations were (this reinforced to me that I was not likeable and was 'bad' – further cementing my negative personal identity);
- Service providers who saw a diagnosis, not a person, when I walked through the doors; and
- Service providers believed everything written in my notes about me and did not seek to discover their perceptions of me through an unbiased lens.

Rachel

For me, personal recovery has been about understanding myself in relation to others. Part of the recovery process involved seeking to understand my own behaviour in the context of relationships within my immediate family. Applying self-knowledge explored through sessions with a trusted psychologist, I began to understand these experiences from different perspectives, which contributed to my overall healing process. It was through this process of healing and self-discovery that I identified the importance of connection with health professionals and service providers.

Connection is the first, most important step in supporting someone in their recovery. If the 'fit' between the person and the health professional is 'good' (built on mutual respect and trust demonstrated in interactions), the person is much more likely to lean into your experience as a health professional and want to work with you. You could have all the professional knowledge in the world, but if you are not able to connect with the person you are working with, you are unlikely to get very far in building a therapeutic relationship with them. Whereas, if you acknowledge that you may not always have all the answers, but are willing to walk alongside the person, this can significantly increase the likelihood of experiencing a more positive therapeutic relationship.

In summary, the factors that helped in my recovery journey were:

- Having a practitioner who took the time to get to know me without assuming they knew my story;
- Having a practitioner who did not assume the people who were in my life were helpful to my recovery (even though they may have presented themselves as this); and
- Having a practitioner who kept pace with me and introduced new ways of thinking and approaches to me, at a time when I was able to understand and accept them.

Factors that did not help were:

- Practitioners who created treatment plans and recovery goals without my input or collaboration;
- Practitioners who read my file and thought they 'knew' me; and
- "Fast food" style practitioners who spent less than 15 minutes with me and were there to 'give me' something rather than build a connection with me.

Citizenship

Beyond the traditional models of recovery discussed above, the concept of citizenship is concerned with a person's societal responsibilities, roles, rights, relationships, and resources, and intersects with the concept of personal recovery (Carr & Ponce, 2022). To be a citizen is to be actively involved in the community through appointment to valued roles and sharing of knowledge and skills. It is not enough to support people experiencing mental health challenges to obtain support or resources in isolation, rather there is a need to integrate them fully into society to ensure they experience the full rights of citizenship. For example, viewed through the lens of citizenship, there is a difference between helping someone to obtain employment and ensuring that person is supported, engaged, and valued in their position.

Citizenship incorporates elements of clinical, societal, and personal recovery, acknowledging that medical and psychological supports may be beneficial (clinical recovery) but that recovery continues beyond the clinical context and is influenced by the person's ability to participate in society (societal recovery) and how this participation brings meaning to their lives (personal recovery). Clinicians can support citizenship using the CHIME framework described below to enable people to enjoy the rights, responsibilities, roles, resources, and relationships that society has to offer (Reis *et al.*, 2022).

RECOVERY FRAMEWORK

A framework that has been adopted in clinical practice to measure and support the process of personal recovery is the CHIME framework (Leamy *et al.*, 2011). CHIME is an acronym representing the following principles of recovery.

Connectedness – this refers to positive feelings of connection facilitated by support from others, either through peer support and social groups, relationships with family, friends, and others, or a sense of belonging to a community.

Hope and optimism – a key principle of recovery is having the hope or belief that recovery is in fact possible. Underpinning this is the motivation to make positive change, engage in hope-inspiring relationships, think positively, and have dreams and aspirations to work towards.

Identity – this refers to rebuilding a positive sense of self and identity beyond mental ill health and overcoming the stigma often associated with mental illness. Learning to celebrate one's unique self and develop the positive aspects of one's own identity can be an important component of recovery.

Meaning – however the person defines a meaningful and purposeful life is entirely up to them. Supporting someone to find meaning in their own mental health experience and in their other life experiences (including their roles and future goals) can help facilitate personal recovery.

Empowerment – encouraging people to take back control of their lives can be an empowering experience. Empowerment is about focusing on the person's strengths, facilitating autonomy, and enabling them to take personal responsibility for their actions and decisions.

Above all else, a recovery-oriented approach to delivering services including occupational therapy should have the best interests of the person at its core.

Taking a recovery-oriented approach requires close collaboration with the individual engaging with services, to ensure their needs and wishes are both respected and met.

Lived Experience Perspective

Rachel

The most supportive and effective person in my personal recovery was a health professional who didn't "seek" to diagnose me but decided to get to know me. I felt a connection by being seen and heard with each interaction. I didn't feel 'helped' as such but rather appreciated the essence of our relationship and his being present alongside me. This connection facilitated my recovery by validating my feelings, as well as creating the safety and trust that allowed our therapeutic relationship to flourish.

The connection we shared was similar to talking to a trusted friend. He modelled what this could look like further and empowered me to create a circle of close and supportive friends that would become my family of choice.

For a very long time, he was the only person who held hope for me, and gradually this promoted optimism for a brighter future. We achieved this by sharing mutually honest conversations about what a life could look like, free from all the current stressors and demands that I was experiencing. We explored strategies that could break the cycle of fatigue that comes with depression, by focussing on self-compassion and repair.

I didn't need to justify or explain, there were no judgements, no rush to "get better" in a set timeframe. I could just be my authentic self, whilst making meaning, whilst safely exploring my new identity of 'mother'. He gave me permission to be kind to myself when others misunderstood me, my needs, my wants, and my behaviour during distress. I received understanding and acceptance, which aided in my progress of healing and recovery.

I enjoyed equal power and respect, regardless of how well or unwell I presented. He believed I possessed the skills and resources to continue to look after myself, which would aid in my recovery. He used the strengths-based approach to support me in pinpointing those qualities that had kept me alive and that I could draw on to aid my future self. It was a turning point with a realisation that I could harness existing inner resources (such as determination, intellect, and resilience).

I still remember how he treated me as a deserving person and, more importantly, how this was cathartic for my soul. It has had a lasting impact. I now realise that it is not so much about the therapeutic strategy that's employed in personal recovery, but more so about the sense of connection built through the therapeutic relationship.

RECOVERY-ORIENTED APPROACH

A National Framework for Recovery-Oriented Mental Health Services (Commonwealth of Australia, 2013) has been developed in consultation with people with lived experience to help guide the delivery of recovery-oriented approaches in Australia. The framework consists of five overlapping practice domains that should be considered in concurrence with each other:

- Promote a culture and language of hope and optimism
- Person-first and holistic
- Support personal recovery
- Organisational commitment and workforce development
- Action on social inclusion and the social determinants of health, mental health and wellbeing

Arblaster *et al.* (2019) developed three core competencies informed by lived experience to guide recovery-oriented occupational therapy practice.

1. Knowing – this relates to the different types of knowledge clinicians require to work effectively, using a recovery-oriented approach, including knowledge of diagnosis, recovery, human rights, lived experience, and practice, and how these can be integrated to understand and support each person in recovery.
2. Doing – this relates to the active processes and behaviours of clinicians supporting people in recovery and includes: building on strengths and connecting to beliefs, hopes and dreams, promoting occupational participation, and using person-centred language.
3. Being/becoming – this relates to a clinician's ability to relate to and work with people in a recovery-oriented way. This involves a journey through reconciliation to authenticity and a journey of lifelong learning, acknowledging the continual shift in 'being' as one reflects on and adjusts their practice with evolving life experience.

Role of Occupational Therapists in Supporting Recovery

Occupational therapists can support recovery (Kelly *et al.*, 2010; Krupa *et al.*, 2009; Nugent *et al.*, 2017):

- Believing that recovery is possible.
- Respecting and valuing the person's expertise – they are experts by lived experience.
- Use of language (words, stories, meaning).
- Holding a consistent sense of hope, compassion, realism, and resilience.
- Including family members and loved ones as partners in recovery.
- Being aware of where the person is at in relation to their recovery and respecting their right to define their own experience and reality.
- Working alongside the person, rather than being directive and inflexible.
- Assessing strengths, and internal and external resources, rather than focussing only on deficits and losses.
- Encouraging self-advocacy and responsibility-taking.
- Ensuring options for choice are made available where possible.
- Challenging stigma and discrimination in services and the wider community.
- Facilitating consumer involvement in service development and service delivery where possible.
- Respecting the person's right to take informed risks.

Recovery-Oriented Assessment and Intervention Process

The Canadian Practice Process Framework (CPPF; Polatajko *et al.*, 2007) is a commonly used approach in occupational therapy practice that can be applied in the mental health context. The framework consists of eight steps that exist within the frame(s) of reference, embedded in the societal and practice context. Examples of a recovery-oriented approach to each of the steps are provided below:

1. **Enter/initiate** – at this stage, the focus should be on building a collaborative and empowering relationship with the person, which may involve establishing trust, acknowledging the person's strengths, experiences, and preferences, and emphasising the collaborative nature of the therapeutic relationship.
2. **Set the stage** – encourage open and honest communication about the person's expectations of recovery, and promote autonomy and empowerment. Actively engage the person in the decisions that affect them.
3. **Assess/evaluate** – explore the person's strengths, values, and goals, as well as identify areas of challenge in which the person may need support.
4. **Agree on objectives, and plan** – collaborate with the person to determine their goals. Ensure these align with their values and what they are hoping to achieve. Develop a plan for support that they are comfortable with, and that incorporates their strengths, interests, and preferred approaches to intervention.
5. **Implement plan** – ensure any interventions have been agreed upon with the person and will help them towards achieving their own personally meaningful

goals. Encourage the development of skills that will enable the person to actively engage in their meaningful occupations and help them integrate actively into society, fostering a sense of belonging and hope.

6. **Monitor/modify** – regularly check in with the person to determine what is and isn't working. Be prepared to modify the plan as the person's priorities may shift. Be flexible and adaptable to the person's changing needs and ensure interventions continue to help the person on their recovery journey. If interventions are no longer serving this purpose, consider alternative strategies to help the person meet their goals.

7. **Evaluate outcomes** – reflect on the outcomes expected at the beginning of the process. Were these outcomes met? Consider the person's experience of mental health challenges but also any indicators of recovery, which may include increased quality of life, sense of hope and purpose, improved social connections and sense of belonging.

8. **Conclude/exit** – celebrate the person's successes and highlight their strengths and resilience. Ensure the person is prepared for what comes next by linking them in with relevant supports and resources.

These steps generally occur in order, with some flexibility allowed, to enable the therapist to tailor their approach to best suit the needs of the person they are working with.

A review evaluating existing measures of recovery in the Australian context identified 22 measures of individual recovery, of which the following five met specific suitability criteria outlined in the article (Burgess *et al.*, 2011):

- Recovery Assessment Scale (Giffort *et al.*, 1995)
- Illness Management and Recovery Scales (Mueser *et al.*, 2004)
- Stages of Recovery Instrument (Andresen *et al.*, 2006)
- Recovery Process Inventory (Jerrell *et al.*, 2006)
- Recovery Orientation (Resnick *et al.*, 2005)

In addition to these, the Mental Health Recovery Star (Lloyd *et al.*, 2016) is a holistic outcome measure supporting recovery by providing consumers with a visual representation of their recovery progress (ten-pronged star) and the ability to plan how they will set about achieving their personally meaningful recovery goals (ladder of change). There is evidence to support the relevance and usefulness of the Mental Health Recovery Star as an outcome measure in recovery-oriented services (Lloyd *et al.*, 2016).

The Recovery Evaluation and Suicide Support Tool (RESST) is another recovery-focused measure that evaluates recovery across four key areas: Self-Worth, Life

Worth, Social Worth, and Self-Understanding, which can be used to guide recovery-oriented assessment and intervention following a suicidal episode (Sokol *et al.*, 2023). The RESST has sound psychometric properties (reliability and validity), enabling clinicians and researchers to quantify progress in personal recovery. Beyond this, it may also be used as a tool to promote hope and empowerment by helping people identify aspects of their own personal recovery and work towards achieving their own recovery goals (Sokol *et al.*, 2023).

PERSON-CENTRED APPROACH TO RECOVERY

Client- or person-centred approaches to care primarily aim to acknowledge the person seeking mental health support as a human first. Within this approach, common themes underpinning person-centred care include a holistic approach, alignment with the person's needs and values, utilising dignity, respect, and compassion, empowering the person, and offering choice, involvement, and collaboration (Boardman & Dave, 2020).

Key components of person-centred approaches:

1. **Rights** – clinicians working with people experiencing mental health challenges must consider their human rights, including freedom, and balance maintaining the person's safety with their right to live their life the way they want to.
2. **Relationship to practice and service organisation** – person-centred approaches align with personal recovery, drawing on the person's history, goals, individual contexts, beliefs, and occupations, to inform decisions regarding intervention and support.
3. **Importance for clinicians** – not only do person-centred approaches improve the experience of mental health consumers accessing services, but they can also improve the experience of clinicians providing support. Clinicians who are encouraged to treat their clients with compassion and respect, and who are afforded the time to consider the person holistically, and use these factors to inform their decision-making processes, are likely to experience greater job satisfaction while improving the outcomes for their client.
4. **Values and evidence** – clinicians seeking to deliver quality, person-centred care should seek to provide evidence-based care that also aligns with the values of stakeholders (including the person, their family, and other health professionals and services involved in supporting them).
5. **Training** – involvement of consumers (clients and carers) in the development and delivery of mental health training

Lived Experience Perspective

Trish

I remember being admitted to a hospital in distress and speaking to an allied health staff member about what I thought was leading to my distress. One of the challenges that I quoted was the fact that my two dogs were continually running in and out of the house, and the house had so much sand in it that it could grow potatoes. His first and only solution was to suggest that I give away my dogs.

He had not considered the protective factors that the dogs held for me including the comfort, companionship, and sense of personal safety that they provided. Neither did he consider the impact of the highly sedating medication that I was prescribed, or consider what supports I might use, nor did he advocate to the doctors that perhaps the dosage of medication was impacting my activities of daily living. He made no connection with the fact that I was a single mum living below the poverty line and perhaps may not have access to nutritious foods which would have the provided energy and vigour required to sweep the floor more frequently. Nor did he assess how the soul-eating stigma of feeling like I was and always would be a 'mental patient' destroyed hope and drained personal efficacy.

He only saw the dogs as the problem. I felt an immediate disconnection from the relationship and anything he had to say to me was received with stony silence. I did not like or trust him. I felt that he did not 'see me' and did not know what I valued. Any partnership with him would risk what I held near and dear. This allied health staff member's focus on the dogs told me that I was incapable of cleaning, that I was broken and degraded beyond repair, and should not hope to have the same access to pets and choice as others did. It eroded my identity and made me fear the power of mental health services.

The problem he saw represented was the dogs and if I got rid of the dogs, my house would be clean and orderly. Of course, the true reason for my challenges with my household chores was my ADHD and all that I needed was to have some understanding of how ADHD impacts tasks and ways in which I could manage this challenge.

I notice that service providers will often go for the 'low hanging fruit' and ignore the higher-level social determinants of health and other factors that contribute to the challenge. What they see as 'the problem' is often not *the* problem. Carol Bacchi's exploration of "What's the Problem Represented to Be" (2009), reminds me of that staff member and his simplistic and erroneous assumptions of my challenges. I urge future OTs to consider that for many of us, our minds and descriptions of our challenges have been colonised by the bio-medical framework provided to us. We have no other way to understand our experiences except through 'mental illness' and as a result, we may not know or be able to express what our 'root cause' of our challenges might be. *Explore outside of this box. Look for what has gone unnoticed and unaddressed!*

In summary, factors that may enhance recovery include:

- Understanding the problem represented may not be the true representation;
- Understanding how clinician bias and the 'clinician's illusion' (Cohen & Cohen, 1984) influence clinical approaches and interventions; and
- Creating approaches that explore language and concepts used by individuals to establish a shared understanding.

Factors that may disengage recovery include:

- Practitioners who assume they know the challenge and disconnect from further exploration;
- Practitioners who exert 'power over' the individual and 'do to' not 'with' the person; and
- Practitioners who cannot adapt their approach when rapport and perceived safety are threatened.

As demonstrated in Trish's story above, the attitudes of clinicians can have an impact on how the consumer experiences their recovery and affect their attitudes towards seeking support in the future. Daya *et al*. (2020) have proposed a conceptual model that incorporates consumers' experiences of treatment and care from multiple perspectives (humanist, facilitator, activist, transformer). The model provides an opportunity for researchers and clinicians to increase their awareness and understanding of diversity among consumers' experiences of treatment and care and respond more effectively to their preferences around language, experiences, and priorities.

Using a Strengths-Based Approach

Historically, approaches to mental health recovery have relied heavily on the medical model, seeking to eradicate features of mental health conditions through the use of pharmacological and psychological treatments. More recently, however, there has been a shift towards a strengths-based approach, moving the focus away from the person's deficits and focusing instead on their strengths and abilities (Xie, 2013). Using a strengths-based approach, clinicians consider the person's positive characteristics and harness these to promote a sense of confidence and hope. A review of strengths-based approaches in mental health found evidence to support that strengths-based approaches were associated with better recovery outcomes, including reduced rates of hospitalisation, improved uptake of employment and education opportunities, and improved intrapersonal outcomes including greater self-efficacy and feelings of hope (Tse *et al.*, 2016). Additionally, it is important to understand that in neurodivergent populations understanding of self, connection to the body, and their use of language may make it difficult to have a shared understanding of strengths and challenges (Sokol *et al.*, 2023). Taking time to explore what a person experiences or means when they use a particular word or phrase will help to build a deeper understanding within the assessment phase.

Collaboration and Shared Decision-Making in Recovery-Oriented Occupational Therapy Practice

The concept of shared decision-making promotes a shift in the power dynamic between clinicians and consumers, facilitating the development of plans to address mental health challenges that actively engage the consumer in the process and therefore incorporate their perspective and priorities (Grim *et al.*, 2016). When the decision-making process is shared between the consumer and clinician, both are considered experts, and decisions are made collaboratively.

Steps involved in shared-decision making:

1. Clinician and consumer work collaboratively, sharing preferences and evidence to support their choices;
2. Clinician and consumer discuss this information and any issues from their perspectives; and
3. Ideally, both parties come to a collaborative decision based on the evidence presented that aligns with the consumer's values and preferences.

Lived Experience Perspective

Rachel

As someone with lived experience who now engages in peer work, a concept that I value strongly is that of 'walking alongside' someone on their recovery journey. As health professionals working in the mental health space, you need to consider the people you are working with as partners in healthcare, as opposed to being someone requiring support. Beyond collaborating with the person themselves, it is also important to consider the person within the context of their own lives. As human beings, we rarely exist in isolation. It is important to consider and support the other key people around us, which may include kin or other family members such as a partner/significant other or caregiver, parent, child or children, *etc*.

In my youth, I flew under the radar for support as my family appeared, outwardly, quite typical. A white, articulate, well-presented, and well-behaved child, who was academically gifted and achieving highly in sports, did not fit the mould of a child requiring support in the low socioeconomic environment I existed in. I felt loved and enjoyed success in school and sports, despite experiencing a home situation that included family domestic violence, alcohol abuse, and crime. Reflecting on this now, I would have benefited from further support at school as my parents lacked the know-how to access resources. It is important to acknowledge that not everyone you come across in need of support will outwardly appear to fit any preconceived notions you have of what someone in distress 'looks' like.

Shared Decision-Making Using Recovery Narratives

Occupational therapists use shared decision-making to promote autonomy and empowerment in mental health consumers' recovery journey (Milbourn *et al.*, 2018). Milbourn *et al.* (2015) described how lived experiences and narratives of mental health consumers should be at the centre of the recovery process for the person. Occupational therapists are required to actively listen to and interpret the stories that people who experience mental illness share about their lives and what they believe helps in moving them beyond the label of being a patient with a mental illness (Milbourn *et al.*, 2017). For example, if during a meeting with a mental health consumer, the person discloses information about themselves (*e.g.*, is having thoughts about suicide or engaging in non-suicidal self-injury), that information may concern the health professional, resulting in an unequal power differential. The OT needs to be aware of the impact and power of their words and actions on the mental health consumer and how they can work together to make a shared agreed decision about the best way forward which respects and supports the person's recovery journey. The OT responding "You need to get help" doesn't support dialogue or exploration. Rather, the OT should validate the person and the emotions that they have shared with them: "That sounds like you are having a difficult time, can I please ask if you feel comfortable to share a little more about how you are feeling and what is happening for you." This approach creates an opportunity to share power and decision-making with the person on how to proceed in addressing the mental health consumer's expressed needs.

Using Soft Skills to Build Recovery Relationships

Occupational therapists work alongside people with lived experience of mental illness to focus on meaningful occupations that facilitate accomplishment and affirmation while respecting the subjective meanings of the mental health consumers' everyday activities (Milbourn *et al.*, 2017). Occupational therapists employ a lens of therapeutic value attached to meaningful activities that act as a conduit to facilitating and building motivation, roles, and routines around everyday activities (Hasselkus, 2011). Occupational therapists are skilled in using interpersonal communication to support emotional and social development recovery along the lifespan (Wilburn *et al.*, 2021).

Soft skills employed in the mental health recovery context include communication, conflict resolution, negotiation, and decision-making (Sancho-Cantus *et al.*, 2023). The development of these skills is important for nurturing opportunities for working alongside mental health consumers with the respect and understanding of their recovery identity (Rønning & Bjørkly, 2019). Underpinning the use of soft skills includes the ability to use empathy as a way of interpreting and understanding the emotional language of the mental health consumer (Moudatsou *et al.*, 2020). Active listening, empathy, and understanding of the person's individual lived experience inform the development of genuine recovery-focused practice (Horgan *et al.*, 2021). For example, rather than asking "what's wrong", an occupational therapist approaching a mental health consumer who is in emotional distress could instead locate themselves with the person in the here and now, informing the person they are here for them, validating the distressed emotion ("I notice you seem upset") and employing curiosity to find out more ("Can we go and sit down and talk more about what's happening for you?").

Working with Culturally and Linguistically Diverse Populations and Mental Health Recovery

Diversity includes differences between people in how they identify on grounds including age, caring responsibilities, disability, gender, sexual orientation, Indigenous status, and cultural and socioeconomic backgrounds (O'Leary *et al.*, 2015). Australia is a multicultural, diverse society with over 33% of Australians being born overseas and speaking more than 300 languages (Australian Bureau of Statistics, 2016). The uptake of recovery-focused mental health practice in Australia has often failed to address the impact of colonialism including discrimination against mental health service users with culturally and linguistically diverse (CALD) backgrounds (Levy-Fenner *et al.*, 2022). Mental health consumers have argued for intersectional-informed care that takes into account and captures the nuances and needs of CALD mental health consumers (Price-Robertson *et al.*, 2017; Talwar, 2010). CALD individuals may define and express mental health needs (including language, expression of feelings, and ability to ask for help) in different ways than are considered or expected in the dominant cultural approaches to mental health care (Plowman & Izzo, 2021). According to Levy-Fenner *et al.* (2022), mental health services remain oriented around individualistic conceptualisations of recovery, which are not always culturally sensitive. People from CALD backgrounds accessing mental health services may be dealing with an increased risk of experiencing psychological distress due to intersecting considerations such as loss of family contact, adjustment to a new country, limited knowledge of the health system, and difficulty with the uptake of English language requirements (O'Brien *et al.*, 2021). Other impacts to be considered include: Indigenous populations are the most incarcerated in the world and most have had experiences of harmful systemic and institutional racism and discrimination (Hamilton *et al*, 2020), all of which impact their trust levels with systems containing power.

It is then important that occupational therapists working alongside mental health consumers with CALD backgrounds consider aspects such as trust, power differential, confidentiality, and communication, all of which impact the quality of the recovery relationship (O'Brien *et al.*, 2021). For example, an occupational therapist working with a CALD mental health consumer may need to consider the religious/spiritual beliefs of family members and the potential stigma of talking about mental health with family if wanting to develop a recovery relationship that embraces and validates a spiritual connection for the person and their family.

The Unique Challenges and Opportunities for Recovery-Oriented Practice when Working with Neurodiverse Individuals

A recent study identified that the leading cause of death for autistic individuals was caused by injury and poisoning, which also included suicide, and non-suicidal self-injury (Hwang *et al.*, 2019). It is estimated that the risk of attempting, and death by suicide is more than three times higher for autistic individuals in comparison to non-autistic individuals (Blanchard *et al.*, 2021). A historical lens viewing autism through a biomedical deficit-focused model may contribute to stigma, increased mental health needs, and subsequent "masking" and "autistic burnout" (Raymaker *et al.*, 2020). Strength-based approaches can be used to promote positive well-being, mental health, and quality of life in autistic populations (Cherewick & Matergia, 2023). Strength-based approaches align with recovery-orientated practices, focusing on the connection between the biopsychosocial aspects of the person, their passions, interests, and the performance arising from interactions between their individual strengths and challenges (Bölte, 2023). For example, an occupational therapist focusing on an autistic individual's passions (*e.g.*, online gaming) may facilitate conversations that plant the seeds of motivation (hope), of socialising with like-minded individuals (connection), which in turn leads to a positive affirmation of self (identity) and foster interest in developing the passion from a leisure consideration into an opportunity for further training and employment (meaning and engagement).

Additionally, it should be recognised that many individuals identifying as LGBQTIA+ also identify as being neurodivergent (Van Der Miesen *et al.*, 2016; Warrier *et al.*, 2020). People identifying as LGBTIA+ are at greater risk of interpersonal, physical, and family domestic violence, displacement, loss of access to housing, schooling, and financial and work opportunities, as well as stigma and prejudicial attitudes (Fedina *et al.*, 2022; Goldsmith & Bell, 2022.). They are also less likely to reach out to services for support (McDermott *et al.*, 2018). People of colour who identify as belonging within the LGBQTIA+ community, and are neurodivergent, are more likely to experience challenges compounded by the intersectionality of belonging to multiple disadvantaged groups (Hutson *et al.*, 2022). These experiences of minority and race stress have been linked to increased risk of self-injury and suicidality (Jackman, 2017). Occupational Therapists, when engaging with members of this population, are encouraged to reflect on how their personal relationship with privilege and intersectionality may either help or hinder their ability to understand and connect with the complexities and injustices experienced by the LGBQTIA+ population. Epistemic and hermeneutical injustice may occur unintentionally within the professional relationship if an occupational therapist does not examine their attitudes, experiences, and beliefs which impact acceptance of narrative and connection.

Lived Experience Perspective

Trish

Throughout my life, I have always felt different. I was severely bullied throughout my schooling and would often measure my thoughts, feelings, and reactions by how much they deviated from 'normal people'. I often described myself as an alien living on a foreign planet trying to understand the customs and ways of a foreign species. I had no connection to 'normal' and no structures to make sense of my experiences. I used to tell myself that the reason I had no friends as a child was because of family violence, homelessness, and caregivers who had alcohol addictions. I thought the other kids did not like me because I was the smelly kid who came to school in rags, with no lunch, and without the 'right' school supplies. It was funny I never noticed that my five other siblings always made friends. Later, as an adult, the story I told myself about why I had such poor interpersonal and social skills was that it was the result of frequently moving schools, bullying and never having access to friends to 'practice' my interpersonal skills with. It has taken me a long time to understand that most people are born with the innate ability to create friendships.

When my distress finally brought me into mental health services, this gave me some comfort. The label of 'mental illness' confirmed my painful alienation from 'normal society' was real but it was the result of a 'brain disorder'. I belonged to a group defined as the 'mentally ill' and that meant I did fit in somewhere, even if I was still marginalised. I wore that label like my life depended on it but somehow it did not draw me closer to understanding myself or managing my distress.

When I was 55 years old, an autistic person asked me: "Have you ever considered that you might be autistic?" Suddenly, meaning was transformed, and life made sense for the first time. For decades I had cried out for help but had the hermeneutical injustice of not having the language or concepts that could support help-seeking that actually helped. I remember trying to explain to a psychiatrist my feelings of being an outlier who could only fake 'normalcy' in short bursts and if I stayed within 'society' for too long my fakeness would be discovered. I did not know that I was describing autistic masking. I did not have the language. I still remember the feelings of rejection and helplessness as I listened to my psychiatrist burst into laughter after I had finished my descriptions. She seemed to feel that such expressions were ridiculous and deserving of instant dismissal. I was reminded that even my attempts to create shared understanding would see me as a deviation from the norm. Nowadays, I have read so much literature about the incredibly high rates of misdiagnosis of 'personality disorders' when it comes to undiagnosed autism and ADHD. It makes me wonder how different my life may have been if *even one person* in all the 'help providers' I had seen had taken the time to assess me for ADHD and Autism (AuDHD).

Having an AuDHD screening tool for all people coming into mental health services would be a 'game changer'. Most importantly, having a screening tool that assesses for the female presentation (including transgender females) of AuDHD is needed. Once we can understand ourselves, we can more effectively understand our needs and, perhaps, manage our distress without needing mental health service support.

In summary, factors that may enhance recovery include:

- Learning about neurodiversity and the silent populations within mental health;
- Developing screening tools that explore neurodivergence (ADHD, Autism, FASD, *etc.*);
- Assuming everyone who is receiving mental health services has some level of neurodivergence and complex trauma (until screening proves otherwise); and

- Recognising that most people who come into services have hyperactive threat systems and are excellent lie detectors (keep communications honest, simple, direct, and clear).

Factors that may disengage recovery include:

- Assuming the social and verbal language used is mutually understood when we share the same spoken language; and
- Assuming individuals all have the same understanding of their bodies, environment, and safety (interoception, exteroception, enteroception, proprioception, nociception, and neuroception).

SUMMARY

This chapter highlighted the complexity of recovery in a mental health context and the important role that occupational therapists can have in facilitating personal recovery and promoting citizenship. This chapter introduced recovery-oriented approaches, including the use of the CHIME framework, recovery-focused assessments, and how the Canadian Practice Process Framework can be applied in a recovery-focused way. This chapter emphasised the role of person-centred and strengths-focused approaches in moving away from the medicalised view of recovery, towards a more holistic and personalised framework of recovery where power is shared between clinicians and consumers to achieve the best outcome for each individual. Some of the unique considerations for culturally and linguistically diverse and neurodivergent populations were also presented to encourage reflection on the varying needs of individuals whose recovery journeys may be influenced by other interacting factors. Finally, this chapter incorporated the lived experience perspective to demonstrate the application of theoretical concepts presented and highlight the deeply personal nature of recovery.

Key Points

- There is no single, universally accepted definition of recovery; the process is as unique as the individual experiencing it – work within the person's framework and reality;
- There are, however, some common themes relevant to personal recovery that are encompassed by the CHIME framework: connectedness, hope and optimism, identity, meaning, and empowerment, all of which are built upon demonstrating genuine respect for skills and capacity (seen and unseen);
- The focus of occupational therapy on activity, participation, and functioning means that occupational therapists are well-placed to advocate for and support

people in their personal recovery journeys, enabling them to set personally meaningful goals and find meaning in their lives.

REFERENCES

Andresen, R., Caputi, P., Oades, L. (2006). Stages of recovery instrument: development of a measure of recovery from serious mental illness. *Aust. N. Z. J. Psychiatry, 40*(11-12), 972-980.
[http://dx.doi.org/10.1080/j.1440-1614.2006.01921.x] [PMID: 17054565]

Anthony, W.A. (1993). Recovery from mental illness: The guiding vision of the mental health service system in the 1990s. *Psychosoc. Rehabil. J., 16*(4), 11-23.
[http://dx.doi.org/10.1037/h0095655]

Arblaster, K., Mackenzie, L., Gill, K., Willis, K., Matthews, L. (2019). Capabilities for recovery-oriented practice in mental health occupational therapy: A thematic analysis of lived experience perspectives. *Br. J. Occup. Ther., 82*(11), 675-684.
[http://dx.doi.org/10.1177/0308022619866129]

Australian Bureau of Statistics. (2016). *Country of birth.* Available from: http://www.abs.gov.au/websitedbs/censushome.nsf/home/quickstatscob?opendocument&navpos=220.

Bacchi, C. (2009). *Analysing Policy: What's the problem represented to be?.* Pearson Education.

Blanchard, A., Chihuri, S., DiGuiseppi, C.G., Li, G. (2021). Risk of Self-harm in Children and Adults With Autism Spectrum Disorder. *JAMA Netw. Open, 4*(10), e2130272-e2130272.
[http://dx.doi.org/10.1001/jamanetworkopen.2021.30272] [PMID: 34665237]

Boardman, J., Dave, S. (2020). Person-centred care and psychiatry: some key perspectives. *BJPsych Int., 17*(3), 65-68.
[http://dx.doi.org/10.1192/bji.2020.21] [PMID: 34287426]

Bölte, S. (2023). A more holistic approach to autism using the International Classification of Functioning: The why, what, and how of functioning. *Autism, 27*(1), 3-6.
[http://dx.doi.org/10.1177/13623613221136444] [PMID: 36330803]

Burgess, P., Pirkis, J., Coombs, T., Rosen, A. (2011). Assessing the value of existing recovery measures for routine use in Australian mental health services. *Aust. N. Z. J. Psychiatry, 45*(4), 267-280.
[http://dx.doi.org/10.3109/00048674.2010.549996] [PMID: 21314238]

Carr, E.R., Ponce, A.N. (2022). Supporting Mental Health Recovery, Citizenship, and Social Justice. *Community Ment. Health J., 58*(1), 11-19.
[http://dx.doi.org/10.1007/s10597-021-00900-y] [PMID: 34716831]

Castelein, S., Timmerman, M.E., van der Gaag, M., Visser, E. (2021). Clinical, societal and personal recovery in schizophrenia spectrum disorders across time: states and annual transitions. *Br. J. Psychiatry, 219*(1), 401-408.
[http://dx.doi.org/10.1192/bjp.2021.48] [PMID: 35048855]

Cherewick, M., Matergia, M. (2023). Neurodiversity in Practice: a Conceptual Model of Autistic Strengths and Potential Mechanisms of Change to Support Positive Mental Health and Wellbeing in Autistic Children and Adolescents. *Adv. Neurodev. Disord.*
[http://dx.doi.org/10.1007/s41252-023-00348-z]

Cohen, P., Cohen, J. (1984). The clinician's illusion. *Arch. Gen. Psychiatry, 41*(12), 1178-1182.
[http://dx.doi.org/10.1001/archpsyc.1984.01790230064010] [PMID: 6334503]

Coleman, R. (2011). *Recovery: An alien concept.* P&P Press.

Commonwealth of Australia. (2013). *A National Framework for Recovery-Oriented Mental Health Services.* Available from: https://www.health.gov.au/sites/default/files/documents/2021/04/a-nationa--framework-for-recovery-oriented-mental-health-services-policy-and-theory.pdf.

Deegan, P.E. (1988). Recovery: The lived experience of rehabilitation. *Psychosoc. Rehabil. J., 11*(4), 11-19. [http://dx.doi.org/10.1037/h0099565]

Fedina, L., Ashwell, L., Bright, C., Backes, B., Newman, M., Hafner, S., Rosay, A.B. (2022). Racial and gender inequalities in food, housing, and healthcare insecurity associated with intimate partner and sexual violence. *J. Interpers. Violence, 37*(23-24), NP23202-NP23221. [http://dx.doi.org/10.1177/08862605221077231] [PMID: 35404722]

Giffort, D., Schmook, A., Woody, C., Vollendorf, C., Gervain, M. (1995). *Recovery Assessment Scale..* Illinois Department of Mental Health.

Glover, H. (2012). Recovery, Life Long Learning, Social Inclusion and Empowerment: Is a new paradigm emerging? In: Ryan, P., Ramon, S., Greacen, T., (Eds.), *Empowerment, lifelong learning and recovery in mental health: Towards a new paradigm..* Palgrave Macmillan. [http://dx.doi.org/10.1007/978-0-230-39135-2_2]

Goldsmith, L., Bell, M.L. (2022). Queering environmental justice: Unequal environmental health burden on the LGBTQ+ community. *Am. J. Public Health, 112*(1), 79-87. [http://dx.doi.org/10.2105/AJPH.2021.306406] [PMID: 34936411]

Grim, K., Rosenberg, D., Svedberg, P., Schön, U.K. (2016). Shared decision-making in mental health care—A user perspective on decisional needs in community-based services. *Int. J. Qual. Stud. Health Well-being, 11*(1), 30563. [http://dx.doi.org/10.3402/qhw.v11.30563] [PMID: 27167556]

Hamilton, S.L., Maslen, S., Best, D., Freeman, J., O'Donnell, M., Reibel, T., Mutch, R., Watkins, R. (2020). Putting 'justice' in recovery capital: Yarning about hopes and futures with young people in detention. *International Journal for Crime. International Journal for Crime, Justice and Social Democracy, 9*(2), 20-36. [http://dx.doi.org/10.5204/ijcjsd.v9i2.1256]

Hasselkus, B. (2011). *The meaning of everyday occupation.* Slack.

Horgan, A., O Donovan, M., Manning, F., Doody, R., Savage, E., Dorrity, C., O'Sullivan, H., Goodwin, J., Greaney, S., Biering, P., Bjornsson, E., Bocking, J., Russell, S., Griffin, M., MacGabhann, L., van der Vaart, K.J., Allon, J., Granerud, A., Hals, E., Pulli, J., Vatula, A., Ellilä, H., Lahti, M., Happell, B. (2021). 'Meet Me Where I Am': Mental health service users' perspectives on the desirable qualities of a mental health nurse. *Int. J. Ment. Health Nurs., 30*(1), 136-147. [http://dx.doi.org/10.1111/inm.12768] [PMID: 32808438]

Hutson, T.M., McGhee Hassrick, E., Fernandes, S., Walton, J., Bouvier-Weinberg, K., Radcliffe, A., Allen-Handy, A. (2022). "I'm just different–that's all–I'm so sorry … ": Black men, ASD and the urgent need for DisCrit Theory in police encounters. *Policing, 45*(3), 524-537. [http://dx.doi.org/10.1108/PIJPSM-10-2021-0149]

Hwang, Y.I.J., Srasuebkul, P., Foley, K.R., Arnold, S., Trollor, J.N. (2019). Mortality and cause of death of Australians on the autism spectrum. *Autism Res., 12*(5), 806-815. [http://dx.doi.org/10.1002/aur.2086] [PMID: 30802364]

Jackman, K.B. Nonsuicidal self-injury among gender minority populations: A mixed methods investigation [Doctoral thesis, Columbia University]. *ProQuest.*Available from: https://www.proquest.com/dissertations-theses/nonsuicidal-self-injury-among-gender-minority/docview/1987552426/se-2. (2017).

Jerrell, J.M., Cousins, V.C., Roberts, K.M. (2006). Psychometrics of the recovery process inventory. *J. Behav. Health Serv. Res., 33*(4), 464-473. [http://dx.doi.org/10.1007/s11414-006-9031-5] [PMID: 16703473]

Kelly, M., Lamont, S., Brunero, S. (2010). An Occupational Perspective of the Recovery Journey in Mental Health. *Br. J. Occup. Ther., 73*(3), 129-135. [http://dx.doi.org/10.4276/030802210X12682330090532]

Krupa, T., Fossey, E., Anthony, W.A., Brown, C., Pitts, D.B. (2009). Doing daily life: How occupational therapy can inform psychiatric rehabilitation practice. *Psychiatr. Rehabil. J., 32*(3), 155-161. [http://dx.doi.org/10.2975/32.3.2009.155.161] [PMID: 19136347]

Leamy, M., Bird, V., Boutillier, C.L., Williams, J., Slade, M. (2011). Conceptual framework for personal recovery in mental health: systematic review and narrative synthesis. *Br. J. Psychiatry, 199*(6), 445-452. [http://dx.doi.org/10.1192/bjp.bp.110.083733] [PMID: 22130746]

Levy-Fenner, E., Colucci, E., McDonough, S. (2022). Lived Experiences of Mental Health Recovery in Persons of Culturally and Linguistically Diverse (CALD) Backgrounds within the Australian Context. *J. Psychosoc. Rehabil. Ment. Health,* 1-26. [http://dx.doi.org/10.1007/s40737-022-00319-y] [PMID: 36533215]

Lloyd, C., Waghorn, G., Williams, P.L. (2008). Conceptualising Recovery in Mental Health Rehabilitation. *Br. J. Occup. Ther., 71*(8), 321-328. [http://dx.doi.org/10.1177/030802260807100804]

Lloyd, C., Williams, P.L., Machingura, T., Tse, S. (2016). A focus on recovery: using the Mental Health Recovery Star as an outcome measure. *Adv. Ment. Health, 14*(1), 57-64. [http://dx.doi.org/10.1080/18387357.2015.1064341]

McDermott, E., Hughes, E., Rawlings, V. (2018). Norms and normalisation: understanding lesbian, gay, bisexual, transgender and queer youth, suicidality and help-seeking. *Cult. Health Sex., 20*(2), 156-172. [http://dx.doi.org/10.1080/13691058.2017.1335435] [PMID: 28641479]

Milbourn, B., Martin, R., Overheu, H., Schalk, D. (2018). Can mental health legal representation and advocacy contribute to personal recovery? *Adv. Ment. Health, 16*(2), 129-140. [http://dx.doi.org/10.1080/18387357.2018.1480397]

Milbourn, B., McNamara, B., Buchanan, A. (2017). A qualitative study of occupational well-being for people with severe mental illness. *Scand. J. Occup. Ther., 24*(4), 269-280. [http://dx.doi.org/10.1080/11038128.2016.1241824] [PMID: 27734712]

Milbourn, B., McNamara, B.A., Buchanan, A.J. (2015). Respecting recovery: research relationships with people with mental illness. *Qual. Res. J., 15*(3), 256-267. [http://dx.doi.org/10.1108/QRJ-12-2013-0071]

Moudatsou, M., Stavropoulou, A., Philalithis, A., Koukouli, S. (2020). The Role of Empathy in Health and Social Care Professionals. *Healthcare (Basel), 8*(1), 26. [http://dx.doi.org/10.3390/healthcare8010026] [PMID: 32019104]

Morrison, L.J. (2009). *Talking back to psychiatry: The psychiatric consumer/survivor/ex-patient movement.* Routledge,.

Nugent, A., Hancock, N., Honey, A. (2017). Developing and Sustaining Recovery-Orientation in Mental Health Practice: Experiences of Occupational Therapists. *Occup. Ther. Int., 2017,* 1-9. [http://dx.doi.org/10.1155/2017/5190901] [PMID: 29097969]

O'Brien, J., Fossey, E., Palmer, V.J. (2021). A scoping review of the use of co□design methods with culturally and linguistically diverse communities to improve or adapt mental health services. *Health Soc. Care Community, 29*(1), 1-17. [http://dx.doi.org/10.1111/hsc.13105] [PMID: 32686881]

O'Leary, J., Russel, G., Tilly, J. (2015). *Building inclusion: An evidence-based model of inclusive leadership.*

Pelletier, J.F., Davidson, L., Giguère, C.É., Franck, N., Bordet, J., Rowe, M. (2020). Convergent and Concurrent Validity between Clinical Recovery and Personal-Civic Recovery in Mental Health. *J. Pers. Med., 10*(4), 163. [http://dx.doi.org/10.3390/jpm10040163] [PMID: 33053639]

Plowman, M., Izzo, S. *Recommendations for a culturally responsive mental health system.* Available from: https://vtmh.org.au/wp-content/uploads/2021/06/Recommendations-for-a-Culturally-Responsive--ental-Health-System-Report_ECCV_VTMH_June-2021.pdf. (2021).

Polatajko, H.J., Crak, J., Davis, J., Townsend, E.A. (2007). Canadian Practice Process Framework. In: Townsend, E.A., Polatajko, H.J., (Eds.), *Enabling occupation 2: advancing an occupational therapy vision for health, well-being and justice through occupation.*. Canadian Association of Occupational Therapists.

Price-Robertson, R., Obradovic, A., Morgan, B. (2017). Relational recovery: beyond individualism in the recovery approach. *Adv. Ment. Health,* *15*(2), 108-120.
[http://dx.doi.org/10.1080/18387357.2016.1243014]

Raymaker, D.M., Teo, A.R., Steckler, N.A., Lentz, B., Scharer, M., Delos Santos, A., Kapp, S.K., Hunter, M., Joyce, A., Nicolaidis, C. (2020). "Having All of Your Internal Resources Exhausted Beyond Measure and Being Left with No Clean-Up Crew": Defining Autistic Burnout. *Autism Adulthood,* *2*(2), 132-143.
[http://dx.doi.org/10.1089/aut.2019.0079] [PMID: 32851204]

Reis, G., Bromage, B., Rowe, M., Restrepo-Toro, M.E., Bellamy, C., Costa, M., Davidson, L. (2022). Citizenship, Social Justice and Collective Empowerment: Living Outside Mental Illness. *Psychiatr. Q.,* *93*(2), 537-546.
[http://dx.doi.org/10.1007/s11126-021-09968-x] [PMID: 35048313]

Resnick, S.G., Fontana, A., Lehman, A.F., Rosenheck, R.A. (2005). An empirical conceptualization of the recovery orientation. *Schizophr. Res.,* *75*(1), 119-128.
[http://dx.doi.org/10.1016/j.schres.2004.05.009] [PMID: 15820330]

Rønning, S.B., Bjørkly, S. (2019). The use of clinical role-play and reflection in learning therapeutic communication skills in mental health education: an integrative review. *Adv. Med. Educ. Pract.,* *10*, 415-425.
[http://dx.doi.org/10.2147/AMEP.S202115] [PMID: 31417328]

Sancho-Cantus, D., Cubero-Plazas, L., Botella Navas, M., Castellano-Rioja, E., Cañabate Ros, M. (2023). Importance of Soft Skills in Health Sciences Students and Their Repercussion after the COVID-19 Epidemic: Scoping Review. *Int. J. Environ. Res. Public Health,* *20*(6), 4901.
[http://dx.doi.org/10.3390/ijerph20064901] [PMID: 36981814]

Sokol, Y., Glatt, S., Levin, C., Tran, P., Rosensweig, C., Silver, C., Hubner, S., Primavera, L., Goodman, M. (2023). Recovery after a suicidal episode: Developing and validating the Recovery Evaluation and Suicide Support Tool (RESST). *Psychol. Assess.,* *35*(10), 842-855.
[http://dx.doi.org/10.1037/pas0001269] [PMID: 37732963]

Talwar, S. (2010). An Intersectional Framework for Race, Class, Gender, and Sexuality in Art Therapy. *Art Ther.,* *27*(1), 11-17.
[http://dx.doi.org/10.1080/07421656.2010.10129567]

Tew, J., Ramon, S., Slade, M., Bird, V., Melton, J., Le Boutillier, C. (2012). Social Factors and Recovery from Mental Health Difficulties: A Review of the Evidence. *Br. J. Soc. Work,* *42*(3), 443-460.
[http://dx.doi.org/10.1093/bjsw/bcr076]

Tse, S., Tsoi, E.W.S., Hamilton, B., O'Hagan, M., Shepherd, G., Slade, M., Whitley, R., Petrakis, M. (2016). Uses of strength-based interventions for people with serious mental illness: A critical review. *Int. J. Soc. Psychiatry,* *62*(3), 281-291.
[http://dx.doi.org/10.1177/0020764015623970] [PMID: 26831826]

Van Der Miesen, A.I.R., Hurley, H., De Vries, A.L.C. (2016). Gender dysphoria and autism spectrum disorder: A narrative review. *Int. Rev. Psychiatry,* *28*(1), 70-80.
[http://dx.doi.org/10.3109/09540261.2015.1111199] [PMID: 26753812]

Warrier, V., Greenberg, D.M., Weir, E., Buckingham, C., Smith, P., Lai, M.C., Allison, C., Baron-Cohen, S. (2020). Elevated rates of autism, other neurodevelopmental and psychiatric diagnoses, and autistic traits in transgender and gender-diverse individuals. *Nat. Commun.,* *11*(1), 3959.
[http://dx.doi.org/10.1038/s41467-020-17794-1] [PMID: 32770077]

Wilburn, V.G., Stoll, H.B., Chase, A., Moring, K., Rohr, A. (2021). Strategies to Occupations in Recovering Youth Enrolled in a Recovery High School. *Occup. Ther. Ment. Health,* *37*(4), 357-369.

[http://dx.doi.org/10.1080/0164212X.2021.1899097]

Xie, H. (2013). Strengths-based approach for mental health recovery. *Iran. J. Psychiatry. Behav. Sci.,*   7(2), 5-10.
[PMID: 24644504]

CHAPTER 18

The Future of Occupational Therapy: Recovery, Participatory Citizenship and the Impact of Technology

Tongai F. Chichaya[1,*], **Bex Symons**[1] and **Phil Morgan**[2]

[1] *Department of Occupational Therapy, Coventry University, Coventry, England, United Kingdom*

[2] *Therapies and Quality (Mental Health), Dorset Healthcare University NHS Foundation Trust, Poole, Dorset, United Kingdom*

Abstract: This chapter was co-authored by a peer researcher with lived experience. People with mental health challenges are often pushed to the margins of society, and experience powerlessness, which prevents them from being able to access their full rights as citizens. The chapter explores the concept of citizenship within the context of mental health and occupational therapy. Limitations of the recovery approach are discussed and opportunities for enacting participatory citizenship to address the limitations are explored. The intersection between participatory citizenship and occupational justice is examined.

The chapter also delves into the impact of technology on citizenship, discussing the opportunities and challenges it presents for individuals with mental health conditions. It highlights the importance of considering technology's role in shaping social norms, facilitating participation, and promoting inclusion. In an increasingly technological society, occupational therapists could play a key role in public health and through 'occupation' support people with their identity and finding meaning. It is essential that occupational therapists engage in promoting digital citizenship, people's interaction with AI, and participation in the virtual world.

The chapter suggests reflective exercises for readers to consider; these can be undertaken individually or collaboratively as part of group activities. These reflections are designed to support a shift in thinking towards a more participatory approach to promote citizenship, address occupational injustice, and create inclusive societies for individuals with mental health challenges.

Keywords: Digital citizenship, Mental health, Occupational justice, Occupational therapy, Participatory citizenship, Recovery.

* **Corresponding author Tongai F. Chichaya:** Department of Occupational Therapy, Coventry University, Coventry, England, United Kingdom; E-mail: chichayatf@gmail.com

Tawanda Machingura (Ed.)

INTRODUCTION

People with mental health challenges are often pushed to the margins of society and experience powerlessness, which prevents them from being able to access their full rights as citizens (Hamer *et al.* 2017). This results in mental health service users being at a significantly higher risk of experiencing occupational injustices such as occupational marginalisation, occupational alienation, occupational inconsideration, or occupational deprivation than the general population (Wilcock and Townsend, 2009; Chichaya, Joubert and McColl, 2019; Khronenberg and Pollard, 2005). To ameliorate the risk, the participatory occupational justice framework (PJOF) is growing in popularity within the field of occupational therapy. The PJOF is a useful conceptual tool when working from an occupational justice lens in occupational therapy practice and is in line with the ethos of citizenship (Whiteford *et al.* , 2017). There is also a drive from within occupational therapy for a focus on participatory citizenship and how we work collaboratively with people with disabilities and mental health services to increase inclusivity and promote social justice (Fransen *et al.* , 2015; Fransen *et al.* , 2013).

Citizenship is an increasingly prominent concept within mental health as a way of promoting the rights, participation, and inclusion of people with mental health challenges within society (Davidson *et al.* , 2021; MacIntyre *et al.* , 2021). This is for two reasons: firstly the social change promised by the Recovery Approach, whilst leading to some changes for people with mental health challenges, has not delivered the transformation of services and communities that had been promised (Rowe and Davidson 2016; Brannelly 2018); and secondly, the nature of citizenship is changing with the rapid uptake of technology (Morgan *et al.* , 2020).

This chapter will first define citizenship in the context of mental health and its relationship with Recovery. This will be followed by a discussion of citizenship within occupational therapy. Following this conceptual exploration, there will be a focus on the key themes from the mental health citizenship research and a discussion of the implications for occupational therapy. The chapter will move on to explore the impact of technology on citizenship and what this means for occupational therapy practice now and in the future. This section is predominantly based on a small-scale research project undertaken by Phil Morgan as part of a PhD, and elements of his thesis are reproduced throughout this chapter. Bex Symons worked with Phil as a peer researcher on this project. The chapter will conclude with a call to action and a proposed approach to implementing citizenship approaches.

In each section, there will be reflective exercises for you to consider as you work through the chapter (these can be undertaken individually or as part of a group activity). These reflections are designed to support your understanding and how you may wish to adopt this thinking in your practice, as well as the challenges and opportunities this will bring.

WHAT IS CITIZENSHIP?

Citizenship in Mental Health

Citizenship is an important and contested concept in mental health (MacIntyre *et al.* 2021). Due to the mental health legislation, for example, the UK Mental Health Act 1983, it could be argued that people with mental health challenges have a unique experience of citizenship as their human rights are dependent on their health status (Hamer and Findlayson 2015; Brannelly 2018). Once you are labelled with mental health challenges, you can be perceived as different, dangerous, and not to be trusted (Hamer *et al.* 2014; Hamer and Findlayson 2015; Vervliet *et al.* 2019; Cogan *et al.* 2021). This, in turn, can lead to a loss of personal power and a collapse in the sense of agency and role in society, which reinforces people's mental health challenges (Hamer *et al.* 2017).

The service user/survivor movement has long fought for full citizenship. However, neither the de-institutionalisation of the 80s and 90s nor the Recovery movement has delivered the level of change that has led to equal citizenship (Rowe and Davidson 2016; Eiroa-Orosa and Rowe 2017). This lack of progress has resulted in social exclusions that perpetuate and sustain inequalities. This is why a focus on citizenship within mental health is being viewed as an important lens through which people's experience of inclusion and exclusion in society can be explored to enhance participation, promote people's rights, and deliver social justice (Rowe and Davidson 2016; Morgan *et al.* 2020; Davidson *et al.* 2021; MacIntyre *et al.* 2021). This is not to say the core principles of Recovery are not important, but rather that exploring citizenship provides a political and social context to understand Recovery and its implementation. Before exploring citizenship, it is important to revisit the concept of Recovery.

Personal Recovery

The Recovery approach evolved out of the survivor/service user movement in the United States, with service user activists such as Pat Deegan promoting the value of lived experience. She aligned the rights of people with mental health challenges alongside those with disabilities in a call for social change (Deegan 1988). The purpose of this was to shift the focus from illness and clinical recovery to one that supported people to build a life and find meaning and purpose. The core components of this were the role of peer support, self-management, valuing the expertise of people with lived experience, and fundamentally people having a sense of citizenship (Davidson *et al.* 2021)

The seminal definition of personal recovery was put forward by Bill Anthony (1993)

Recovery is a deeply personal, unique process of changing one's attitudes, values, feelings, goals, skills and/or roles. It is a way of living a satisfying, hopeful, and contributing life even with limitations caused by the illness. Recovery involves the development of new meaning and purpose in one's life as one grows beyond the catastrophic effects of mental illness (p15)

Based on this, Anthony put forward a new vision for mental health services that put personal recovery at their heart, which required a fundamental shift in focus away from biomedical approaches and greater involvement of people with lived experience. This then saw Personal Recovery being adopted in mental health policy, initially in English-speaking countries and now across the globe (Slade *et al.* 2017).

However, as Recovery was beginning to be adopted more widely, service-user activist Mary O'Hagan (2008) warned against the increasingly individualised approach to Recovery. She was concerned about an approach that neglected the social, political, and economic aspects of Recovery and stressed the importance of service-user/survivor leadership in the implementation of Recovery to counterbalance this.

Leamy *et al.* (2011) undertook a systematic review and identified 5 core elements that supported personal recovery, which created the acronym CHIME. These are Connectedness, Hope, Identity, Meaning, and Empowerment. All of these elements are core to occupational therapy practice. The wide-scale adoption of the Recovery approach led to an increased focus on initiatives such as a focus on Individual Placement and Support (employment support), peer support workers, and the development of Recovery Colleges. There is clear evidence that these approaches have benefits for some people (Slade *et al.* 2014).

However, despite these benefits for some, the implementation of the Recovery approach has been criticised for benefiting those who are white, have social and/or economic capital, have an increasingly individualised approach, ignore the impact of neo-liberalism and rationing of mental health services, and are colonised by mental health services, excluding those with lived experience from shaping the direction. (Rose 2014; Recovery in the Bin [RiTB] 2016). Therefore, the anticipated transformation of mental health services did not occur; however, it is being proposed that citizenship may have a central role in transforming mental health care and reconnecting Recovery to its radical and social roots (Davidson *et al.* 2021; Carr and Ponce 2022). Davidson *et al.* (2021) describe it as 'Recovering Citizenship'. It is, therefore, important to understand how citizenship is conceptualised.

Citizenship and Social Class

Theories of citizenship within Western Democracies have been shaped by the seminal work of T.H. Marshall's 1949 (1987), *Citizenship and Social Class*. This saw the birth of the welfare state within the United Kingdom and described the rights and obligations between the state and its citizens. Marshall describes how people have:

- Civil Rights- right to assembly, freedom of speech
- Political Rights- right to vote or stand for election
- Social rights- access to welfare, healthcare, and education

These rights were balanced with obligation, for example, taxation or, at the time, conscription to the military. The extent and balance of these rights varies from country to country. Whilst Marshall described these rights as universal, they are based on a heterosexual, white, and masculine archetype, and because of this, they do not address citizenship in a way that is fully inclusive, nor do they explore whose voice is heard or excluded. This 'normative' approach to citizenship does not consider the needs of people with disabilities and mental health challenges (Atterbury and Rowe 2017) and has been criticised by feminists and post-colonialists for its gendered and ethnocentric stance (Lister 2007; Hamer *et al.* 2017). Therefore, without a more critical perspective on citizenship, it sustains oppression and exclusion (Atterbury and Rowe 2017; Vervliet *et al.* 2019).

Marshall's definition and citizenship developed out of Aristotle's (1995)*Politics* 4 B.C. (Hamer 2012; Rowe and Pelletier 2012). Aristotle views citizenship as the relationship between a person and the city-state. According to him, people can expect to flourish within the city-state, and the state can expect people to fulfill their duties. This is balanced through the concept of *Justice.* However, due to self-interest, struggles for power, and the prioritisation of different rights, justice becomes distorted. This struggle for justice is described by Aristotle (1995) as *politics.* For Aristotle, the rights of citizenship were only available to men. Thousands of years later, the issues relating to balancing rights, power, and inclusion are still pertinent to citizenship.

Over the centuries, within Western societies, the legal rights of citizenship have been passed to increasing numbers of citizens. Within UK legislation, examples include the Abolition of Slavery Act 1838, the Representation of the People Act

(Equal voting rights for men and women over 21) 1928, the Sexual Offences Act 1967 (which decriminalised homosexuality), and the Representation of the People Act 2000 (giving the right to vote to people detained under the Mental Health Act). However, people such as asylum seekers and undocumented migrants are excluded and are unable to access many of the legal benefits of citizenship.

Two 19th-century thinkers, De Tocqueville (2002) and Durkheim (2014), also played a significant role in developing the concept of citizenship. De Tocqueville studied the French and American revolutions and examined how new laws and morals were generated. He argued that through social movements, there is a march to greater equality. Therefore, citizenship can shift and change and is understood beyond the legal definition alone. Durkheim (one of the founders of sociology) also argues that citizenship is not just enacted through legal rights but through how morals, attitudes, and democratic structures are buried deep into individual consciousness. This creates a sense of what is considered normal within a cultural context. This, in turn, constructs what is considered to be citizenship within that context. It is through this process of normalcy can lead to people with mental health challenges being excluded (Hamer *et al.* 2014).

Despite the legal changes that have been won, the legacy and continued prejudice of structural racism, homophobia, ableism, and sexism continue to exclude people's participation in society (Atterbury and Rowe, 2018). This includes the discrimination people with mental health challenges experience and how this intersects with other forms of discrimination (Fagrell Tryff *et al.* 2019). This discrimination can lead to people feeling like second-class or 'non-citizens' (Hamer 2012).

De Tocqueville highlighted the importance of social movements as important in representing the views of those who are marginalised (and) this being a key component of citizenship. He warns against what J.S. Mill described as the 'tyranny of the majority' in ensuring that the views of people who are disadvantaged are taken into consideration. Durkheim views this solidarity as both natural and important to citizenship; he views excessive individualism as pathological and highlights the importance of new social movements to bring people together via civic participation and community groups. However, despite this, increasingly individualistic approaches have shaped citizenship.

Lived experience perspective – what citizenship means to me

Bex Symons, our co-author and peer researcher with lived experience, describes citizenship as follows:

Citizenship means to me that 'we' all have a voice. 'We' have a right for our voice to be heard. Every voice carries equal weight. 'We' should care about as many people being included as possible. 'We' should be willing to be involved in involving as many participants as possible. If 'we' witness or are made aware of limitations or discrimination, everyone should feel the weight of speaking up to challenge actions. Ultimately, 'we' are not stagnant participants, 'we' are active contributors.

> **Reflective Exercise:**
> What does citizenship mean to you? For some people, it means being part of a nation state; for others, it can be belonging to a group, community, or club, having rights and responsibilities, or it can be about justice. How might your experience of citizenship be different than other people?

Neoliberalism and Recovery

In the later 20th and 21st centuries, citizenship has increasingly been shaped by the individualistic philosophy of 'neoliberalism'. This philosophy is so embedded in Western society that it is presented as 'common sense' or the way of the world. There is not a single definition of neoliberalism, but its defining features are free markets, individualism, and decentralisation. Therefore, they are concerned with shrinking the role of the state, increasing the role of businesses and corporations, and reducing regulation (Gabe 2020).

Neoliberals suggest that social rights are no longer important as the welfare state is no longer relevant as funding has been diminished and that there is now greater emphasis on individuals taking responsibility for their own health and social needs. The value of an individual's citizenship is determined by their economic contribution (Atterbury and Rowe 2017). Cruickshank (1999) described the 'new technologies of citizenship' [p2], which seek to secure the compliance of people by directing their attention to consumption, monetizing their participation, and directing their agency to be passive within this process. Therefore, the targets of resistance become harder to find and, therefore, to challenge. For example, within the UK and the US, there are fewer people voting; however, instead of encouraging more people to vote, there are increased constraints on people being able to vote, or people are encouraged through the media to focus on who is deserving or undeserving of welfare. There is increasing anxiety about immigration or encouraging people to give up their data to companies such as Meta (Zuboff 2019; Isin and Ruppert 2020).

One of the reasons that the implementation of the Recovery Approach has been criticised is that mental health services have not been sufficiently engaged in understanding the impact of neoliberalism on people with mental health challenges. The UK-based service user/survivor activist group Recovery In the

Bin (RITB) argues that as mental health services have taken the lead on implementing Recovery, rather than people with lived experience, the original tenets of Recovery have been lost. This has led to a more individualised approach to Recovery focusing on personal responsibility and engagement, which masks the underfunding of mental health services and does not acknowledge the intolerable social and economic conditions such as poor housing, poverty, stigma, and discrimination, which in turn result in greater coercion. They have developed the un-recovery star, which highlights the impact of poverty and discrimination on attempts to 'recover' and argues that it is unfair to locate Recovery in an individual in the context of cuts to services and marginalisation. Hammel (2020) argues that it is important for occupational therapists when offering choices to their clients that they understand the context within which people are making choices and the factors that can have an impact on that. This highlights the importance of understanding intersectionality (the impact of multiple forms of discrimination) in occupational therapy practice.

These concerns raised in the mental health literature in relation to the impact of neo-liberalism are similar to those raised by critical occupational therapists (Whiteford and Townsend 2011; Hammel, 2015) and, more broadly, the World Federation of Occupational Therapy (WFOT), whose revised position statement on human rights reiterates the concern of upholding human rights by pursuing occupational justice for everyone (WFOT, 2019). The concept of occupational justice, while not having a single definition, is generally about promoting social, economic, and political change to create occupational opportunities that enable people to engage in diverse and meaningful occupations of their needs and choices (Townsend and Wilcock, 2004; Wilcock and Townsend 2009). When conditions for occupational justice are met, the occupational rights of people to engage in diverse, meaningful occupations are upheld. When engagement in meaningful occupations is barred, confined, restricted, segregated, prohibited, disrupted, alienated, marginalised, or exploited, occupational injustice occurs (Townsend and Wilcock, 2004; Kronenberg and Pollard 2005). This means that promoting Recovery and citizenship is not just a case of delivering care and treatment but is part of a struggle for social change and justice.

There are two main authors who have driven the citizenship agenda within the mental health literature; these are Rowe (Rowe *et al.* 2007; 2009; 2012; Rowe and Pelletier 2012; Clayton *et al.* 2013; Rowe and Davidson 2016, Atterbury and Rowe 2017) and Hamer (2012; Hamer and Finlayson 2015; Hamer *et al.* 2014, 2017, 2019). Hamer's (2012) initial focus was the lived experience of citizenship of people with mental health challenges. This research captured people's sense of exclusion and alienation and also the elements that supported inclusion and participation. The work of Rowe and colleagues developed out of the mental health and homeless sector in the United States when they noticed that when people were housed, they did not go on to integrate with their communities. They set up a randomised control-trial that offered mentoring, citizenship training, and community participation. The findings of this trial of those on the experimental side saw an increased quality of life and a reduction in the use of substances and reoffending (Clayton *et al.* 2013). Thus, highlighting citizenship is not just a useful way of conceptualising people's experiences but an intervention in its own right.

5Rs of Citizenship

Their conceptualisation of citizenship was based on what they defined as the 5 Rs (Rowe and Pelletier 2012; Atterbury and Rowe 2017), which are:

- Rights
- Responsibilities
- Roles
- Resources
- Relationships

They focus on how the interplay of the 5Rs shapes people's ability to access citizenship. These 5Rs are informed by De Tocqueville and Durkheim's conceptualisation of citizenship, for example, how people's resources and relationships helped and hindered their access to full citizenship alongside their access to rights and opportunities to participate in roles and undertake responsibilities.

> **Reflective Exercise:**
> How can you use the 5 Rs of Citizenship alongside occupational therapy models to incorporate a greater focus on citizenship in your work?

Increasingly, Rowe and colleagues have collaborated internationally with colleagues in New Zealand, Norway, Scotland, and Spain to develop a citizenship research base. The focus of subsequent research has used participatory approaches to define citizenship alongside people with lived experience (MacIntyre *et al.* 2021), exploring how to develop citizenship-focused mental health services and the role of professionals (Rowe and Davidson 2016; Hamer *et al.* 2019; Carr and Ponce 2022; Flanagan *et al.* 2023; Eiroa Orasa 2023), the development of citizenship measures (O'Connell *et al.* 2017; Cogan *et al.* 2022) and community participation and collective action (Quinn *et al.* 2020; Danielsen *et al.* 2021; Nesse *et al.* 2021; Reiss *et al.* 2022).

Alongside the 5Rs work, there has been an increased focus on 'collective citizenship' (Quinn *et al.* 2020; Reiss *et al.* 2022), which involves people with lived experience coming together with health professionals and people from community groups and organisations to drive social change. For example, people with mental health challenges work alongside a poverty action group or participate in community arts projects (Reiss *et al.* 2022). It is through this participation that people then enact their citizenship and can drive change and resist some of the forces of neoliberalism. It also has much in common with the critical approaches to citizenship, such as 'Acts of Citizenship.'

Act of Citizenship

Hamer's (2012) theoretical framework was 'Acts of Citizenship' (Isin and Neilsen 2008). The focus of critical citizenship is uncovering and challenging the dominant discourses that shape social norms (for example, what is considered mad or the likelihood of someone receiving a diagnosis based on their gender or ethnicity) and seeking social justice. Critical citizenship sees people in their geographical and historical context, which is dynamic and contested (Isin and Neilsen, 2008)

Isin and Neilsen (2008) argue that citizenship is a dynamic process that citizens can shape as well as be shaped by. They argue that acts undertaken by individuals or communities that rupture and challenge social norms are, in themselves, the act of citizenship, and citizens come into being by performing these political acts (Isin and Ruppert 2020). The focus of citizenship then becomes the striving for rights. Lister (2007) argues that citizenship is not just about having rights but also recognition, and this is a form of cultural citizenship. People have the right to be different and fully participate and be valued. The acts of participation and drive for a social model of madness that Hamer describes can be considered 'acts of citizenship'.

Critical citizenship also recognises that citizenship is broader than the relationship between the individual and the state, although this has been under-recognised within mental health literature (Morgan *et al.* 2020). It also has a relationship with supranational organisations such as corporations or bodies like the European Union. In addition, the internet means people have global connections that spread beyond national borders (Isin and Ruppert 2020). It is important that these broader forms of citizenship, such as global citizenship (where people see themselves a part of the world rather than a nation), consumer citizenship (where people view that you exercise power through how you spend), and digital citizenship (our interactions in cyberspace) are acknowledged (Isin and Ruppert 2020). Digital citizenship is particularly important, especially as technology is rapidly shaping our lives (Morgan *et al.* 2020). This has only been exacerbated through the COVID-19 pandemic and the rapid introduction of technology across all elements of our lives (Morgan, 2023).

This attention to people's participation across all aspects of their lives, both in the virtual and personal world, is also key to occupational therapy. The sense of justice and promoting social change is rooted in the origins of occupational therapy as a profession, and connecting with participatory citizenship provides the profession an approach to engaging with these social and political dimensions.

Citizenship and Occupational Therapy

The origins of occupational therapy can be traced back to the moral treatment movement, which emerged in the late 18th and early 19th centuries (Keilhofner, 2009). The moral treatment movement was a reaction to the harsh and inhumane treatment of people with mental illness at the time. Proponents of moral treatment believed that people with mental illness could be cured by providing them with a humane and therapeutic environment (Scull, 1979).

People with mental illness were encouraged to participate in a variety of activities, such as work, education, and recreation. This was based on the belief that engagement in meaningful occupations could help to improve mental health and well-being. The moral treatment movement had a significant impact on the development of occupational therapy. Early occupational therapists were influenced by the moral treatment movement's emphasis on meaningful activity and its belief in the potential of people with mental illness to recover (Ikiugu, 2007). In its broad sense, citizenship includes aspects like the legal status of belonging to a state, the right to participate in political processes, social identity, and the duty to contribute to the common good of a society (Fransen *et al.* 2013). However, citizenship in the context of occupational therapy and promoting occupational justice goes beyond legal and political definitions with emphasis on meaningful social and community participation, as well as the elimination of discrimination and stigma against others. This includes people with mental health conditions, as they are often stigmatised and discriminated against. Therefore, it is through occupation that human beings can demonstrate their citizenship. When thinking about this in a 21st-century context, it is important to consider how we would collaboratively create humane and therapeutic communities and societies both in person and online.

The relationship between occupational therapy and citizenship is complex and political. Traditionally, occupational therapy has focused on helping people with mental illness to develop the skills and abilities needed to function independently in society. Such a limited focus has led to the development of critical occupational therapy challenging the status quo (Whiteford and Townsend 2011; Hammel, 2015). Critical occupational therapy emerged as a response to the recognition that traditional occupational therapy practices did not always consider the broader societal and systemic issues that impact individuals' abilities to engage in meaningful occupations. In recent years, there have been calls for a progressive shift towards a more social and political perspective (Pollard, Sakellariou, and Kronenberg, 2009). This focus aligns with the principles of critical citizenship, such as 'Acts of Citizenship' or 'collective citizenship' . From a critical occupational therapy perspective, citizenship is not simply a set of rights and obligations but also a process of struggle and empowerment (Kronenberg, Pollard and Sakellarioiu 2011). People with mental health conditions have the right to be full citizens within their communities, but they often face a number of challenges to achieving this right. The challenges include discrimination, stigma, and lack of access to resources and services, and these challenges have only increased since the COVID-19 pandemic (Marmot *et al.* 2020).

Occupational therapists are increasingly recognising the importance of citizenship for people with mental illness and are increasingly working to support them to engage in their communities and participate fully in society (Whiteford *et al.* 2017). However, this work is often hindered by the health and social systems in which occupational therapists work, thereby creating the notion of 'good intentions being overruled' (Townsend, 1998).

Citizenship is underpinned by a human rights-based approach, which is important in 'levelling the playing field' for persons with disabilities, including those with mental health conditions, so that they have equal access to livelihood, education, health, and other services within the community. In addition, it is about removing physical and social barriers and bringing about attitude adjustment among service decision-makers, service providers, family members, and society at large. In essence, the human rights model caters to both civil and political rights, as well as economic and cultural rights. This model can be considered an enhancement beyond the social model of disability. The social model clearly articulates discrimination against people with disabilities within society and argues for society to adapt to people's needs rather than locating the problem within individuals with disabilities or mental health challenges; however, it does not provide the moral principles and values as a base, which the human rights model does (Degener, 2014). People with mental health conditions are equal citizens and, therefore, have the same rights as everyone else. All actions to enable people with mental health conditions to flourish as equal citizens must be rights-based.

Fransen *et al.* (2015) argue that the key task for occupational therapists is to promote the expression of citizenship through occupation and acts to counter dis-citizenship. Essential to this is viewing health as a societal issue, something that needs to be addressed beyond the individual. In adopting a participatory citizenship approach in occupational therapy, a three-stage approach is suggested (Fransen *et al.* 2013):

- **Forming Partnerships:** to work collectively and transdisciplinary with all stakeholders to promote citizenship
- **Establish spaces to practice citizenship:** creating an inclusive environment (physical, social, and virtual) to enable equal participation.
- To embrace **participatory citizenship as a way of being in the world with others** by challenging injustice and promoting inclusion.

When we come to look at how we embed citizenship approaches in mental health, these three elements are key.

Reflective Activity:
You have been introduced to a range of theoretical approaches to citizenship, which one makes the most sense to you? Why do you favour that approach?
How will you embed Fransen et al. (2013)'s three stage approach in your practice?

Occupational Justice and Participatory Citizenship

The WFOT position statement on occupational therapy and human rights outlines the key tenets of occupational justice as the rights for all to have a choice in occupations, to participate in a range of occupations, and to freely engage in occupations (WFOT,2019). From an occupational therapy perspective, it is important to note that addressing the different forms of occupational injustice faced by people with mental health conditions is a complex and multi-faceted process. We advocate that this begins with occupational therapists having an understanding of citizenship from an occupational perspective. The premise upon which these actions are built is the understanding of the potency and use of occupation as a vehicle for enacting citizenship.

A recent publication on citizenship and occupational therapy provides a valuable resource for educating occupational therapy students and occupational therapists about participatory citizenship from an occupational perspective with some guided activities (Fransen-Jaïbi *et al*, 2021). The publication offers a number of practical activities. In this chapter, to demonstrate how these activities can be applied by occupational therapists to promote citizenship, we have selected the activity focusing on the role of media in shaping the representation of citizenship and how media influences public opinion. This includes the impact of social media, where algorithms and bots can manipulate information and contribute to misinformation. In this activity, participants are asked to identify newspapers and other print or electronic media with articles on living with mental health conditions. Participants will then need to think about the impression being made about people with mental health conditions in the media and how these representations are likely to promote inclusion or worsen their exclusion. The activity involves cutting out news headlines, taking pictures and stories that depict the misrepresentation created by the media, and presenting this in a poster format. Participants will then work together to co-create a counter-narrative that redresses the misrepresentation. Variations to producing counter-narrative media can be through film clubs or writing books. Access Dorset in the UK provides an example of citizen journalism in which a university collaborated with people with disabilities to co-create a short film to illustrate the challenges faced by people who use wheelchairs when trying to access public transport (BBC, 2014; Access Dorset 2014). This was a powerful way to bring out marginalised voices to the attention of the mainstream media, and the resource remains available on social media (Access Dorset 2016). This approach links strongly with acts of citizenship and collective citizenship and the importance of people with lived experienced participating to drive change. This shifts the focus of occupational therapy practice to not just on the individual and their functioning but supporting groups to take action in the work and to enhance peoples' opportunity to participate.

The participatory occupational justice framework (PJOF; Whiteford *et al*, 2017) is also a key tool. The PJOF aligns with critical occupational therapy practice, especially when working with disadvantaged and oppressed people (Whiteford and Townsend, 2011). This makes the PJOF ideal for use when working with people with mental health conditions. The PJOF (Fig. **1**) consists of six enabling collaborative processes that can be used for taking action to promote engagement in meaningful occupations. The processes are embedded in a local, regional, national, and global context.

The PJOF is a tool for addressing the gap between the vision for all people being able to engage in desired meaningful occupations and the current practices. While the PJOF is not linear, generally, the process starts with raising consciousness about occupational injustice. In mental health, this step might include raising consciousness on how people with mental health conditions are excluded or restricted from participating in meaningful occupations. This practice requires *critical reflexivity* in which occupational therapists consider the power relations between them and their service users and other stakeholders. *Co-creation,* in which occupational therapists work collaboratively with service users to delineate and raise consciousness about identified occupational injustices, can be more beneficial. The other four processes are more fluid and can overlap or be implemented simultaneously. These collaborative processes include engaging collaboratively with partners, mediating an agreed plan, strategising resource funding, supporting implementation, and continuous evaluation of the plan. Ultimately, the sixth process is about inspiring advocacy for sustainability or closure. Of importance to note when using the POJF is the notion that professionals can act as catalysts to inspire sustainability allowing individuals and groups of people to continue engaging in meaningful occupations as citizens without necessarily continuing to have professional input where possible. Based on this, it is now important to turn to the core themes within the mental health citizenship literature and explore how these relate to occupational therapy practice.

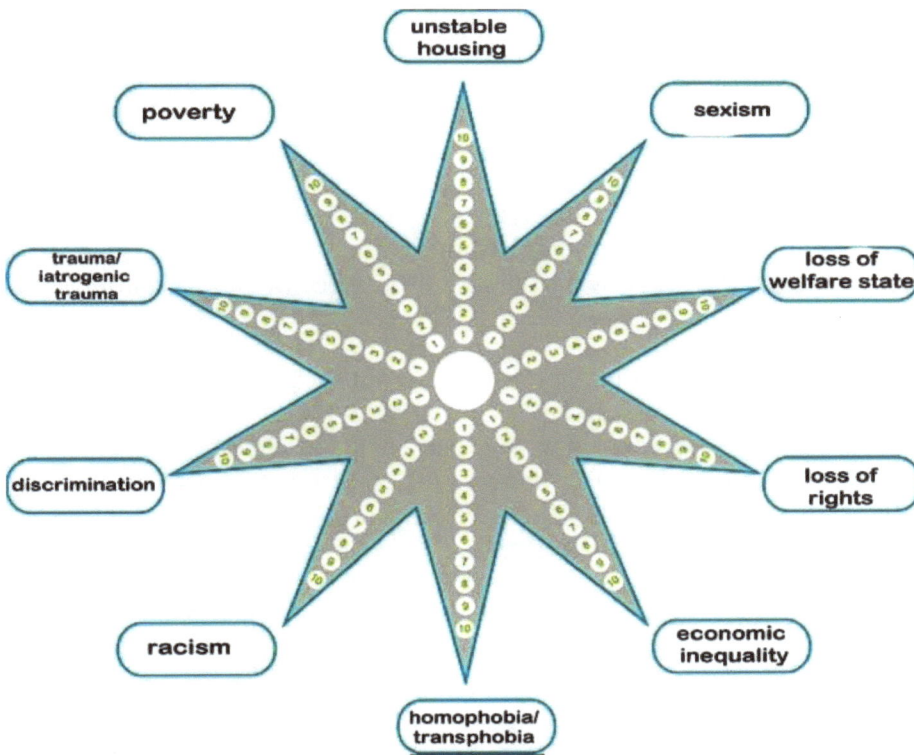

Fig. (1). Participatory Occupational Justice Framework Source: Whiteford *et al.* 2017.

Key Themes from the Mental Health Citizenship Literature

Four core themes from the mental health citizenship literature will be focused on as they are most pertinent to Recovery and Occupational Therapy; these are: belonging and participation; having a voice and co-production; the role of mental health services and allyship of mental health professionals; the role of technology and future impacts.

'Belonging' and participation as Citizenship

One of the key findings across the research literature is that engaging in activities and opportunities to participate in society, such as employment, people's sense of citizenship increased (Hamer and Finlay 2015; Harper *et al.* 2017; Hamer *et al.* 2019; Danielsen *et al.* 2021; MacIntyre *et al.* 2021; Nesse *et al.* 2021; Reiss *et al.* 2022). Hamer *et al.* (2017) describe the notion of *homo occupacio*, the persona of the citizen, as the self-directed, self-initiated occupational human who takes possession of his or her world through a repertoire of occupations located within the rules and norms of society. However, for those who have been labelled with a psychiatric diagnosis, the ability to participate and exercise the rights and responsibilities as citizens can be conditional, often interrupted, and, at times, denied. Therefore, it is important that reasonable adjustments are in place to make communities more accessible and support participation (Hamer *et al.* 2017). Fundamental to this is adopting a 'social model of madness', which moves away from a biomedical approach dominating understandings of mental health challenges to one that focuses on the importance of societal change in terms of attitudes, support, and opportunity (Beresford 2010; Hamer *et al.* 2017). This is a key finding for occupational therapists in taking a role in promoting citizenship and being aware of barriers to participation on a political dimension as well as a physical and social one.

It is also important to note that increasingly, a number of Rowe's collaborators are focusing on 'collective citizenship' (Quinn *et al.* 2020; Reis *et al.* 2022), where people with lived experience are engaged in leading community projects that contribute to social justice, e.g., working with poverty action groups, peer support, or art-based activism, thus moving away from a paternalistic approach to one where people are supported to undertake actions for themselves. Therefore, when considering occupations and citizenship, occupational therapists should consider working collectively in partnerships with people who access services and community groups for people to develop their own projects and collaborations.. This aligns strongly with POJF and participatory citizenship in emphasising the importance of trying to create a just society and create a context where all people can flourish.

Having a voice and making a change

Quinn *et al.* (2020)andReis *et al.* (2022), as described above, demonstrate how people collectively participating can shape their sense of citizenship and change. This chimes strongly with the POJF in OTs working as a catalyst for change and the importance of moving away from predominately individual-focused work to work with groups and communities focused on transformation.

Interestingly, according toMorgan (2023), people from a service user/survivor-led organisation saw citizenship as more than a sense of belonging and viewed it as being an activist and making a difference.

For me it's about community, belonging, connectedness, rights, being able to participate, being able to have a voice and being part of a broader whole.

Participant 1

I think citizenship goes beyond that [Belonging]. It's almost like you're working towards a common good.

Participant 2

Participants also highlighted the importance of mental health professionals in sharing power with people with lived experience in co-producing approaches to citizenship (Morgan, 2023). Therefore, it is fundamental that occupational therapists effectively engage in partnerships with peer workers, survivor-led organisations, and wider community organisations to support people's participation and having a voice. Again, from a critical perspective, understanding the barriers to this (incorporating intersectional perspectives) includes some of the practices of mental health services themselves.

Reflective Activity:
'Acts of Citizenship' is about challenging injustice; according to Morgan (2023), those with lived experience see their role as activists; what role do health professionals have in being activists?

How can occupational therapists share power and build alliances with service user/survivor organisations (or other groups promoting social justice)?

The Role of Mental Health Services and Allyship of Professionals

Hamer *et al.* (2019) describe 'acts of citizenship' as being important for professionals in supporting citizenship. They describe the role of mental health professionals in bending the institutional rules to facilitate citizenship for their service users. These can be small acts such as going above and beyond to help people have a bus pass but also challenging the attitudes of colleagues (Hamer *et al.* 2019). There are calls for mental health professionals to work as allies. However, it is important to note that allyship is complex as it requires the repositioning of power. Mental health professionals are trained to intervene, whereas being an ally is about creating space and enabling the priorities and actions of others; this is likely to include dismantling existing power structures. Russo *et al.* (2018) warn against mental health professionals trying to help but inadvertently not seeing people with lived experience as equals. It is important as practitioners we engage in reflexivity to examine whether we are really sharing power.

To effectively promote citizenship, mental health professionals will need comprehensive training on how to promote justice and rights (Eiroa-Orosa, 2023). Similar training should also be offered to people who access services and their families. There have been concerns raised by mental health professionals on how realistic it is to promote citizenship when there is a focus on fast-paced work and preoccupation with risk. (Bellamy *et al.* 2017; Clayton *et al.* 2020). To address this as well as training programmes (Eiroa-Rosa 2023), Flanagan *et al.* (2023) have established a learning collaborative and resources to bring about organisational change, both of which have the potential to address some of these barriers.

There are more fundamental difficulties in implementing citizenship approaches when mental health services maintain existing power structures, which subject people to detention and restrictive practices alongside promoting citizenship (Brekke *et al.* 2021). Considering the role of mental health services to be aligned with citizenship approaches would involve a shift away from the biomedical paradigm. It would be important to increase the roles of people with lived experience in shaping them. To consider the extent of mental health services, social problems such as poverty and housing should be addressed, considering a radical overhaul of legislation such as the Mental Health Act to promote greater elements of autonomy, advocacy, and choice. As a participant in Morgan (2023) states:

It's a system that is created because the Mental Health Act and because of the way society treats mental health. It isn't about keeping the person well; it's about managing of behaviour and the behaviours connected to the absence of actual support and human connection. The system is necessary because of the system. It's self-perpetuating...It isn't about making people feel safe it isn't even about safety. It's about control. If it was about safety, you'd be asking people what happened to you to make you feel like this...what is the pain?

Within the mental health citizenship literature, there are calls for a radical reorganising of mental health services (Davidson and Rowe 2016; Carr and Ponce 2022); however, there is a pragmatic acknowledgement that mental health services will need to drive this change forward. It is essential to avoid some of the pitfalls of the implementation of the Recovery approach, which is undertaken in partnership with people with lived experience and is aligned with other marginalised groups (such as anti-racist, disability, and LGBT+ organisations) (Davidson and Rowe 2016; Brannelly 2018; Carr and Ponce 2022).

Reflective Activity:
What would a radically redesigned mental health system, which promoted citizenship, Recovery, and occupational justice, look like (how would you involve people with lived experience and share power)?

Alongside citizenship in mental health services, it is important to address the importance of social policy to support societal change. This work is being undertaken in Scotland, where the research into citizenship is shaping social policy (MacIntyre *et al.* 2019; 2021.) To effectively implement citizenship approaches, it will require a sharing of power and a focus on the promotion of citizenship at the micro (individuals and their networks), meso (communities and services), and macro levels (local and national government). Fundamental to this, as stated above, is creating participatory spaces for people with lived experience to undertake acts of citizenship to co-produce future citizenship (Nouf and Ineland 2023). Occupational therapists have a role to play in each of these spaces.

Impact of Technology on Mental Health Citizenship

One theme in the citizenship and mental health literature that has been relatively neglected is the impact of digital technology (Morgan *et al.* 2020). Eiroa-Orosa and Tormo-Clemente (2022), in their study analysing the impact of the COVID-19 pandemic on rights and citizenship for people with mental health challenges, state that the *"digital divide is wreaking havoc"* (p10), highlighting the importance of urgent attention to this area.

Whilst benefits such as greater connectivity and accessibility have been identified (Fry 2018), there remain concerns about the harms to society, whether this is greater surveillance (Zuboff 2019), the harm to mental health due to social media (reference), the undermining of democratic institutions, current inequalities being hard-baked into Artificial Intelligence (AI) and algorithms (Petersen *et al.* 2019; Mohamed *et al.* 2020), or in more extreme cases, AI replacing large numbers of jobs, leading to mass unemployment (Susskind, 2020), or even AI taking over the world (Future of Life Institute 2023). There are concerns about the role of government and who is setting the agenda for social change, especially as the overarching goal of technology companies is to have greater involvement and oversight of our lives to maximise their profits (Zuboff 2019). Whilst these harms and benefits will impact all citizens, it is likely that those already marginalised, such as people with mental health challenges, will experience the greatest impacts. People with mental health challenges are already one group who are more likely to be digitally excluded (do not have access to the internet) (Greer *et al.* 2019), and this will potentially lead to further exclusions, particularly as people are increasingly being required to access public services online (Jaegar 2021). These changes are raising new ethical questions about the current and future rights of citizenship in relation to privacy, data, and AI. Therefore, this is an important consideration for citizenship in mental health and for occupational therapy practice.

As technology is changing society so rapidly, Morgan (2023) argues that it is important not just to look at citizenship in the present but also in the future. Alongside three peer-researchers, they undertook a small-scale research project (14 participants), which worked with a digital technology company and a peer-led mental health organisation through a series of interviews, focus groups, co-production workshops, and creation of a film to explore what inclusive future citizenship may look like and what benefits and opportunities there might be for people with mental health challenges. The data was analysed using Braun and Clarke's (2019) reflexive thematic analysis. The key themes are highlighted in bold below. Please note this study is on a very small scale; therefore, it is important to be aware of the limitations of this study and be cautious about generalising these findings. However, this is an under-researched and significant area; therefore, the findings have been included to promote further discussion rather than be seen as definitive.

The key concerns were the **divide** in society, how this would potentially grow, and whether this was between the global south and the rest of the world, young and old, rich or those in poverty, or those who had access to technology. The importance of **agency and power** is for people to have digital rights, choices over how and whether they engage in technology, and the role in democracy for people being able to shape citizenship. Linked to this was the importance of **having a voice** and being able to contribute to discussions about citizenship, especially from a lived experience perspective. Co-production was seen as central to being able to represent the needs and views of people with mental health challenges and people from other marginalised groups, and this would need to take place not just with health and social care services but also with corporations and governments. The final theme was the question about whether interaction in a digital space was changing, what it meant to be **human in a digital world** in terms of connection, and how we find meaning, purpose, and identity.

Participants felt it was important for health and social care professionals and for people who access services and their networks to be able to access education on citizenship, rights, and digital rights. This is another opportunity for occupational therapists to be involved in co-producing and co-delivering this training.

The four themes identified by participants align with concerns in terms of critical occupational therapy and participatory citizenship in seeking to support people's sense of agency, having a voice, and challenging existing power dynamics. It is essential that as occupational therapists engage in promoting citizenship, they focus on digital citizenship or people's participation in the virtual world as key to this. Not only that, they also work with people with lived experience and industry to explore how technology can enhance people's sense of connection and participation in society. It is interesting to note the concerns raised about what it means to be a human in an increasingly digital world, in particular, how people will find connection, meaning and purpose. In an increasingly technological society, occupational therapists can play a key role in public health and, through 'occupation', support people with their identity and finding meaning.

Reflective Activity:
What is your understanding of the role of technology in shaping citizenship? What are the opportunities and challenges?
How can you incorportate digital citizenship into your practice?

Conclusion: Citizenship and Future Occupational Therapy Practice

There is an increasing focus on citizenship both in mental health and within occupational therapy. This creates an opportunity for occupational therapy to continue to reconnect with its roots by challenging injustice and promoting participation. It is essential that any development consider the role of technology and digital citizenship, and as a profession, occupational therapists support people with their digital rights and also enable them to shape the technological inputs in their lives.

For our approaches to align with the principles of citizenship and Recovery, it is essential that we develop our approaches in partnership with people with lived experience. It is fundamental that we do not see ourselves as having the answers but co-create spaces to collectively develop solutions. In undertaking co-production, we need to be aware of the pernicious impact of neoliberalism and avoid the pitfalls suffered by the implementation of the Recovery approach. This will require a shift in focus away from biomedical approaches to the delivery of healthcare to sharing power with the people we are supporting and working to create opportunities for participation. The activities proposed by Fransen-Jaïbi *et al.* (2021) will play an important role in this.

As we look to progress the profession, the change of approach will be a challenge and require courage. It is anticipated that this will take time. It is important for each of us to look at the things we are able to change and influence. It can be on a micro level, working with individuals to participate as citizens, on a local or community level, developing projects, or on a macro level, working with governments and corporations to seek wider social change and policy change to support the participation of not just people with mental health challenges but all marginalised groups. The POJF provides useful guidance in addressing local, national, and global approaches to citizenship from an occupational perspective.

In simplifying our next steps, it may be worth considering this three-stage approach, which incorporates Fransen *et al.* 's (2013) three approaches and the layered approach promoted in the citizenship literature (Nouf and Ineland 2023). This involves promoting citizenship on three levels: individual (working with the person and their network to participate as citizens), community (working to develop community projects and inclusive communities), and justice (focus on acts of citizenship that promote justice, whether this is on a small or large scale). If each of us undertakes this as core to our occupational therapy practice, it could lead to a radically different mental health system and significantly improved quality of life for the people we serve.

REFERENCES

Anthony, W.A. (1993). Recovery from mental illness: the guiding vision of the mental health service system in the 1990s. *Psychosoc. Rehabil. J., 16*(4), 11.

Aristotle, (1995). *Aristole's Politics.*

Atterbury, K., Rowe, M. (2017). Citizenship, community mental health, and the common good. *Behav. Sci. Law, 35*(4), 273-287.
[http://dx.doi.org/10.1002/bsl.2293] [PMID: 28631834]

(2014). *Dorset wheelchair users record access problems.*https://www.bbc.co.uk/news/uk-england-dorst-27903477

Bellamy, C.D., Kriegel, L., Barrenger, S., Klimczak, M., Rakfeldt, J., Benson, V., Baker, M., Benedict, P., Williamson, B., MacIntyre, G. (2017). Development of the citizens measure into a tool to guide clinical practice and its utility for case managers. *Am. J. Psychiatr. Rehabil., 20*(3), 268-281.
[http://dx.doi.org/10.1080/15487768.2017.1338064]

Beresford, P., Nettle, M., Perring, R. (2010). *Towards a social model of madness and distress. Exploring What Service Users say.* (pp. 27-41). York: Joseph Rowntree Foundation.

Brannelly, T. (2018). An ethics of care transformation of mental health service provision: creating services that people want to use.*Ethics From the Ground Up: Emerging Debates, Changing Practices and New Voices in Healthcare..* London: Palgrave MacMillan.
[http://dx.doi.org/10.5040/9781350495494.ch-002]

Braun, V., Clarke, V. (2019). Reflecting on reflexive thematic analysis. *Qual. Res. Sport Exerc. Health, 11*(4), 589-597.
[http://dx.doi.org/10.1080/2159676X.2019.1628806]

Brekke, E., Clausen, H.K., Brodahl, M., Lexén, A., Keet, R., Mulder, C.L., Landheim, A.S. (2021). Service user experiences of how flexible assertive community treatment may support or inhibit citizenship: a qualitative study. *Front. Psychol., 12*727013
[http://dx.doi.org/10.3389/fpsyg.2021.727013] [PMID: 34566813]

Carr, E.R., Ponce, A.N. (2022). Supporting mental health recovery, citizenship, and social justice. *Community*

Ment. Health J., 58(1), 11-19.
[http://dx.doi.org/10.1007/s10597-021-00900-y] [PMID: 34716831]

Chichaya, T.F., Joubert, R.W.E. (2019). Applying the occupational justice framework in disability policy analysis in Namibia. South African Journal of Occupational Therapy Clayton, A., Miller, R., Gambino, M., Rowe, M. and Ponce, A.N., 2020. Structural barriers to citizenship: a mental health provider perspective. *Community Ment. Health J., 56*, 32-41.

Clayton, A., O'Connell, M.J., Bellamy, C., Benedict, P., Rowe, M. (2013). The Citizenship Project part II: impact of a citizenship intervention on clinical and community outcomes for persons with mental illness and criminal justice involvement. *Am. J. Community Psychol., 51*(1-2), 114-122.
[http://dx.doi.org/10.1007/s10464-012-9549-z] [PMID: 22869206]

Cogan, N., MacIntyre, G., Stewart, A., Harrison-Millan, H., Black, K., Quinn, N., Rowe, M., O'Connell, M. (2022). Developing and establishing the psychometric properties of the Strathclyde Citizenship Measure: A new measure for health and social care practice and research. *Health Soc. Care Community, 30*(6), e3949-e3965.
[http://dx.doi.org/10.1111/hsc.13789] [PMID: 35344232]

Cogan, N.A., MacIntyre, G., Stewart, A., Tofts, A., Quinn, N., Johnston, G., Hamill, L., Robinson, J., Igoe, M., Easton, D., McFadden, A.M., Rowe, M. (2021). "The biggest barrier is to inclusion itself": the experience of citizenship for adults with mental health problems. *J. Ment. Health, 30*(3), 358-365.
[http://dx.doi.org/10.1080/09638237.2020.1803491] [PMID: 32762384]

Cruikshank, B. (1999). *The Will to empower; democratic citizens and other subjects..* United States: Cornell University Press.
[http://dx.doi.org/10.7591/9781501733918]

Dorset, A. (2014). *Make Pokesdown Station.*https://www.youtube.com/watch?v=KDtKvvHVFVo&t=5s

Dorset, A. (2016). *Access to the future.*https://www.youtube.com/watch?v=_gPNx6QKbTs&t=443s

Danielsen, K.K., Øydna, M.H., Strömmer, S., Haugjord, K. (2021). "It's More Than Just Exercise": Tailored exercise at a community-based activity center as a liminal space along the road to mental health recovery and citizenship. *Int. J. Environ. Res. Public Health, 18*(19), 10516.
[http://dx.doi.org/10.3390/ijerph181910516] [PMID: 34639815]

Davidson, L., Rowe, M., DiLeo, P., Bellamy, C., Delphin-Rittmon, M. (2021). Recovery-oriented systems of care: a perspective on the past, present, and future. *Alcohol Res., 41*(1), 09.
[http://dx.doi.org/10.35946/arcr.v41.1.09] [PMID: 34377618]

(2002). *Democracy in America..* Chicago: University of Chicago Press. (Original work published 1835)

Deegan, P.E. (1988). Recovery: The lived experience of rehabilitation. *Psychosoc. Rehabil. J., 11*(4), 11-19.
[http://dx.doi.org/10.1037/h0099565]

Degener, T. (2014). A Human Rights Model for Disability.*Disability Social Rights..* Cambridge University Press.

Durkheim, E. (2014). *The division of labor in society.* New York: Simon and Schuster. (Original work published 1893)

Eiroa-Orosa, F.J., Rowe, M. (2017). Taking the concept of citizenship in mental health across countries. Reflections on transferring principles and practice to different sociocultural contexts. *Front. Psychol., 8*, 1020.
[http://dx.doi.org/10.3389/fpsyg.2017.01020] [PMID: 28680412]

Eiroa-Orosa, F.J., Tormo-Clemente, R. (2022). Recovery, citizenship, and personhood of people with lived experience of mental health problems during the pandemic: two expert focus groups. In *Medical. Sci. Forum, 4*(1), 42. [MDPI.]

Eiroa-Orosa, F.J. (2023). Citizenship as mental health. A study protocol for a randomised trial of awareness interventions for mental health professionals. *J. Public Ment. Health, 22*(3), 117-126.

[http://dx.doi.org/10.1108/JPMH-09-2022-0089]

Fagrell Trygg, N., Gustafsson, P.E., Månsdotter, A. (2019). Languishing in the crossroad? A scoping review of intersectional inequalities in mental health. *Int. J. Equity Health, 18*(1), 115.
[http://dx.doi.org/10.1186/s12939-019-1012-4] [PMID: 31340832]

Flanagan, E., Tondora, J., Harper, A., Benedict, P., Giard, J., Bromage, B., Williamson, B., Acker, P., Bragg, C., Adams, V., Rowe, M. (2023). The Recovering Citizenship Learning Collaborative: a system-wide intervention to increase citizenship practices and outcomes. *J. Public Ment. Health, 22*(3), 127-132.
[http://dx.doi.org/10.1108/JPMH-12-2022-0125]

Fransen, H., Kantartzis, S., Pollard, N., Viana Moldes, I. (2013). http://www.enothe.eu/index.php?page = activities/meet/ ac13/default

Fransen, H., Pollard, N., Kantartzis, S., Viana-Moldes, I. (2015). Participatory citizenship: Critical perspectives on client-centred occupational therapy. *Scand. J. Occup. Ther., 22*(4), 260-266.
[http://dx.doi.org/10.3109/11038128.2015.1020338] [PMID: 25937095]

Fransen-Jaïbi, H., Kantartzis, S., Pollard, N., Viana-Moldes, I. (2021). *Educational materials on citizenship from an occupational perspective.*
[http://dx.doi.org/10.17979/spudc.9788497498142]

Fry, H. (2018). *Hello world: how to be human in the age of the machine..* London: Random House.

(2023). https://futureoflife.org/open-letter/pause-giant-ai-experiments/

Gabe, J., Cardano, M., Genova, A. (2020). *Health and Illness in the Neoliberal Era in Europe..* United Kingdom: Emerald Publishing Limited.
[http://dx.doi.org/10.1108/9781839091193]

Greer, B., Robotham, D., Simblett, S., Curtis, H., Griffiths, H., Wykes, T. (2019). Digital exclusion among mental health service users: qualitative investigation. *J. Med. Internet Res., 21*(1)e11696
[http://dx.doi.org/10.2196/11696] [PMID: 30626564]

Hamer, H.P. (2012).

Hamer, H.P., Kidd, J., Clarke, S., Butler, R., Lampshire, D. (2017). Citizens un-interrupted: Practices of inclusion by mental health service users. *J. Occup. Sci., 24*(1), 76-87.
[http://dx.doi.org/10.1080/14427591.2016.1253497]

Hamer, H.P., Finlayson, M. (2015). The rights and responsibilities of citizenship for service users: some terms and conditions apply. *J. Psychiatr. Ment. Health Nurs., 22*(9), 698-705.
[http://dx.doi.org/10.1111/jpm.12258] [PMID: 26271209]

Hamer, H.P., Finlayson, M., Warren, H. (2014). Insiders or outsiders? Mental health service users' journeys towards full citizenship. *Int. J. Ment. Health Nurs., 23*(3), 203-211.
[http://dx.doi.org/10.1111/inm.12046] [PMID: 24147764]

Hamer, H.P., Kidd, J., Clarke, S., Butler, R., Lampshire, D. (2017). Citizens un-interrupted: Practices of inclusion by mental health service users. *J. Occup. Sci., 24*(1), 76-87.
[http://dx.doi.org/10.1080/14427591.2016.1253497]

Hamer, H.P., Rowe, M., Seymour, C.A. (2019). 'The right thing to do': Fostering social inclusion for mental health service users through acts of citizenship. *Int. J. Ment. Health Nurs., 28*(1), 297-305.
[http://dx.doi.org/10.1111/inm.12533] [PMID: 30152193]

Hammell, K. W. (2020).

Hammell, K.W. (2015). Occupational rights and critical occupational therapy: rising to the challenge. *Aust. Occup. Ther. J., 62*(6), 449-451.
[http://dx.doi.org/10.1111/1440-1630.12195] [PMID: 25871425]

Harper, A., Kriegel, L., Morris, C., Hamer, H.P., Gambino, M. (2017). Finding citizenship: What works? *Am. J. Psychiatr. Rehabil., 20*(3), 200-217.

[http://dx.doi.org/10.1080/15487768.2017.1338036]

Ikuigu, M. (2007).

Isin, E.F., Nielsen, G.M. (2008). *Acts of Citizenship..* London: Zed Books.

Isin, E.F., Ruppert, E.S. (2020). *Being digital citizens..* Lanham: Rowman & Littlefield Publishers.

Isin, E.F., Nielsen, G.M. (2008). *Acts of Citizenship..* London: Zed Books.

Jæger, B. (2021). Digital Citizenship–A review of the academic literature/Digital Citizenship: eine systematische Literaturanalyse. *dms–der moderne staat–Zeitschrift für Public Policy. Recht und Management, 14*(1), 5-6.

Keilhofner, G. (2009). *Conceptual Foundations of Occupational Therapy Practice 4thedition..* Philadelphia: F.A Davis Company.

Kronenberg, F., Pollard, N., Sakellarioiu, D. (2011). *Occupational Therapy without borders II: towards an ecology of occupation-based practices..* Edinburgh, New York: Churchill Livingstone/Elsevier.

Kronenberg, F., Pollard, N. (2005). Overcoming occupational apartheid: A preliminary exploration of the political nature of occupational therapy.*Occupational Therapy without Borders: Learning from the Spirits of Survivors..* London: Elsevier Churchill Livingstone.

Leamy, M., Bird, V., Le Boutillier, C., Williams, J., Slade, M. (2011). Conceptual framework for personal recovery in mental health: systematic review and narrative synthesis. *Br. J. Psychiatry, 199*(6), 445-452. [PMID: 22130746]

Lister, R. (2007). Inclusive citizenship: Realizing the potential. *Citizensh. Stud., 11*(1), 49-61. [http://dx.doi.org/10.1080/13621020601099856]

MacIntyre, G., Cogan, N., Stewart, A., Quinn, N., O'Connell, M., Rowe, M. (2022). Citizens defining citizenship: A model grounded in lived experience and its implications for research, policy and practice. *Health Soc. Care Community, 30*(3), e695-e705. [PMID: 34155710]

MacIntyre, G., Cogan, N.A., Stewart, A.E., Quinn, N., Rowe, M., O'Connell, M. (2019). What's citizenship got to do with mental health? Rationale for inclusion of citizenship as part of a mental health strategy. *J. Public Ment. Health, 18*(3), 157-161.

Marmot, M., Allen, J., Goldblatt, P., Herd, E., Morrison, J. (2020). *Build Back Fairer: The COVID-19 Marmot review. The pandemic, socioeconomic and health inequalities in England. London: Institute of Health Equity Marshall, T.H. (1987), Citizenship and Social Class..* London: Pluto Press.

Marshall, T.H. (1987). *Citizenship and Social Class.*

Mohamed, S., Png, M.T., Isaac, W. (2020). Decolonial AI: decolonial theory as sociotechnical foresight in artificial intelligence. *Philos. Technol., 33*, 659-684.

Morgan, P. (2020).

Morgan, P. (2023).

Morgan, P., Brannelly, T., Eales, S. (2020). Future studies, mental health and the question of citizenship. *Ment. Health Soc. Incl., 24*(1), 23-32.

Nesse, L., Aamodt, G., Gonzalez, M.T., Rowe, M., Raanaas, R.K. (2021). The role of occupational meaningfulness and citizenship as mediators between occupational status and recovery: a cross-sectional study among residents with co-occurring problems. *Adv. Dual Diagn., 14*(3), 99-118.

Nouf, F., Ineland, J. (2023). Epistemic citizenship under structural siege: a meta-analysis drawing on 544 voices of service user experiences in Nordic mental health services. *Front. Psychiatry, 141*156835 [PMID: 37333919]

O'Connell, M.J., Clayton, A., Rowe, M. (2017). Reliability and validity of a newly developed measure of citizenship among persons with mental illnesses. *Community Ment. Health J., 53*(3), 367-374.

[PMID: 27714484]

O'Hagan, M. (2008). Recovery: the true meaning of recovery. *Ment. Health Today,* •••, 16-17.
[PMID: 19189473]

Petersen, A., Tanner, C., Munsie, M. (2019). Citizens' use of digital media to connect with health care: Socio-ethical and regulatory implications. *Health, 23*(4), 367-384.
[PMID: 31045440]

Pollard, N., Sakellariou, D., Kronenberg, F. (2009). *A Political Practice of Occupational Therapy.* Churchill Livingstone.

Ponce, A.N., Rowe, M. (2018). Citizenship and community mental health care. *Am. J. Community Psychol., 61*(1-2), 22-31.
[PMID: 29323416]

Ponce, A.N., Rowe, M. (2018). Citizenship and community mental health care. *Am. J. Community Psychol., 61*(1-2), 22-31.
[PMID: 29323416]

Quinn, N., Bromage, B., Rowe, M. (2020). Collective citizenship: from citizenship and mental health to citizenship and solidarity. *Soc. Policy Adm., 54*(3), 361-374.

(2016). https://recoveryinthebin.org

Reis, G., Bromage, B., Rowe, M., Restrepo-Toro, M.E., Bellamy, C., Costa, M., Davidson, L. (2022). Citizenship, social justice and collective empowerment: living outside mental illness. *Psychiatr. Q., 93*(2), 537-546.
[PMID: 35048313]

Rose, D. (2014). The mainstreaming of recovery. *J. Ment. Health, 23*(5), 217-218.
[PMID: 24988317]

Rowe, M. (2015). *Citizenship and Mental Health..* New York, NY: Oxford University Press.

Rowe, M., Davidson, L. (2016). Recovering Citizenship. *Isr. J. Psychiatry Relat. Sci., 53*(1), 14-20.
[PMID: 28856875]

Rowe, M., Davidson, L. (2016). Recovering Citizenship. *Isr. J. Psychiatry Relat. Sci., 53*(1), 14-20.
[PMID: 28856875]

Rowe, M., Bellamy, C., Baranoski, M., Wieland, M., O'Connell, M.J., Benedict, P., Davidson, L., Buchanan, J., Sells, D. (2007). A peer-support, group intervention to reduce substance use and criminality among persons with severe mental illness. *Psychiatr. Serv., 58*(7), 955-961.
[http://dx.doi.org/10.1176/ps.2007.58.7.955] [PMID: 17602012]

Rowe, M., Benedict, P., Sells, D., Dinzeo, T., Garvin, C., Schwab, L., Baranoski, M., Girard, V., Bellamy, C. (2009). Citizenship, community, and recovery: A group-and peer-based intervention for persons with co-occurring disorders and criminal justice histories. *J. Groups Addict. Recovery, 4*(4), 224-244.
[http://dx.doi.org/10.1080/15560350903340874]

Rowe, M., Clayton, A., Benedict, P., Bellamy, C., Antunes, K., Miller, R., Pelletier, J.F., Stern, E., O'Connell, M.J. (2012). Going to the source: creating a citizenship outcome measure by community-based participatory research methods. *Psychiatr. Serv., 63*(5), 445-450.
[http://dx.doi.org/10.1176/appi.ps.201100272] [PMID: 22549531]

Russo, J., Beresford, P., O'Hagan, M. (2018). Commentary on: Happell, B. & Scholz, B (2018). Doing what we can, but knowing our place: Being an ally to promote consumer leadership in mental health. International Journal of Mental Health Nursing, 27, 440–447. *Int. J. Ment. Health Nurs., 27*(6), 1877-1878.
[http://dx.doi.org/10.1111/inm.12520] [PMID: 29984890]

Scull, A.T. (1979). Moral treatment reconsidered: some sociological comments on an episode in the history of British psychiatry. *Psychol. Med., 9*(3), 421-428.

[http://dx.doi.org/10.1017/S0033291700031962] [PMID: 384444]

Slade, M., Amering, M., Farkas, M., Hamilton, B., O'Hagan, M., Panther, G., Perkins, R., Shepherd, G., Tse, S., Whitley, R. (2014). Uses and abuses of recovery: implementing recovery-oriented practices in mental health systems. *World Psychiatry, 13*(1), 12-20.
[http://dx.doi.org/10.1002/wps.20084] [PMID: 24497237]

Slade, M., Oades, L., Jarden, A. (2017). *Wellbeing, recovery and mental health..* New York: Cambridge University Press.
[http://dx.doi.org/10.1017/9781316339275]

Susskind, D. (2020). *A World Without Work: Technology, Automation and How We Should Respond..* Great Britain: Random House.

Townsend, E., Wilcock, A.A. (2004). Occupational justice and client-centred practice: a dialogue in progress. *Can. J. Occup. Ther., 71*(2), 75-87.
[http://dx.doi.org/10.1177/000841740407100203] [PMID: 15152723]

Townsend, E. (1998). *Good Intentions Overruled: A Critique of Empowerment in the Routine Organization of Mental Health Services..* University of Toronto Press.
[http://dx.doi.org/10.3138/9781442675414]

Vervliet, M., Reynaert, D., Verelst, A., Vindevogel, S., De Maeyer, J. (2019). "If You Can't Follow, You're Out." The perspectives of people with mental health problems on citizenship. *Appl. Res. Qual. Life, 14*(4), 891-908.
[http://dx.doi.org/10.1007/s11482-017-9537-4]

Whiteford, G., Townsend, E. (2011). Participatory occupational justice framework.*Occupational therapy without borders.* (pp. 64-84). London: Elsevier.

Whiteford, G., Townsend, E., Hocking, C. (2000). Reflections on a renaissance of occupation. *Can. J. Occup. Ther., 67*(1), 61-69.
[http://dx.doi.org/10.1177/000841740006700109] [PMID: 10695170]

Whiteford, Townsend, Bryanton, Wicks (2017).

Wilcock, A.A., Townsend, E.A. (2009). Occupational justice.*Willard & Spackman's occupational therapy.* (11th ed., pp. 192-199). Baltimore: Lippincott Williams& Wilkins.

Zuboff, S. (2019). *The age of surveillance capitalism..* London: Profile Books.

SUBJECT INDEX

www.ingramcontent.com/pod-product-compliance
Lightning Source LLC
Chambersburg PA
CBHW050802220326
41598CB00006B/100